The Real CdC

COVID FACTS FOR REGULAR PEOPLE

JOHN PAUL BEAUDOIN, SR.

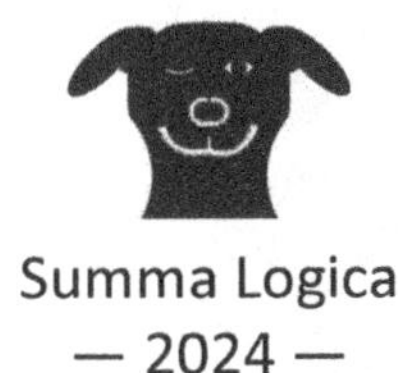

Summa Logica
— 2024 —

Copyright © 2024 Summa Logica LLC

All rights reserved.

Except as permitted under U.S. Copyright Act of 1976, no part of this publication may be reproduced, distributed, or transmitted in any form or by any means, except for brief quotations and reviews, without the prior written permission of the copyright owner. Please purchase only authorized electronic editions and abstain from electronic piracy of copyrighted materials. Consider the author's rights to his labor and your own personal integrity.

Disclaimer
The factual information provided in this book is believed to be accurate at the time of publication and was gleaned from official state records and from sources listed in the References section. The opinions of the author throughout this book are his own and they in no way construe medical or legal advice. The author is neither a medical nor legal professional and is not licensed in either capacity in any jurisdiction. Readers should consult with medical and legal professionals for advice before acting on any opinion or fact expressed in this book.

Limitation of Liability and Warranty Disclaimer
This book is provided to the public for informational and educational purposes. The author and publisher shall not be liable for the use of any information or opinions expressed herein.

Paperback ISBN: 979-8-9900220-0-3
Ebook ISBN: 979-8-9900220-1-0
Library of Congress Control Number: 2024902837

Edited by Richard Kramer

John Paul Beaudoin, Sr.
The Real CdC: Covid Facts For Regular People

First Edition

Published by
Summa Logica LLC
9 Julia Court
Winchester, New Hampshire, USA 03470

TheRealCdC.com
CoquindeChien.substack.com
ViaVeraVita.com
X: @JohnBeaudoinSr

Printed in the United States of America

In Memory

of

John Paul Beaudoin, Jr.

and with tribute to his

brothers,

Charlie & Henri

Dedicated to the fallen and injured,
their families and friends.
May those affected have the strength
to righteously fight the good fight
to protect humanity from inhumanity.

TABLE OF CONTENTS

PRAEFATIO

This book is for anyone open to truth. Cut through all the BS from both sides of covid and vaccine issues. Become informed in order to make your own decisions. Your life may depend on it.

Learn facts derived from official record-level source data (RLSD) not published elsewhere. The Centers for Disease Control and Prevention (CDC) and state health departments publish data that is not capable of being collated across variables. Only source data at the record-level can be easily analyzed for important changes at the margins. What happened? When? To whom? The answers are in this book.

If you believe covid vaccines work or don't work, read this book. Learn not the opinions of biased researchers beholding to their funding sources. Learn rigorous truth irrespective of your own or others' preconceptions.

The word *externality* appears often throughout this book. In this context, *externality* means an input or condition that interrupts the normalcy of a system. Examples are a new pathogen, a new government policy, or a new drug administered en masse.

CONCLUSIONS

Beaudoin's analyses are more robust than those from any state health department or the CDC. How can that be? There are only two possible reasons. Either 1) all states and the CDC are simultaneously incompetent, or 2) they are all simultaneously hiding this information from the public.

In this book, Beaudoin uses death certificate RLSD, obtained through a Massachusetts Public Records Request (state version of a FOIA), to provide far more pertinent and useful information than any report as yet issued by government entities.

What occurred in 2020 was starkly different from what subsequently occurred in 2021 and 2022. When you strip away what is normal, as determined from the data for 2015 through 2019, from the corresponding data for 2020 through 2022, that which remains reveals what occurred differently over the latter three years, aka 'the signal.' The excess or deficits after removing the expected normal baseline events is what people want to know: what happened; to whom it happened; when it happened.

Examination of the Massachusetts death certificates in conjunction with the records available in the national Vaccine Adverse Event Reporting System (VAERS) exposed evidence of fraudulent death certificates. In August 2022, Beaudoin filed a lawsuit in the United States District Court, District of Massachusetts, seeking to correct the fraudulent death certificates together with other remedies.[1] This book includes comments on portions of the lawsuit's foundational evidence, which was submitted to the Court in *Exhibits F, G,* and *H* of the complaint.

BOOK SUMMARY

2020 Massachusetts Causes, Ages, and Seasonality Profiles

1) Greater excess respiratory deaths
2) Excess deaths average age matched covid deaths average age within 1.0 year
3) Highly seasonal – ON from March to June, OFF from June to November, ON from November through December

2021 & 2022 Massachusetts Causes, Ages, and Seasonality Profiles

1) Greater excess circulatory system and blood-related deaths
2) Excess deaths average age differed greatly from covid deaths average age by 12.5 and 7.1 years, respectively
3) Not seasonal, but rather linearly increasing to steady-state

This book dives deeply into individual causes of death such as arrhythmia, stroke, heart attack, lymph and marrow cancers, pulmonary emboli, and other thromboembolic (clot) related deaths. Acute renal failure stood out with one of the highest increases (100% increase) in 2022, likely due, in large part, to the Emergency Use Authorization (EUA) drug remdesivir.

Commentary on how this all happened will be interspersed throughout this book.

No matter how many expert witnesses one side puts on a debate panel or in a courtroom, the opposing party will bring an equal number. Complex statistical analysis is often only persuasive rather than conclusive. After hearing the statistical analyses, the debate judges or courtroom juries are often left more confused than before they heard debate or testimony. Then they often revert to their preconceived notions because the expert testimonial analyses of one party canceled the other's.

Fortunately, an understanding of the facts presented in this book does not require special expertise. This book empowers regular people with the comprehensible facts they need to claim agency and make their own decisions about public health policy.

More important than impersonal data and graphs are the human suffering and death they reveal. The deaths of real people are explored in the early chapters through inspection of their death certificates and corresponding VAERS reports. Chapter 2 includes the stories of two Massachusetts women and one teenager who suffered strokes within hours of receiving a covid shot, resulting in death within days of the shots. One of these unfortunate deaths is the subject of a published case report authored by six doctors. The report implicates a covid modified messenger RNA (mRNA) injection in her death.

THESIS

The ***symptom spectrum profile***, ***age spectrum profile***, and ***seasonality profile*** of *excess* deaths all changed starkly on a year boundary (2020/2021) coincident with the introduction of covid vaccines (so-called).

Please continue reading to learn the facts and truth. The lives of your children depend on it.

ADGNITIONES (ACKNOWLEDGMENTS)

Rich Kramer first told me I should write a book

Then, Ed Dowd told me I should write a book

(So I wrote a book. Much thanks to Rich and Ed.)

A special thanks to Dr. Meryl Nass for promoting my work and giving me confidence

Nick Hudson asked me to join PANData Analytics, then prodded me to begin writing articles on Substack instead of only my Twitter memes of covid data analyses

My sister and brother-in-law, Margot and Jim Carpenter, told me to keep going when many others discouraged me from investing time in covid data

Dr. Henry Ealy recognized the importance of my analyses and invited me into the Grand Jury Investigation Planning Group. Thanks to all in that group, some wanting to remain anonymous

Charles Kovess and Dr. Stephen Frost for the invitation to speak and subsequently participate in weekly zoom calls on Medical Doctors for COVID Ethics International. Charles is a superb moderator

Thanks to the Thursday crew from Steve Kirsch's Vaccine Steering Committee where we discussed weekly new research and findings for Steve to use on his VSRF show a couple hours later: Steve Kirsch, Jonathan Couey, Kevin McKernan, Stephanie Seneff, Ira Bernstein, Jessica Rose, Marc Girardot, Mathew Crawford, Chris Masterjohn, Karen Stewart, Hilary Grant-Valdez, Byram Bridle with drop-ins from Peter McCullough and Paul Marik

Friends from *Bagels and Bibles* Saturday morning Bible study group who put up with me talking about covid for years and who supported my efforts to save children

Mary Holland and all the crew at CHD for the support and speaking opportunities

Dr. Madhava Setty for his friendship and article featuring my lawsuit and work

Professor Retsef Levi for his words of encouragement, which give me further confidence in bringing truth and new analysis techniques

Michelle Orfanos for prodding me to get the book done and for setting up meetings with publishers, book designers, and editors

Maria Nardi for the early support of my writing and for urging me to keep writing and don't let up

Dr. Drew Pinsky and Dr. Kelly Victory for bringing me up on his show simulcast to a Twitter space, treating me with respect, and listening to difficult facts theretofore unheard

Michael Levitt, Ben Martin, Joel Smalley, Martha, Mundy brothers Liberty Monks, Daniel Horowitz, Dr. Leigh Vliet for supporting my work

Professor Norman Fenton and Doc Malik (Dr. Ahmad Malik) for offering their podcast platforms for me to spread needed truth

Aaron Hertzberg for supporting the methodology, obtaining another state's records, and working together with me toward truth derived from vital records

Jason Gerhard and Yury Polozov, members of New Hampshire's General Court, for sponsoring me to meet with various New Hampshire state officials and politicians

Mark Kulacz, for appearances on *Housatonic.Live*, and Scott Schara, for an appearance on *Deprogramming with Grace's Dad*, and most importantly for understanding and sharing a special kind of loss, unfair and unending

Thank you to all the organizations that invited me to speak and to the many podcasters and news venues who interviewed me

There are so many others who have supported and helped me. I feel badly ending the list here as some will feel omitted. The TRUTH movement is full of many good souls on a righteous campaign to prevent maiming and death caused by government and oligarchs

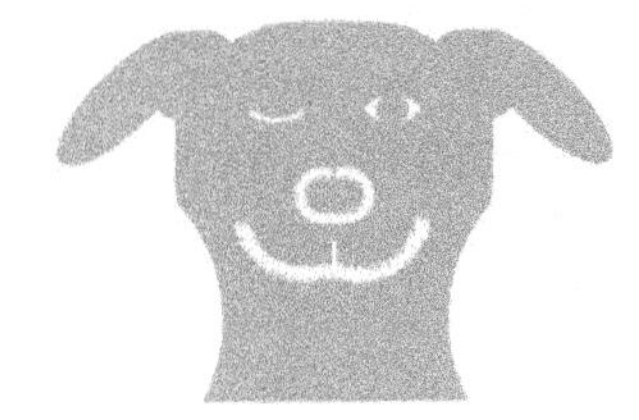

INTRODUCTION

On Saint Patrick's Day 2020, a friend invited me for beers at a bar named Finnegan's Wake. Since the loss of my eldest son, John Jr., in a motorcycle accident at age 20 in July 2018, I hadn't been social at all. Going out for beers on St. Patrick's Day was an opportunity to get off the couch and rejoin the world.

In the weeks leading up to March 17, 2020, there was a rising feeling of dread stemming from news of a killer virus spreading around the world.

As I sat in the crowded bar, beer in hand, I felt a type of claustrophobia set upon me; but not from walls, rather from people around me. They were too close. And we were all breathing the same air. I remember that I was worried about not being alive for my other two sons, Charlie, then 19, and Henri, then 17. So I left my beer and my friends; and I went home to sit on my couch and watch YouTube, since I had canceled cable TV in an attempt to depart the couch.

When Charlie entered the room, I told him I was worried about the virus and that he should be careful. Charlie responded by saying that it's all bullshit and people were worrying needlessly. As a parent, even though I had an inkling Charlie was right, I felt the need to correct him and tell him that he should be considerate of others. I wanted to ensure that Charlie took the health threat seriously, at least for a little while. I knew that he would only listen to facts, not television reporters or politicians ... or Dad. Thus began my journey for truth in the covid era.

In search of truth, the first thing I did was download New York City (NYC) Department of Health data. In mid to late March 2020, NYC had the most purported covid deaths of any place in the world; and their data portal was publicly available online. I learned the ages, co-morbidities, and dates of death of purported covid victims. Something did not seem right.

My paternal grandmother died in the Spanish flu pandemic of 1918. When I was a child, elderly relatives spoke of funeral processions going from St. James Church, past the end of their street, to St. James Cemetery in Haverhill. I was young and it's a distant memory, but what I clearly remember is that they said there were at least four funerals a day, every day, for several months. That is what a pandemic looks like.

What I found in the NYC data, in those early covid days, was that nearly all covid deaths had multiple co-morbidities, the great majority of which were diabetes and obesity. Overall, covid deaths skewed very old in age, not like the Spanish flu, which killed at an average age of around 28. I remember that because my grandmother was 28 upon her death and had four young children, my father being only six months old.

There were some younger people in their 40s dying in March 2020 in NYC, but only those who were morbidly obese and diabetic. It seemed that 92-year-old healthy people without co-morbidities were not dying from covid, but the younger obese were dying from covid.

It seemed evident that it was not age that was the issue, but rather that the elderly were more likely to have co-morbidities. Thus, I thought that age per se was not to blame, but rather the co-morbidities.

Hubris is the Achilles heel of most researchers. Ergo, I fully admit that I was wrong in characterizing co-morbidities as the only contributing factor. I soon learned that age correlates to declining ability to produce an immune system response. Accordingly, age can be a factor in addition to co-morbidities.

Whenever the news media reported something that did not seem right to me, I investigated the data. Of course, I found my way to CDC data, which I thought at the time was primary source data. I was completely wrong about that. Most of the data from the CDC or Johns Hopkins is sourced from state health systems and vital records data. This is not a reliable primary source of data. For death data, the death certificates are the best source of primary, Record Level Source Data (RLSD). The only way to dive deeper into more granular data than what death certificates provide would be to inspect hundreds to thousands of pages of medical history and treatment for each decedent.

During the first weeks of covid, I ran math operations on CDC data to determine if the news media was telling the truth or misinforming. One of the first data sets I analyzed came in two files. *Weekly Counts of Deaths by State and Select Causes 2014–2018* and *Weekly Counts of Deaths by State and Select Causes 2019–2020.*[1] The years 2014–2019 would define a baseline of "normal mortality."

My early work with those two online files revealed that the 2014–2018 data file was incorrectly assembled. The discrepancy was evident because the pneumonia and influenza numbers did not add up in some of the cells. This exacerbated the 2020 covid numbers in relation to the pneumonia and influenza numbers that year.

I wrote to the CDC keeper of that specific file, whose e-mail address was on the screen with the link to the file. After sending him an explanation of the issue, I received no reply. Instead, the 2014–2018 file had disappeared from the website. About a day and a half later, the 2014–2018 file reappeared. I still had no reply via e-mail. However, when I rechecked the 2014–2018 file for the inconsistency I had discovered earlier, it was gone. The 2014–2018 file data had been altered. To be clear, it was not the method of aggregation of pneumonia and influenza that changed, but rather the cell data itself was changed without any posted explanation.

I was taken aback. The CDC just changed official historical data after an e-mail from a random citizen. How can they just do that? These are public records. The point here is that I lost trust in the CDC cause-of-death data in that moment. Whether I'd made a mistake, or the CDC committed data mischief does not matter. I became a covid skeptic right at that moment. This is what motivated me to continue data studies in order to truth test the narratives being fed to us by news media and politicians.

I had little patience listening to people denying that covid exists or denying viruses exist. If someone could not back up statements with hard facts, to me their opinions were just noise. Nine months later, the same thing happened with the covid vaccines. People took sides without any actual factual knowledge, and it was difficult to sift through the media noise to find truth.

All I want is truth. I learned rather quickly that research papers and articles were corrupted by biases regardless of how many times an author wrote, "None" in the "Conflicts of Interest" field. My trust in doctors also ebbed when many unquestioningly fell in line with the nonsensical propaganda that masks prevent the spread of SARS-CoV-2 (SCV2) virus.

The mask issue is not the focus of this book, but any engineer worth anything knows from studying fluid dynamics that neither surgical masks nor N95 masks are rated to filter the type of aerosol carrying SCV2. Doctors rarely have education or experience in medical device design or manufacturing, yet they pretend to be authorities on mask effectiveness. Sadly, the average patient will blindly trust a doctor's groundless opinion no matter how absurd it may be.

NIOSH and OSHA are government organizations that have qualified engineers who study and report on mask effectiveness in context of aerosolized virus. Staff from those organizations had little to say about masks in the early covid era when masking was forced upon us. Their silence was obvious to those of us who know which profession is expert in which science. NIOSH and OSHA personnel seemed gagged and prevented from commenting on the mask subject.

In March 2021, in response to a *Public Records Request,*[2] I received some twelve hundred pages of internal e-mails and reports from the Department of Public Health of Massachusetts (MA DPH). Within those pages, I found internal e-mails among agents of MA DPH and Professor Gregory Rutledge of the Massachusetts Institute of Technology (MIT). The MA DPH contracted Rutledge to test samples pulled from the 1.2 million masks that Governor Baker had flown in from China on the New England Patriots jet.[3] In a set of e-mails dated April 20, 2020, the MA DPH was informed by Rutledge that most of the samples came nowhere near the specification of 95% filtration efficiency (FE). The e-mails basically confirmed that masks don't work against aerosolized SARS-CoV-2 (SCV2) virus. To see e-mail excerpts and learn more, please refer to my article entitled, *The Baker Knew*.[4]

Governor Baker instituted the Massachusetts mask mandate effective May 6, 2020, despite knowing that masks do not prevent spread of SCV2.[5]

In the first few months of the covid era, I wrote eleven papers. I stuck to hard facts and tried not to rely on source papers that were underpowered, biased, or those that made conclusory statements after the body of data therein demonstrated near zero confidence in findings.

Over the first covid year, I tracked the purported covid deaths per capita of every nation and U.S. state having populations of more than three million, 168 jurisdictions in all. For this purpose, I relied on real time data published on the Worldometer website, https://www.worldometers.info/coronavirus/country/us/ and https://www.worldometers.info/coronavirus/.

In May 2020, Massachusetts ranked third in the world in per capita covid deaths. New Jersey and New York ranked first and second, respectively. Sweden did not mandate masking, recommended social distancing of an arm's length, closed no bars, clubs, discos, or schools, and allowed people to manage their fear and mitigation based on individual choice. When other nations instituted mandates around May 2020, Sweden ranked tenth in the world in per capita covid deaths.

One year later, in May 2021, Massachusetts ranked fifth in the world in per capita covid deaths while Sweden dropped to forty-third. Despite all of the mandates imposed in Massachusetts, including masking, school closures, epidemiolog(y)(ist) small business closures, and foreclosures, Massachusetts remained among the worst in the world for covid mortality. Sweden fared far better thanks to its respect for the freedom of its citizens to make their own decisions about how to deal with the risks from covid.

I also studied the issue of covid seasonality by tracking temperature and humidity data from https://weatherspark.com against purported covid deaths in fifty world locations. I found covid to be a highly seasonal respiratory virus. This clear result contradicted the faulty analyses by most government recognized epidemiologists. The reason for the disparity is simple. Government epidemiologists used faulty data aggregation. They confounded the seasonality present in the data by failing to properly segregate it by climactic regions. By combining data from regions with different climates into overly large groups, the clearly evident seasonality was completely obscured. The claim that covid is not a seasonal virus is easily proven false by proper data aggregation and analysis.

I did very little with data for purported numbers of cases. There was no point in looking at cases because of the widespread gross misuse of PCR based testing of asymptomatic people. A cursory look at the data for purported cases vs. purported covid deaths did show general correlations, but there were outliers which were indicative of either low quality data or outright fraudulent data. I also looked at covid hospitalizations and ICU patient counts when a jurisdiction had too few deaths to permit statistical analysis. The vast majority of my data analyses were based on numbers of deaths, especially All-Cause deaths (total deaths from any cause).

During that first summer (2020), the vast majority of my analyses examined data for All-Cause deaths. All-Cause is the one variable that cannot easily be manipulated by governments. Governments can manipulate causes of death through solicitous or coercive policies, but they cannot change the fact that someone died or did not die.

In the summer of 2020, I became active on Twitter and posted an analysis of Massachusetts All-Cause deaths data. Nobel Prize winner Professor Michael Levitt repeated my analysis and publicly stated my work was correct,[6] which gave me a boost of confidence. Covid, as an epidemic, only lasted about nine weeks in Massachusetts, from mid-March to mid-June 2020. Levitt stated the end date was June 14, precisely. I remember that because it is John Jr.'s birthday. He would have been 22.

In July 2020, at the age of 56, I decided to apply to a local law school. After being accepted, I wrote an e-mail to the Director of Admissions stating that I will not get the covid vaccine when available because I fully lost the hearing in my right ear upon getting an injection in 1968 for the Hong Kong flu. He e-mailed back to me that because I'm over 30, the school will not require covid vaccination. I then entered law school mid-August 2020.

I put most of the covid data analysis aside to concentrate on school work. In the second semester, the Torts professor asked me to do a required ten-minute video on economics and tort law because he felt I was most qualified to understand economics. A month earlier, I became aware of the CDC's official vaccine vigilance system for monitoring and reporting adverse outcomes from vaccines. In February 2021, I loaded the Vaccine Adverse Event Reporting System (VAERS) data into a spreadsheet and began to forensically analyze it.

I wrested value from VAERS by filtering for character strings. I made a table of strings of letters and the number of times each string appeared in VAERS in 2021. Examples are "clot," "thrombo," "headache," "embolism," "aneurysm," "carditis," "deaf," "vertigo." As it happened, from February and each month thereafter until July, some of the highest frequency strings were four conditions from which I suffer or have suffered: "tinnitus," "deaf," "dvt," (deep vein thrombosis), and "vertigo."

I incorporated the VAERS data into my economics and tort law video by showcasing the immunity shield given to the manufacturers for any adverse outcomes of the covid vaccines. The liability (L) was driven to zero dollars ($0) for the pharma manufacturers. This shifted the burden of precautions from the Least Cost Avoiders (manufacturers) to the Most Cost Avoiders (injection recipients). In the case of the experimental covid injections, the injection recipients are also, in every sense of the term, the experimental subjects, effectively in this case the guinea pigs, or lab rats.

This terminology is not hyperbole. It is rigorously accurate. Time cannot be accelerated or slowed. Where, normally, vaccines are first tested with extensive animal trials, animal trials of the covid injections were bypassed by the Department of Defense (DoD) *Operation Warp Speed* (OWS).[7] The human population was injected in place of the animals.

The burden of precautions to the manufacturers is pecuniary (financial). However, in shifting that burden to the Most Cost Avoiders (the people), the burden manifests not financially, but rather in reduced health of the injected. *Id est*, injury, disability, and death are the expected results. Driving liability to zero by government mandate broke the market mechanism and resulted in tremendous human losses as any good economist should expect.

You can find my Torts video on YouTube entitled *The Hand Formula; Economics of Torts; Importance of Torts; Vax tort immunity.*[8] I don't think the professor liked my video.

The law school enacted a covid immunization mandate in the spring of 2021 at the end of my first (1L) year. I applied for a religious exemption. To this day, the law school has neither accepted nor rejected my application for exemption. Instead, the school rebuffed multiple requests to know the status, went unresponsive, then sent me a letter stating that I was un-enrolled and should begin to repay my student loans. I received that letter hours before the registration deadline for classes in August 2021 for my second (2L) year of law school. They effectively kicked me out of their school after taking tens of thousands of dollars from me in tuition and a year of my life studying law.

At 57, I had no job, no law degree, and I felt betrayed, abused, and cheated. I needed some time to dwell on what happened before engaging in a lawsuit.

I do now have a lawsuit pending against the school for breach of contract. Ironically, I received an "A" in Contracts class that second semester.

There was something that really bothered me about researching VAERS. I missed my son so much and I had read several VAERS reports of children, mostly teens, who died shortly after taking the covid vaccines. Some deaths were clearly caused by vaccination. One, age 21, was listed as having had a clotting issue at the age of 16, only five years earlier.

I wondered why vaccine clinic staff did not ask screening questions of the young man to simply ascertain whether he had a clotting problem. I knew in February 2021, after only two months of covid vaccine roll-out, that thromboembolic (clotting) issues were prevalent, lethal, and caused by covid vaccines.

Another young man was found by his father in his car, dead, in the parking lot where he worked. He had not come home from work, so his father went looking for him. I also went looking for my son one night and when I arrived home after not finding him, the police were waiting there to tell me the worst news of my life.

I knew I had to do something to bring truth and facts to The People who were being propagandized by news media, politicians, and celebrities. The public was told that the experimental mRNA technology, never before used in humans en masse, was "safe and effective." No one could know that without results from comprehensive safety trials. I do not purport that

I knew then that the shots were unsafe and ineffective. Rather, I knew the government could not know that they were safe and effective. I just wanted them to stop lying to everyone and stop programming people to risk their lives as chattel for experimentation.

In the fall of 2021, I joined a small zoom call group of mostly scientists and doctors led by Steve Kirsch. Someone on Twitter had noticed my analyses and recommended that I join them.

Weeks later, based on my Twitter posts, Nick Hudson of Pandemics Data & Analytics (PANDA) at https://pandata.org also asked me to join PANDA's weekly zoom calls of about thirty people, mostly doctors and scientists. Shortly after joining, in early 2022, Nick prodded me to begin writing articles and not just post my data analyses on Twitter. Thus, I began writing substack articles on March 9, 2022, under the name "Coquin de Chien." (https://coquindechien.substack.com/)

Around that same time, Dr. Henry Ealy asked me to listen in on group zoom calls that he led to effect grand jury investigation of the CDC and FDA. In the span of a few months, I was in three groups and my weeks were filled with at least six hours per week of conference calls, two days per week researching and writing articles, and other days creating Twitter posts to push truth out to the public.

Regardless of how many analyses I performed or how many analyses I read, there was never going to be any resolution until someone got substantial RLSD. Signals cannot be teased out without RLSD.

In January 2022, I heard on the car radio on my way to the gym that a girl, age 7, in Massachusetts died from covid. Given all my data studies, I knew there was no way a healthy child died from covid. It just does not happen. This is where the story really begins.

Members of Team Reality MA, a group of Massachusetts residents who value freedom, were kind enough to take some of my public records requests, put their names on them, and then file them with the Commonwealth of Massachusetts.

Most of the requests were denied. One notable request was for the resume and other background information of Girish Navani, a member of Governor Baker's Reopening Advisory Board. The request was denied. The Commonwealth wrote that they had no information on Navani. I'd found that he ran a company in the telemedicine business. The company paid $155 million to the U.S. Department of Justice in 2017 to settle False Claims Act allegations.[9] It was inappropriate and wildly conflicting for Navani to be on the Governor's board. The state government website listed him being on the board, yet they denied having any information on Navani. Corrupt is the Commonwealth.

One request was fulfilled, however. The entire death certificate database from 2015 through 2021 was provided in February 2022. Approximately 420,000 death certificates were provided with all details and no redactions. Updated 2022 data files have since brought the total number of death certificate records in my possession to around 500,000. This may be the largest set of RLSD relevant to covid which has been released publicly.

Accordingly, this book is an introduction to discoveries and truths learned from the largest, most robust RLSD that made its way to a member of the public for analysis. From the RLSD, I created multiple presentations, each containing ~100 slides. They comprise tens of hours of presentation time and would fill a series of books.

Between September 2022 and April 2023, I delivered more than thirty presentations to thousands of medical doctors, lawyers, and research biologists. More than one million (1M) people viewed my data compilations and heard the true facts resulting from my investigations.

In my presentations, I generally review the data first, and conclude with some detailed accounts of individual victims of the covid shots. This book flips that order. The early chapters describe some of the immense human loss and suffering which the untested, and manifestly unsafe covid injections have caused. The extensive data and analytical results follow the human story.

You will learn that the ***symptom spectrum profile***, ***age spectrum profile***, and ***seasonality profile*** of excess deaths in 2020, prior to the availability of the covid injections is completely disparate from those in 2021 and 2022.

And you will learn that life-years-lost from the covid vaccines far surpasses the life-years-lost from covid per se.

Please take this information to heart. Pass it around to family and friends. Share it widely.

IMPORTANT NOTE

For many months, I struggled with the decision on whether or not to use real names in my Substack articles. Now, as I write this book, again I struggle with this decision. My discussions with many people at various events and seminars I attended have persuaded me that it is important to include the real names of those impacted by the devastating effects of the covid injections.

If I used real names in my articles earlier than I did, would I have been able to prevent at least one child from dying from covid vaccines? Evidence favors an affirmative answer to that question, which adds to the guilt I carry for not including the names sooner. I am now a citizen journalist and have a duty to the people to report facts important to the public interest.

In a balance of harms analysis, the loss of another child because the truth is hidden weighs substantially heavier than an aggrieved parent learning from this book that the real cause of their child's death was government malfeasance manifest in official policies to hide the truth about the lethality of the covid shots.

I'll not apologize. For I know the anguish. And if someone wanted to use information from my son's death to save other children, I would gladly endure the sadness and relentless guilt in reliving my failure to prevent his decision to buy a motorcycle. That scab is perpetually picked every day I wake up, especially on days I don't want to. Can anyone argue against the importance of trying to save living children by exposing the true cause of death of those who passed?

DEATH CERTIFICATE FORMAT

Death certificates have two (2) parts. Following is an example found on the CDC website.[10]

Examples of properly completed medical certifications

CAUSE OF DEATH (See instructions and examples)

32. **PART I.** Enter the chain of events—diseases, injuries, or complications—that directly caused the death. DO NOT enter terminal events such as cardiac arrest, respiratory arrest, or ventricular fibrillation without showing the etiology. DO NOT ABBREVIATE. Enter only one cause on a line. Add additional lines if necessary.

		Approximate interval: Onset to death
IMMEDIATE CAUSE (Final disease or condition resulting in death) →	a. Rupture of myocardium	Minutes
Sequentially list conditions, if any, leading to the cause listed on line a. Enter the **UNDERLYING CAUSE** (disease or injury that initiated the events resulting in death) **LAST**	Due to (or as a consequence of): b. Acute myocardial infarction	6 days
	Due to (or as a consequence of): c. Coronary artery thrombosis	5 years
	Due to (or as a consequence of): d. Atherosclerotic coronary artery disease	7 years

PART II. Enter other significant conditions contributing to death but not resulting in the underlying cause given in PART I.

Diabetes, Chronic obstructive pulmonary disease, smoking

33. WAS AN AUTOPSY PERFORMED? ■ Yes ☐ No

34. WERE AUTOPSY FINDINGS AVAILABLE TO COMPLETE THE CAUSE OF DEATH? ■ Yes ☐ No

35. DID TOBACCO USE CONTRIBUTE TO DEATH?
■ Yes ☐ Probably
☐ No ☐ Unknown

36. IF FEMALE
■ Not pregnant within past year
☐ Pregnant at time of death
☐ Not pregnant, but pregnant within 42 days of death
☐ Not pregnant, but pregnant 43 days to 1 year before death
☐ Unknown if pregnant within the past year

37. MANNER OF DEATH
■ Natural ☐ Homicide
☐ Accident ☐ Pending investigation
☐ Suicide ☐ Could not be determined

Figure Intro.1

Part I is broken into Cause A, Cause B, Cause C, Cause D. Cause A is the "immediate cause" and should generally represent the last relevant cause that occurred before death. Since everyone's heart stops upon death, it is not relevant unless someone's heart stopped from something associated with the heart or the combination of the heart and impaired breathing. Thus, cardiopulmonary arrest is a common Cause A listing, but it is not relevant if someone fell ten stories from a building and his heart stopped upon impact.

Causes B, C, and D are considered underlying causes of death (UCOD). The UCOD should be listed in reverse time order with the root cause that set off the causal chain of events being the last one listed in A, B, C, or D. An example is Cause A "CARDIOPULMONARY ARREST," Cause B "PNEUMONIA," Cause C "COVID-19 VIRAL INFECTION." A covid infection caused pneumonia that worsened until the heart stopped because the lungs could not transfer enough oxygen to the blood (pulmonary failure).

Part II comprises causes or conditions that are thought to have contributed, or to have possibly contributed, to the person's death. While DIABETES and ASTHMA are common contributing conditions, a positive flu test or positive covid test six months earlier should not be listed if the person dies from a fall down stairs, automobile accident, or drug overdose.

ICD-10 codes are international codes applied to death certificates to match all Parts I and II causes and conditions listed. ICD-10 codes are important for tracking conditions and diseases. Causes or conditions listed in Parts I and II should not be omitted from the ICD-10 codes.[11]

One of the most important material facts to understand is that death certificates are sent from states, Massachusetts included, to the CDC without ICD-10 codes. To the best of my knowledge, the CDC then feeds the death certificates into a software parser that automatically applies ICD-10 codes to the death certificate records. Those that are unable to be coded are then manually coded. When completed, death certificate records are returned to the states with the codes for each record.

The death certificates I obtained for Massachusetts contained ICD-10 codes. The death certificates another person obtained from Minnesota and shared with me contained ICD-10 codes. the death certificates yet a third person obtained from Vermont and shared with me did not contain ICD codes.

The conversion system (parser) is at the CDC. As a central authority, the CDC becomes a single point of failure. If the CDC parser errantly interprets a word or string, the error carries through all states. Also, the fidelity of data for any nuanced situation cannot be high considering that the certifier is not in communication with an automatic software program in Atlanta, Georgia or wherever the ICD-10 parser is.

The system has flaws. But information can be derived by tracking codes over time as long as the researcher understands that the behavior of the death certifier and the function of the automatic parser are points of failure.

PRIMA PARS

People

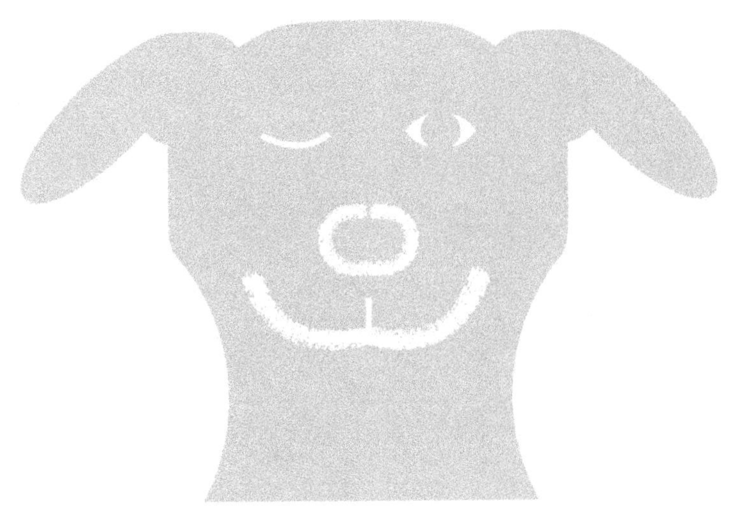

WHAT THEY WON'T TELL YOU ... TELLS YOU

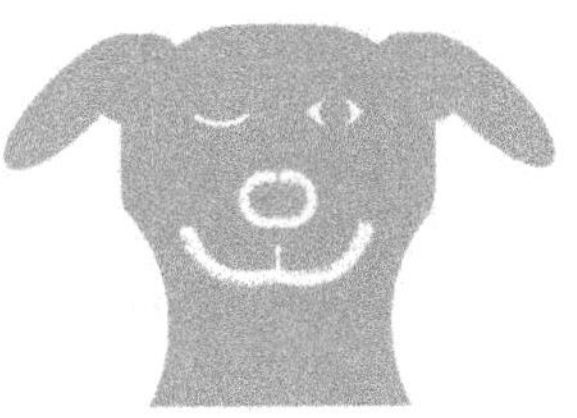

Chapter 1
Cassidy

Several publicly available webpages display the obituary and pictures of a smiling 7-year-old girl holding her dog in her arms. Her name is Cassidy Patrice Baracka, and she died on January 18, 2022.[1.2.3.4.]

The obituaries, news articles, and news video clips found online report that Cassidy died as a result of "*complications from Covid-19*." They also state that Cassidy was active in gymnastics, dance, Brownie Scouts, attended numerous NHL Boston Bruins hockey games, and traveled to Disney World.

Cassidy is the reason I sought death certificates in Massachusetts. Contrary to all media reports, and to the extent of my then-current knowledge, no healthy child died from covid in Massachusetts before Cassidy. I wanted evidence because I don't trust either side of the vaccine argument: media, politicians, and bureaucrats on one side, or fringe antivaxxer wing nuts on the other side.

The death certificate for Cassidy confirms what the news media stated: Cassidy died on January 18, 2022. The "Immediate Cause of Death" (Cause A in Part I) is listed as "*COMPLICATIONS OF CORONAVIRUS-19 VIRAL INFECTION*" in "*DAYS*." This is consistent with the obituary and news reports in the use of "*complications*" in context of covid. But what does that mean? There are no further Underlying Causes of Death ("UCOD," or Causes B, C, or D of Part I) listed on her death certificate. What "*complications*" did Cassidy have? The medical examiner omitted the "*complications*" causing the death of a healthy 7-year-old girl.

A document entitled, *COVID-19 Alert No. 2*, dated March 24, 2020, and published by the National Vital Statistics System (NVSS), which is part of the CDC, states, "*... the rules for coding and selection of the underlying cause of death are expected to result in COVID-19 being the underlying cause more often than not.*" It also states:

"COVID-19 should be reported on the death certificate for all decedents where the disease caused ***or is assumed to have caused or contributed to death****. Certifiers should include as much detail as possible based on their knowledge of the case, medical records, laboratory testing, etc. If the decedent had other chronic conditions such as COPD or asthma that may have also contributed, these conditions can be reported in Part II."* [5]

It appears that covid should not be put in Cause A as it appeared on Cassidy's death certificate. This is more clearly outlined in a subsequent document published by NVSS in April 2020 entitled, *Report No. 3 - Guidance for Certifying Deaths Due to Coronavirus Disease 2019 (COVID-19)*. In the "*Conclusion*" section of this document, it states:

"An accurate count of the number of deaths due to COVID-19 infection, which depends in part on proper death certification, is critical to ongoing public health surveillance and response. When a death is due to COVID-19, it is likely the UCOD and thus, it should be reported on the lowest line used in Part I of the death certificate." [6]

Clearly, covid should not have been placed in Cause A as it was in Cassidy's case. The real immediate cause of death, whether a hemorrhage, respiratory failure, sepsis, multi-organ failure, or something else immediate, remains unknown to the public based on Cassidy's death certificate.

Part II is defined as "*Other significant conditions contributing to death.*" Cassidy's death certificate Part II states, "*FUNGAL AND BACTERIAL PLEURITIS; ASTHMA.*"

The following international diagnostic codes (ICD-10 codes) were applied to Cassidy's death certificate:

U07.1 "COVID-19"
A49.9 "Bacterial infection, unspecified"
B49 "Unspecified mycosis"
J45.9 "Asthma, unspecified"
R09.1 "Pleurisy"

Despite conditions contributing to Cassidy's death, it is still unclear what she immediately died from on January 18, 2022. The conditions listed in Part II appear not to be from covid. In fact, they are fungal ("mycosis") and bacterial, not viral. SARS-CoV-2 is a virus, not a bacterium or a fungus. And if they were secondary to covid and causal in the death, they should have been listed in Part I before covid.

The Vaccine Adverse Event Reporting System (VAERS) is built and maintained by the U.S. Department of Health and Human Services (HHS). One can report to VAERS or search VAERS online. HHS also has a portal from which files can be downloaded.[7]

In a search for age 7 girls who might have been reported to VAERS around the time Cassidy died, I applied the search criteria "F" for female, "7" for age in years, and "MA" for Massachusetts to the 2022 file downloaded from VAERS on February 3, 2023.

There are thirteen age 7 girls from Massachusetts reported to VAERS in 2022. Only four of the thirteen have vaccination dates prior to Cassidy's death.

One of those four (4), reported March 5, 2022, had symptoms of "*Diarrhea*" and "*PRODUCT ADMINISTERED TO PATIENT OF INAPPROPRIATE AGE.*" She received an adult dose. The ONSET_DATE and VAX_DATE are both "*12/16/2022.*" That seems not to fit Cassidy's death certificate information, which states that Cause A occurred in "*DAYS,*" not "*WKS*" or "*MOS.*"

The second of the four was also covid-vaccinated in December 2021. Her VAERS report stated, "*on Feb 22, 2022 patient felt the need to spit... bright red blood came out. No known illness or symtpoms* [sic] *at the time whatsoever, she continued to spit blood and a large clot from her mouth. Again at the end of May 2022 child felt the need to spit and tasted blood in her mouth...a few drops of bright red blood and a small clot came up.*" This text mentions February and May 2022 symptom dates, which were after Cassidy died, thus, this child's report cannot possibly be Cassidy.

The third of the four was injected on December 4, 2021, had onset of symptoms on December 5, 2021, and was reported to VAERS on March 5, 2022. She had symptoms of "chills; fever; headache;...Since the report was made in March, it is highly unlikely to be Cassidy's VAERS report. One can assume that the reporter would have reported death as "Y" in the proper field if this report was about Cassidy. Cassidy's death was robustly reported in the news as a covid death. Cassidy's death certificate also states that it happened in "DAYS," whereas this VAERS report states the onset occurred more than a month before Cassidy died.

That leaves but one 2022 VAERS report of an age 7 girl injected before Cassidy died. Here is the record of VAERS_ID 2038120:

- *RECVDATE 01/15/2022*
- *VAX_DATE 01/13/2022*
- *ONSET_DATE 01/15/2022*
- *PRIOR_VAX "Severe nausea and vomiting from 5 min post vaccination and for the next 8-10 hours"*
- *SYMPTOM_TEXT "Spiked a 103 fever, severe stomachache, has not had a bowel movement since the day before vaccination, which makes today 3 days without one. First vaccine caused severe nausea and vomiting from 5 minutes post injection and for the next 8-10 hours."* [8]

Cassidy died on January 18, 2022. VAERS_ID 2038120 was reported to VAERS on January 15, 2022, as having been vaccinated January 13, 2022, only 5 days before Cassidy died. The reader can infer if Cassidy and VAERS_ID 2038120 are the same age 7 girl from Massachusetts.

The VAERS report clearly states there was a prior vax in which the girl reacted in five minutes. That indicates that this VAERS report is about a subsequent injection, likely dose 2. The girl in report ID 2038120 spiked a 103F fever, developed a severe stomach ache, and did not have a bowel movement for three days. Cassidy died three days after this VAERS_ID 2038120 report was filed and five days after the injection date stated in the VAERS report.

The Massachusetts death certificate database shows there are only seven age 7 girls who died in Massachusetts in 2022. Three died in January, and one each in March, April, May, and July. Of the January deaths, one was a "*RESPIRATORY FAILURE*" in "*2 WKS.*" and "*BRAINSTEM GLIOMA*" in "*13 MOS.*," one was "*SEVERE SEPSIS WITH MULTIORGAN FAILURE*" in "*33 DAYS,*" "*ARDS*" in "*33 DAYS,*" "*COVID-19 PNEUMONIA*" in "*33 DAYS,*" and the third, Cassidy's death certificate, is the most likely candidate to match with VAERS_ID 2038120.

The death certificates stating "13 months" and "33 days" do not comport with the onset of symptoms field in the VAERS_ID 2038120 report. Interestingly, the death certificate of the girl who died with multiorgan failure and covid was not mentioned in any news media as Cassidy was, though this little girl died only four days after Cassidy. Was this other little girl covid vaccinated? Was she given remdesivir, considered by many to cause kidney failure and multi-organ failure?

Given the exhaustive evaluation of both death certificates and VAERS reports, it is highly likely that Cassidy is the girl described in VAERS_ID 2038120, which raises the issue of how all the reported "facts" can be true.

In the case of Cassidy, if she indeed did receive a covid vaccine on January 13, 2022, reacted soon after, and died five days later, then the school nurse, the school principal, the school superintendent, all doctors and nurses involved in her case at the Nashoba Valley Medical Center, and likely some of the teachers and administrative staff at her school would all know those facts and timing.

Surely, if the VAERS report accurately describes Cassidy's covid vaccine experience, then any one of these many people could come forward to assert that the news media and government are misinforming the public by stating that Cassidy died from covid whereas the true cause of her death is a covid vaccine.

If VAERS_ID 2038120 pertains to Cassidy, then the death certificate needs to be corrected to properly and rightly inform the public.

A 15-year-old boy effectively died on a basketball court in Massachusetts only one month after Cassidy died. If Cassidy is VAERS_ID 2038120, and if someone had publicly spoken up about her death caused by a covid vaccine, perhaps that 15-year-old boy would be alive today.

A 12-year-old girl died from a stroke in Massachusetts in August 2022 only days after receiving a covid vaccine. Perhaps she would be alive today if Cassidy is VAERS_ID 2038120 and if someone would have publicly made known the true cause of Cassidy's death.

From one viewpoint based on facts, it seems highly likely that Cassidy and VAERS_ID 2038210 are the same girl; and from another viewpoint based on emotion, it seems highly unlikely that several tens of mandatory reporters in the school system and the hospital may have violated ethics and law by remaining quiet about the true cause of Cassidy's death.

In fact, when the medical examiner and the media reported that Cassidy died from covid, many parents became frightened of covid and then brought their children to be vaccinated against covid. If Cassidy is VAERS_ID 2038120, then the irony is palpable; and the malfeasance by the medical examiner and the silence of mandatory reporters comprise a heinous crime, which put additional children in harm's way.

One way to clarify the facts is to publish the covid vaccination date of Cassidy Baracka that is in the Massachusetts Immunization Information System (MIIS). The results of a simple five-minute query would empower people to make a more informed decision about covid injections. Either

Cassidy is VAERS_ID 2038120 and parents would decide, on a more informed basis, to protect their children from a covid injection Death Lottery; or Cassidy is not VAERS_ID 2038120 and the concerns of some parents could be alleviated by this information, thus reducing their vaccine hesitancy.

On March 24, 2022, Coquin de Chien (my 'nom de plume') wrote an article entitled, *Tragedy in Groton, Massachusetts,*[9] which detailed the same information herein noted. If Cassidy is not VAERS_ID 2038120, then any person could have contacted me in the past year to tell me I made an error in correlation. No one has contacted me to tell me that.

Only a few minutes of effort by a state employee to look up Cassidy's immunization record and tell the truth would prompt me to drop my federal lawsuit against officials of the Commonwealth of Massachusetts to obtain Cassidy's vaccination record.[10]

Please consider the souls involved in this matter. If Cassidy is VAERS_ID 2038120, then many tens of people involved in the cover-up have the opportunity to come forward with the truth, save their souls, and alleviate the enduring guilt of participating as accessories after-the-fact in the unnatural deaths of more children and adults who died because they were misinformed of Cassidy's true cause of death.

Americans have always been forgiving people. Anyone coming forward with truth will cleanse their soul and save other children and adults who are contemplating a covid vaccine. Whistleblowers nearly always feel relief despite any pecuniary or career losses.

As people on both sides of the issue bicker, debate, and verbally attack each other, there exists the most elegant and simple solution of data transparency waiting for government legislatures to enact.

When someone dies in a car accident, details of the crash are reported publicly. The types of injuries, age and gender of decedents, times of death, and sometimes other health conditions are mentioned. When the investigation is completed, the public is then told information such as the toxicology report, blood alcohol level, fractures that occurred, and other medical information. However, if you ask for the vaccination date of the deceased, the state will deny you the information and claim it is a medical privacy issue.

Purported to be in the public interest, courts will uphold vaccine mandates for five-year-old children to attend public kindergarten. That means a child is coerced to divulge vaccination status and date of vaccination in order to receive public education. Yet, the vaccination status of a child who may have died from the vaccine with onset of symptoms five minutes after injection, followed by death within five days, is considered private information not to be released to the public.

The state steps into a position of protecting the privacy of a deceased child to ensure no one finds out their vaccination date. That same state will demand to know the vaccination date of a living child to attend public schools.

Irrespective of political inclinations, should not every member of the public be able to access the vaccination dates of the deceased? The simple solution to the issue of Cassidy's death, and the deaths of millions of others, is for states to provide the vaccination dates of the deceased upon their deaths. This takes less than five minutes to look up the records in each state's Immunization Information System registry. In service to the public interest, all medical examiners should have access to that registry so that they can correctly assess the causes of death.

Death certificates that do not show a vaccine as a cause of death when someone reacts and dies in five minutes are criminally fraudulent death certificates. When someone dies from a fentanyl overdose, the decedent does not have the privacy to omit it from the death certificate as a cause of death. Vaccines are another type of injected drug that, if causal in the death, should be listed as a cause of death.

There is no excuse for any state to omit the true cause of death, if indeed that cause is a vaccine. Many federal felonies apply to such an omission and will be described in a later chapter.

The government will tell you if someone died from an injection containing fentanyl, or benzodiazepine, or methamphetamine, or bleach, or gasoline, or even air (air embolism). Yet, that same government will not tell you if a product, which was injected into a person, caused a heart attack and death within five minutes. That same government invokes privacy laws to prevent the public from learning if a death was caused by a product produced by a specially protected entity such as a pharmaceutical manufacturer. Does that make any sense? Why are high priced, high profit pharmaceuticals protected while cheap drugs are not?

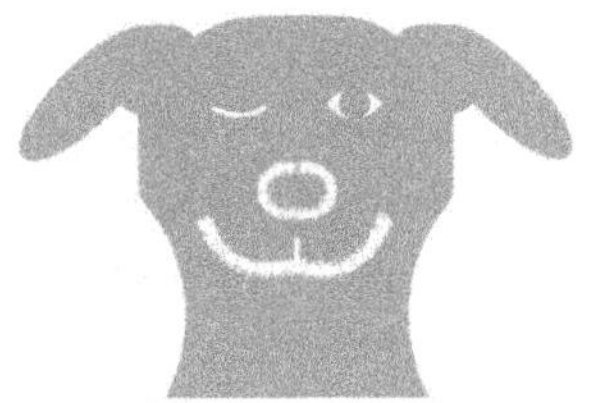

Chapter 2
Three Strokes, Three Months

Diane Claire Dubois (Guerette) died from a hemorrhagic stroke at the age of 62 years old on March 18, 2021, in Massachusetts. Her death certificate states:

- Cause A "*ACUTE INTRACRANIAL HEMORRHAGE IN THE SETTING OF THROMBOCYTOPENIA*"
- Cause B "*IN A PERSON TREATED WITH COVID 19 VACCINATION 11 DAYS PRIOR*"
- Cause C "*TO PRESENTATION*" in "*DAYS*."

ICD-10 codes applied to Diane's death certificate are:

- I62.9 "*Intracranial hemorrhage (nontraumatic), unspecified*"
- D69.6 "*Thrombocytopenia, unspecified*."

Although the causes of death are written in a sentence that is broken up and entered across Causes A through C, notice that there are three causes listed in the fields, but only two in the ICD-10 codes. The *hemorrhage* and *thrombocytopenia* were coded. The covid vaccination, clearly written in Part I, was not coded as a cause of death despite it being the likely root cause of death.

This death certificate is important because the Medical Examiner, Dr. Julie Hull, listed covid vaccine in the lowest line of UCOD (underlying cause of death), which is where the root cause is supposed to be. Clearly, Dr. Hull wishes for it to be known that the covid vaccine is likely the root cause of Diane's death, yet the CDC applied no ICD-10 code associating Diane's death with the covid vaccine. Without an ICD-10 code attribution to the vaccine, the CDC has no mechanism to track covid vaccine-caused deaths such as Diane's stroke death.

From Diane's obituaries online, I learned about her and subsequently wrote about her in my substack article on January 7, 2023, entitled *Massachusetts Anecdrokes.*[1] That substack article reports on a total of three people who died from strokes induced by the covid vaccines. The shots were responsible for ending the lives of two women and a teenage girl over a three-month span. Here is an excerpt from my article about Diane:

Diane is obviously what we called "French-Canadian" when I was growing up. I know better now. We are québécois. Someone wrote nice memories about Diane in her obituary. She was a mother and grandmother and was truly loved by friends and family. One interesting thing that caught my eye was the term "French Meat Stuffing." I still have this every Thanksgiving. My grandfather, René Thibault, taught my mother, Dotty, and she taught my sister, Margot. Whatever bread became stale throughout the year was put into a bag and into the bread drawer without closing the lid. Every year growing up, just before Thanksgiving, I would take out the grinder, clamp it to the table, and grind all the stale bread into breadcrumbs to be used in what my family just called "Stuffing." If any québécois are reading this, then let's be authentic and call it what it is or what it was derived from ... Tourtière. If you look it up, you won't find my family's recipe. And I doubt you will find Diane's recipe. However, there is no doubt that Diane's family loved having her French Meat Stuffing at Thanksgiving every year. I'm so sorry they will miss Diane each Thanksgiving and I hope they carry on the French Meat Stuffing tradition in her memory as we do in my mom's, Dotty's, memory.

Please remember that Diane died on March 18, 2021, about ten months before Cassidy. If only someone had investigated or reported Diane's stroke from vaccine, perhaps Cassidy would be alive today.

Twelve days after Diane died in Massachusetts from a root cause of "COVID-19 VACCINATION," Brianna Mary McCarthy was injected in Massachusetts on March 30, 2021, with a single dose of Moderna covid vaccine. Fifteen days later, Brianna died in Massachusetts. Had the

Massachusetts officials, who are entrusted with protecting the public health and ensuring the safety of medical intervention, timely investigated and reported on the connection between Diane's covid injection and her death, perhaps Brianna would be alive today.

Brianna died at the age of 30 years old on April 15, 2021. Her death certificate states:

- Cause A "*NONTRAUMATIC CEREBRAL HERNIATION*" in "*DAYS*"
- Cause B "*ISCHEMIC STROKE*" in "*DAYS*"
- Cause C "*COVID-19*" in "*MOS.*"

The ICD-10 codes applied to Brianna's death certificate are:

- G93.5 "Compression of the brain"
- I64 "Stroke, not specified as hemorrhagic or infarction"
- U07.1 "COVID-19"

The last cause mentioned in the UCOD causes, Cause C in this case, is "*COVID-19*" in months. Certifier of death, Dr. Steven Schwartz, certified Brianna's death certificate on September 29, 2021. Schwartz essentially certified by signature authority under penalties for fraud on public records that Brianna's root cause of death was covid, which it states she'd had "*MOS.*" (months) earlier.

Brianna's VAERS record was brought to my attention by its author. After waiting six weeks for the doctors to report to VAERS, the author was disgusted that the doctors did not report Brianna's fatal adverse event; so she filed the report herself. Despite a legal duty to report to VAERS, doctors on Brianna's case never filed a VAERS report.

Brianna's VAERS_ID is 1368271, and the report states:[2]

- *RECVDATE 06/02/2021*
- *DATE_DIED 04/15/2021*
- *VAX_DATE 03/30/2021*
- *ONSET_DATE 04/02/2021*
- *Vaccine Type MODERNA*
- *Symptom "BRAIN DEATH, CENTRAL NERVOUS SYSTEM LESION, CEREBROVASCULAR ACCIDENT, CRANIOTOMY, DEATH, ENCEPHALITIS, ENDOTRACHEAL INTUBATION, HEADACHE, HEMIPLEGIA, INTRACRANIAL PRESSURE INCREASED, LUMBAR PUNCTURE, MAGNETIC RESONANCE IMAGING HEAD ABNORMAL, MEDICAL INDUCTION OF*

COMA, MEMORY IMPAIRMENT, MIGRAINE, NAUSEA, SEIZURE, VENTRICULO-PERITONEAL SHUNT, VOMITING, WITHDRAWAL OF LIFE SUPPORT"

- *Adverse Event Description "On April 15th, the otherwise healthy 30 year old daughter of my cousin passed away in a hospital from a massive stroke and seizures related to encephalitis of unknown cause. She recovered easily from Covid19 back in November of 2020, along with several of her close friends and family members with no lingering effects. On March 30th, she was given a single dose of the Moderna vaccine along with her teaching colleagues at a local high school. She initially complained of mild nausea and vomiting but quickly developed a severe headache prompting her to visit the local ER where she received treatment for a migraine. She returned to the ER at least one more time after no relief from the headache. By April 3rd, Saturday, she no longer recognized her sister nor knew what a mask was for. Her family rushed her again to the same ER and she was subsequently transferred the following day to a Hospital. Due to dangerously high intracranial pressure, she suffered a stroke with paralysis of her left side and a seizure. Multiple lesions were noted on her brain via MRI. A shunt was inserted to relieve the pressure, she was intubated and placed into a deep coma from which she would never awaken. Despite these medical interventions and pharmacological interventions, the pressure did not subside. A craniotomy was performed the following Saturday as a last ditch effort to relieve the unrelenting pressure in her brain. The craniotomy was able to reduce the pressure but it was too late. There was no longer any brain activity and my cousin's daughter was removed from life support after they were able to say their goodbyes. The medical examiner will be examining her brain to attempt to find a cause but that report may take 6 months."*

Brianna was a young high school English teacher in the Methuen Public School system. The local news announced on March 9, 2021, that Methuen teachers were to get the vaccine the following week.[3] This was about 5.7 miles from the law school I was attending at the time. Soon after Brianna's death, the law school announced a covid vaccine mandate. Would the law school have put in place a vaccine mandate if they learned that a 30-year-old woman died from the vaccine and did not die from covid as the death certificate fraudulently stated?

Coquin de Chien wrote a substack article on January 11, 2023, entitled *Massachusetts Anecdrokes,* telling more details about Brianna:[4]

> *Brianna is from a special area of Massachusetts. You have to have grown up there to know what I mean (or have several hundred relatives there as I do every holiday was a 2.5 hour drive from Connecticut to Haverhill for Tourtière). Brianna went off to college in New York, but returned home to be part of the community where she was raised. Her obituary claims support for the Bruins and Patriots - not a surprise. And I'm happy to report that Brianna enjoyed more NFL and NHL championships in her short life than* [any season ticket holder at East Rutherford stadium or Madison Square Garden]. *That makes Brianna a winner ... and New Yorkers ... well, you pick the word. Brianna coached women's hockey where she taught English at Methuen High School. The obituary states that she was very family-oriented, typical for that area. That means she was loved by all her family and it also means she will be missed by them as well. The grief will never pass for her parents and sister. I cannot explain the anger I feel as I type this and wipe the tears away. Knowing what I know and seeing what I've seen since John Jr. died, there is no doubt in my mind that Brian, her father, will embrace Brianna again after this life. He may or may not know it yet. But God is real, His love is everlasting, Brianna is there and not even waiting because there time does not exist beyond this Earthly life. She is and always will be surrounded by all souls of family and friends in God's presence. God bless the families of Diane, Brianna, and Eden.*

Eden Grace MacDonald died from a stroke on June 11, 2021, in Massachusetts. Eden was only 17 years old. She was injected a little more than five weeks after Brianna died from a stroke and two months after Diane died, also from a stroke.

If timely investigations had uncovered the serious safety signals represented by Diane's stroke death, proximate to her covid vaccination, or Brianna's stroke death, proximate to her covid vaccination, Massachusetts officials would have had the critical information needed to enable them to make a timely decision to pause administration of the deadly covid vaccines. Had the Massachusetts public health officials dutifully performed their jobs, Eden would likely be alive today.

Eden only had one cause of death on her death certificate. Cause A "*COMPLICATIONS OF CEREBRAL VENOUS SINUS THROMBOSIS.*" Only one ICD-10 was applied, G08 "Intracranial and intraspinal phlebitis and thrombophlebitis."

VAERS_ID 1388042 was found among one hundred seven reports of 17-year-old females from Massachusetts in 2021, many describing horrific reactions to the covid vaccines, but only ID 1388042 noting that death occurred.[5]

VAERS_ID 1388042 states:

- *RECVDATE 06/10/2021*
- *DATE_DIED [empty]*
- *VAX_DATE 05/23/2021*
- *ONSET_DATE 06/07/2021*
- *Event Categories: Death - Yes*
- *Vaccine Type PFIZER\BIONTECH*
- *Symptom "BRAIN OEDEMA, CEREBRAL INFARCTION, CT HEAD ABNORMAL, DECOMPRESSIVE CRANIECTOMY, HAEMORRHAGE INTRACRANIAL, INTRACRANIAL PRESSURE INCREASED, INTRAVENTRICULAR HAEMORRHAGE, VENTRICULAR DRAINAGE"*
- *Adverse Event Description "Patient had massive acute intracranial hemorrhage. Was found down in bathroom. In ED CT scan showed large intraventricular hemorrhage, EVD placed, patient progressed to massive brain swelling and infarctions, decompressive craniectomy, unable to control intracranial pressure, parents agreed to DNR status and patient is not expected to survive."*
- *Current Illness "Headache started around 3 weeks prior to event that delayed dose of second vaccine. Headache was very severe and she saw PCP for it twice and it lasted a week. It then resolved and she got her second vaccine."*

If VAERS_ID 1388042 corresponds to Eden's death certificate, which seems highly likely considering the time of covid vaccination, time of death, and causes of death being a hemorrhagic stroke on each, then a total of three females ages 62, 30, and 17 all died from a stroke within three months in a single state—Massachusetts. Yet there is no evidence that a single Massachusetts official with a legal duty to act in the interest of public health engaged to investigate or report on these major safety signals. It appears that they purposely and intentionally misled the public by avoidance of their legal duties.

Brianna went to the emergency room with a severe headache twice before degrading into a full ischemic stroke, which ended her life. The VAERS record matched to Eden's death certificate stated that she went to her primary care physician twice for a severe headache after her first covid vaccine dose. Then, after her headache resolved over the course of a week, she was administered the second dose, which ended her life.

The same questions raised in Chapter One about Cassidy's death apply to these tragic, untimely deaths. How can these vaccine-induced deaths be completely overlooked by the people and systems which are supposed to protect public health from dangerous medical interventions? In Diane's case, no VAERS report was submitted by any of the medical professionals who are legally mandated to submit such reports. Brianna's VAERS record was entered by a nurse six weeks after her death. If Eden is the girl in VAERS_ID 1388042, then someone acted righteously and justly in timely reporting Eden's case to VAERS. However, there is no evidence that any Massachusetts Public Health official utilized VAERS for its intended purpose by monitoring it for safety signals. In two cases, the root cause of the deaths, clearly covid vaccines, was omitted from the death certificates.

Not one of the three death certificates was assigned an ICD-10 code implicating a covid vaccine in the death. One of the death certificates was assigned an ICD-10 code fraudulently, implicating a covid infection in the death instead of the vaccine. Are these errors and omissions the result of gross malfeasance, or deliberate fraud?

It is not merely the opinion of a nurse who wrote Brianna's VAERS report that Brianna's stroke death is causally linked to a Moderna covid vaccine.

Brianna died at the "BETH ISRAEL DEACONESS MEDICAL CENTER-WEST CAMPUS." Six doctors affiliated with Beth Israel Deaconess Medical Center and Harvard Medical School penned a *Brief Report* about Brianna's case. The title, *Fatal Post COVID mRNA-Vaccine Associated Cerebral Ischemia*, published on December 5, 2022, in *The Neurohospitalist Society* journal, tells us that Brianna's death by ischemic stroke is associated with, or caused by, mRNA covid vaccination.[6]

Nearly every paragraph in Brianna's *Brief Report* associates the vaccine as causing Brianna's stroke and furthers that clots, bleeds, and strokes are not uncommon with covid vaccines.

However, contrary to all prior paragraphs in Brianna's *Brief Report*, the authors switch characterization one hundred eighty degrees in the summary, which is the only paragraph many people read. In the summary, they deem the resultant covid vaccine-caused death to be "extremely rare." Unfortunately, this form of editorial dishonesty has become the rule rather than the exception in most publications concerning covid.

Many highly published scientists and doctors have been asked by journal editors to make changes to soften any implications that paint covid vaccines in a negative light. Oftentimes, they are asked to summarize the paper in a manner contradictory to all the evidence brought forth in the paper's body. Those who fail to comply with this form of self-censorship are censored by outright rejection of papers without a reason stated.

Brianna's *Brief Report* further expresses that Brianna reacted to the Moderna covid vaccine with a severe headache within hours of injection. She degraded quickly until there was a lack of brain activity in days.

Brianna tested positive for covid more than three months before her covid vaccination and was deemed asymptomatic for covid at that time. In other words, she tested positive asymptomatically months earlier and her death was certified as a covid death. Yet, she reacted within hours to the vaccine, which was not mentioned on her death certificate. This is fraud.

Brianna's death certificate, at time of publication of this book, still states that covid is the root cause of death and makes no mention of the covid vaccine as a cause of her death.

Agents of the Commonwealth of Massachusetts were given notice on or before September 9, 2022, via summonses in a Complaint for Injunctive and Declaratory Relief. Having been given notice of Brianna's erroneous death certificate, agents of the Commonwealth had a reasonable time to make changes. They have not corrected the erroneous information in more than ten months and, thus, are now in violation of several federal felony offenses.

Notably, the authors of Brianna's *Brief Report* go out of their way to state that Brianna's ischemic stroke is not a Cerebral Venous Sinus Thrombosis (CVST) type of stroke, which "*has been previously associated with COVID-19 vaccination.*" As noted above, 17-year-old Eden died from a CVST stroke weeks after Brianna died and only about twenty (~20) miles away. The authors of Brianna's *Brief Report* also add to the prior quote, "*... where thrombocytopenia is frequent ...*" Remember that 62-year-old Diane died from an intracranial hemorrhagic stroke in the setting of thrombocytopenia only weeks before Brianna was injected.

Three strokes occurred in two women and one teenage girl in three months in one state. If the VAERS pharmacovigilance system was working properly, if mandatory reporters were making reports, if doctors and medical examiners were completing death certificates properly instead of fraudulently, and if public health officials were doing their jobs dutifully, then these bleeding and clotting deaths from covid vaccination could have been prevented.

Honest presentation of facts to the public is all that is required from government. The public's acceptance or rejection of covid vaccines should derive from honest informed consent and not government slogans and commercials.

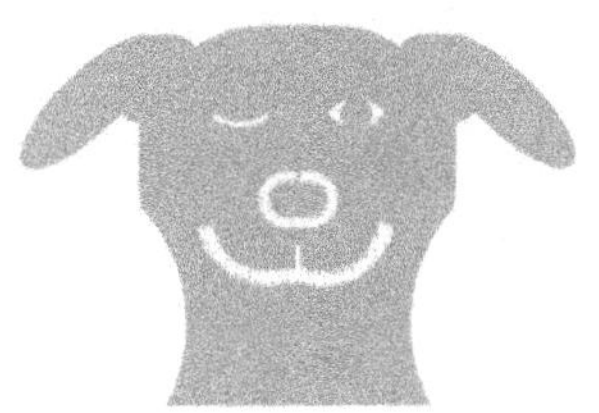

Chapter 3
From Acquaintances

People sought me out to make me aware of the deaths in this chapter. The accounts deserve to be heard and read. The bringers of these accounts care about others, and they want others to know about their friends, extended family members, work mates, or acquaintances.

Holly Renee (Earley) Hodgdon died at the age of 42 on September 13, 2021, at home in Massachusetts.[1] Holly's death left a hole in the lives of a great many people, including her husband, two sons, both her parents, and others.

Holly's brother, Daniel Earley, posted in June of 2021 on social media (as I recall from reading) that he was worried about his sister's internal bleeding. Upon reading Holly's obituary online, I was confused when I read that Holly's brother, Dan, had died before her.

Daniel Earley died at the age of 37 on June 29, 2021, a couple weeks after posting that he was worried about his sister, Holly. The obituary online states that Dan "*passed unexpectedly and peacefully in the comfort of his home with the love of his wife near.*"[2]

Since Dan died in New Hampshire, I do not have his death certificate record. Holly's death certificate states only one cause or condition contributing. There is nothing else listed for this otherwise healthy wife and mother of two young boys. Cause A states, "*COVID-19 INFECTION.*" How does someone die from covid without any listed symptoms whatsoever, and at such a young age?

The Earley parents lost both of their children at the ages of 37 and 42 from "*COVID-19*" "*unexpectedly and peacefully*" and without any follow-up investigation by medical professionals or public officials. Holly's death certificate feloniously lacks a cause of death.

Intentional omission of root cause of death is a federal felony because death certificates are used in federal CDC records.

When were Holly and Dan vaccinated for covid? The public interest so demands this information.

One day in town I was approached by someone who asked if I was the guy who writes about covid on Twitter. I answered affirmatively. He then told me that he follows my work and that he wanted to tell me about his brother's friend.

The man told me the friend's first and last names, place of employment, age, date of death, and job function. He also told me that the friend's employer, Bose Corporation, mandated covid vaccination. Bose was going to terminate his employment if he didn't take a covid vaccine. I was told that the man did not want to take a covid vaccine and that he contemplated quitting his job. On the last day before being fired, the friend relented because he financially needed his job. He received a covid vaccine injection.

The friend, Charles Casella, died November 16, 2021, at the age of 48 in Massachusetts. He was found in bed deceased the morning after his covid vaccine injection. The gentleman who told me this information had everything correct. I sent him a message to let him know the cause of death listed on the death certificate.

Charles' death certificate states that Cause A (the immediate cause) is "*COVID-19.*" There are no underlying causes listed in Part I. Part II Conditions Contributing lists only "*OBESITY.*" There is a big difference between the use of "*OBESITY*" and "*MORBID OBESITY,*" the latter of which is common among real covid deaths.

The public interest so demands that we should know Charles' vaccination date, especially in relation to his death date. The Commonwealth of Massachusetts was notified of the information herein on September 9, 2022. Failure to cure mistakes in a reasonable time manifests in intent to misinform, which is felony fraud.

Abigail (Abby) Sarom Fitzgerald died on December 22, 2021, at the age of 20 in Massachusetts. According to her obituary, Abby was a civil engineering major at a private Massachusetts college, though she maintained New Hampshire as her place of residence where she was raised. More personal information found in the obituary is, of course, heart-wrenching to read. Abby participated in varsity athletics, dance, music performance, and a multitude of other activities. By all accounts, Abby was a healthy, accomplished, intelligent, athletic young woman.

Abby's death certificate states Cause A is "*EOSINOPHILIC MYOCARDITIS*" in "*3 WKS,*" and Cause B is "*ACUTE SYSTOLIC HEART FAILURE*" in "*3 WKS.*"

College mandates for covid vaccination were ubiquitous at the time Abby died. Most schools did not allow exemptions. In fact, the law school I attended is 5.4 miles from the college Abby attended. It is highly likely that Abby had been recently vaccinated for covid; and it is certain that Abby died from a condition widely known to be causally linked to covid vaccines.

There does not appear to be a VAERS report for Abby. If Abby was vaccinated for covid and died shortly thereafter from a known deadly side effect, then many people associated with this case violated several felonies of fraud and inaction concurrent with a legal duty to act, to report to VAERS, and to proffer an accurate death certificate.

Amaya McDonough-Rocha died on August 29, 2022, at the age of 12 in Massachusetts.

I asked Albert Benavides of the VAERSAware.com website to send any suspicious Massachusetts VAERS reports to me. In February 2023, Albert sent me the VAERS report of a young girl. VAERS_ID 2582749 reports on a girl, age 12, who received her third (3rd) dose of Pfizer covid vaccine, HPV Gardasil 9 vaccine, Sanofi Meningococcal Conjugate Menactra, and Sanofi TDAP Adacel—all on August 3, 2022. Here is the record of VAERS_ID 2582749:[3]

- *Date Report Received 02/15/2023*
- *Date Vaccinated 08/03/2022*
- *Date of Onset 08/30/2022*
- *Date Died 08/30/2022*
- *Age "12.00"*
- *Sex "Female"*
- *Symptom "BLOOD ELECTROLYTES NORMAL, BRAIN HERNIATION, BRAIN OEDEMA, HEADACHE, SUDDEN DEATH, TOXICOLOGIC TEST NORMAL"*

- *Adverse Event Description "Sudden Death after a headache episode Post shows Cerebellar tonsillar and bilateral uncal herniation in the setting of 'mild' cerebral edema No fever No rash."*

Notice that the report date to VAERS is 2/15/2023, but the date of death is 08/30/2022. That's about six months apart. Someone did the right thing by reporting, but why did it take so long? During those six months, many more children died. It can take about six months for some death certificates to be finalized, especially those of children. It seems likely that someone received Amaya's death certificate and then filed a VAERS report using the death certificate as the text for adverse event input.

VAERS_ID 2582749 matches the death certificate of Amaya McDonough-Rocha, though there is one small mistake on the VAERS report. The death certificate states that the death occurred on August 29, 2022, a day before the VAERS report death date. The death certificate also states that Amaya was a 12-year-old female. Cause A states, "*SUDDEN CARDIAC DEATH IN A PERSON WITH DILATION OF THE FRONTAL,*" Cause B states, "*HORNS OF THE LATERAL VENTRICLES, CEREBRAL EDEMA, AND,*" Cause C states, "*CEREBELLAR TONSILLAR AND BILATERAL UNCAL HERNIATION.*" There are no Conditions Contributing in Part II.

Notice that the UCOD, or root cause, Cause C, is verbatim from the VAERS report. There is no question that this is the same girl.

If anyone from the CDC or state health department had fulfilled their legal duty to investigate the deaths of Diane, Brianna, Eden, Holly, Dan, Charles, Abby, Cassidy, or Amaya, then perhaps Ian would be alive today.

Ian Robert Shumaker, age 11, died on December 3, 2022. His death certificate states Cause A is "*COMPLICATIONS OF CARDIAC DYSRHYTHMIA OF UNKNOWN,*" Cause B is "*ETIOLOGY IN THE SETTING OF ACUTE UPPER RESPIRATORY,*" and Cause C is "*INFECTION.*" This is another example wherein the death certifier extended a single sentence across multiple "Cause of Death" fields in Part I, in this case, Causes A through C.

Although the following is a word of mouth account comprising second-hand information, I believe it is completely reliable. Ian is said to have felt chest pain and difficulty breathing shortly after receiving a covid booster vaccine. I was told he was brought to a hospital and quickly put on a ventilator. Ian is said to have died shortly after ventilation. I was also told that upon organ donation and removal of his heart for potential transplant, the heart was rejected because it was full of clots.

Of course, child deaths did occur before covid. However, given the correlation of death certificates to VAERS records and the *Brief Report* published by six doctors, one would have to twist his mind into a pretzel of willful ignorance to dismiss all the evidence provided thus far. And there are many more detailed accounts of human tragedy in the following chapters.

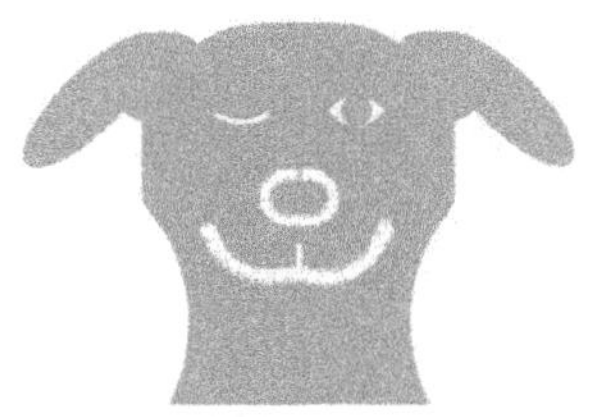

Chapter 4
Vermont

A gentleman by the name of Aaron Hertz obtained the Vermont death certificates from the State of Vermont. However, Vermont did not provide Aaron a database with ICD-10 codes. Instead, we had to use character string searches in Parts I and II to perform data analyses. Two of the Vermont reports are presented here to show that Massachusetts is not the only state with deaths that were almost certainly caused by covid vaccines.

Karyn Samantha Slack died in Vermont on November 21, 2021, at the age of 45. Her online obituary states that she passed away "due to natural causes" and that she was a mother, wife, and friend to many.[1]

Karyn's death certificate states Cause A is "*Pulmonary Thromboembolism*" in "*days,*" Cause B is "*Multifactorial (See Part 2)*" in "*days-years,*" and Part II states, "*Recently Sedentary, Obesity (Body mass index 46.9), Desogestrel/ethinyl estradiol use, and COVID-19 and Influenza vaccinations on 11/11/2021.*"

Given that the word "*COVID*" is in Part II of Karyn's death certificate, CDC's parser might apply the U07.1 code to this death certificate even though "COVID" is used in context to note the type of vaccine given to Karyn on November 11, 2021. Because the ICD-10 codes applied by the CDC's parser are not included on the Vermont death certificates, I do not know if the CDC included U-071 on Karyn's death certificate. If the CDC did so, it would be a systemic error that likely causes massive overcounting of covid deaths. The certifier should have included a vaccine or immunization code on Karyn's death certificate. In fact, by the rules of how to complete death certificates, the covid vaccine should be mentioned in Part I of Karyn's death certificate. Karyn died from a pulmonary embolism, which is somewhat common among covid vaccine side-effects. Most concerning is that a software ICD-10 code parser may be so poor that it could assign

Karyn's death as a U07.1 covid death while omitting any vaccine-related codes.

"*Recently sedentary*" might indicate that Karyn could not walk across the room without feeling tired and out of breath, which is a sign of pulmonary embolism. The drug mentioned is simply prescribed for birth control and menopausal symptoms. However, contraindications include anything that causes thrombosis including DVT (deep vein thrombosis—usually in the calf muscle) and pulmonary embolism. Obesity is common among covid victims and covid vaccine victims, but is also common among Americans, in general.

Having the vaccination date on Karyn's death certificate makes the search of VAERS much easier. There are no entries in the 2021 VAERS database for a 45-year-old female from Vermont vaccinated on November 11, 2021. Remembering that Amaya's VAERS report was entered six months after her death, a search of 2022 VAERS database was performed.

VAERS_ID 2317423 is the only report of a Vermont woman, age 45, vaccinated on November 11, 2021. Here is the record of VAERS_ID 2317423.[2]

- *Date Report Received 06/13/2022*
- *Date Vaccinated 11/11/2021*
- *Date of Onset 11/20/2021*
- *Date Died 11/21/2021*
- *Age "45.00"*
- *Sex "Female"*
- *Symptom "AUTOPSY, DEATH, EXERCISE LACK OF, FATIGUE, MALAISE, PULMONARY EMBOLISM, RESPIRATORY DISORDER, UNRESPONSIVE TO STIMULI"*
- *Adverse Event Description "Decedent was reportedly feeling unwell with respiratory complaints for several days to week prior to death, progressively became more "wiped out" and tired, staying in bed most of the time. She was found unresponsive in the bathroom where she was pronounced dead by EMS. Autopsy confirmed bilateral pulmonary thromboemboli as cause of death, with multiple risk factors including obesity (BMI 46.9), recently sedentary, COVID-19 and Influenza vaccinations, and Desogestrel/ethinyl estradiol."*

Again, more than six months elapsed between death and the VAERS report; and the VAERS report resembles closely the language in the death certificate, but with a few more notables. Clearly, this VAERS_ID 2317423 corresponds to Karyn.

The pulmonary embolism was bilateral, meaning that she had clots in both lungs at the same time. Symptoms of pulmonary embolism are shortness of breath and feeling tired as described in Karyn's VAERS report.

A look at the timing shows that Karyn received a dose of Moderna covid vaccine and a dose of Seqirus quadrivalent influenza vaccine on November 11, 2021. Karyn died ten days later. Although the onset of symptoms is listed in VAERS as November 20, 2021, the day before Karyn died, the text of the VAERS report states that Karyn complained of respiratory issues for days up to a week prior to death. Thus, the onset of symptoms was long before November 20, 2021, and very close to Karyn's vaccination date.

This case notes again the importance of individual record investigation. Six month reporting lag, incorrect onset of symptoms dates, yet reaction in a couple days and death in ten days from a known side-effect of the covid vaccines is extremely important to report to the public. However, the government does not report these deaths to the public. It is left to ordinary citizens to investigate and inform the public, while the government attempts to impede citizen investigation.

Martin Aloysius Joyce, IV died in Vermont on April 23, 2021 at the age of 52.[3] Martin's death certificate states Cause A is "*Cardiopulmonary arrest*," Cause B is "*Congestive Heart Failure*," Cause C is "*Non-ST segment elevation myocardial infarction*," Cause D is "*Arteriosclerotic cardiovascular disease*," and Other Contributing Conditions are "*Obesity, Chronic obstructive pulmonary disease (type unspecified).*"

VAERS_ID 1247687 represents the only 52-year-old man from Vermont who is listed as having died on April 23, 2021. Here is the record of VAERS_ID 1247687:[4]

- *Date Report Received 04/23/2021*
- *Date Vaccinated 04/20/2021*
- *Date of Onset 04/21/2021*
- *Date Died 04/23/2021*
- *Age "52.00"*
- *Sex "Male"*
- *Adverse Event Description "Patient presented early this morning with increasing shortness of breath, chest tightness and associated*

chills. Treated with laboratory studies, xray and CT for PE studies, EKG x2, BIPAP, decline in status, intubated, CPR , expired."

If the VAERS report represents Martin, then he reacted within one day and died from a heart attack within three days of covid vaccination.

Martin's obituary notes that he "died unexpectedly" and had a wife, family, friends. Martin grew up on the Jersey Shore.[3]

Vermont is a very small state with fewer than one tenth the population of the Commonwealth of Massachusetts. The population size only matters to the extent that signals in data are more difficult to find by researchers. A more in-depth data analysis is presented in subsequent chapters. *PRIMA PARS* focuses on relating the tragic stories of individual people.

Karyn and Martin were young. They had families and friends who loved them. It is highly likely that they were killed by the same deadly medical interventions that killed Cassidy, Abby, Ian, Diane, Brianna, Eden, Charles, and the many other human beings whose untimely deaths are related in upcoming chapters.

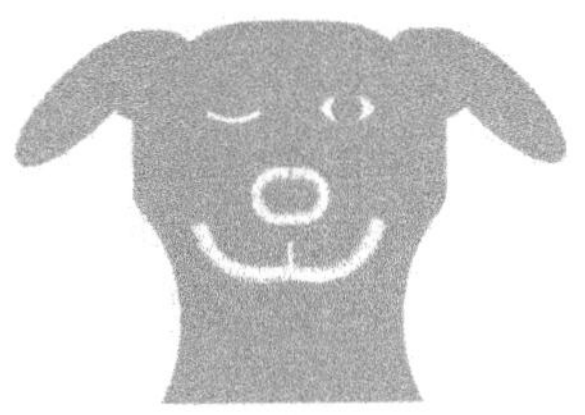

Chapter 5
Fraud of Commission

"Fraud," in a legal sense, is a serious crime. It means far more than a simple lie or misrepresentation. This chapter and the next are not light accusations in a colloquial use of the word "fraud."

Under the Common Law, conviction for fraud requires that the prosecution prove beyond reasonable doubt that 1) the actor made a false representation, 2) the actor knew or should have known that the representation was false at the time he made it, 3) that the actor intended that the recipient of the falsity rely upon it, 4) that the recipient did indeed rely upon the falsity, and 5) that the reliance upon the falsity did bring some harm to the recipient, or another.[1]

There are several specific state and federal statutes involving fraud. Many of these statutes are applicable to the factual evidence reported in these pages. False statements in healthcare matters, fraud in disaster relief, and fraud by wire are but a few of the specific federal felony statutes predicated on fraud.

"Fraud of commission" refers to representations made that are false, as opposed to "fraud of omission," discussed in the next chapter, which refers to representations knowingly and intentionally not made while there exists a duty of the actor to make such representations.

Brianna's death (Chapter 2) was labeled a "covid" death. Covid was the last cause listed in the underlying causes of death (UCOD), which is reserved for the root cause that kicked off the causal chain of events. Knowing that Brianna reacted to the covid vaccine within twenty-four hours and knowing that her condition deteriorated rapidly to cessation of brain activity in just a few days, the certifier of death for Brianna likely committed a fraudulent act upon certification of her death.

One conceivable defense would be that a covid vaccine causes strokes in some people if they previously were infected by covid. In order to invoke this defense, the death certifier would have to openly state factually that those who previously had covid are at a higher risk of dying from the vaccine. The "complication" from COVID-19 would be the covid vaccine, though not listed on the death certificate.

Thus, either there was a fraud committed on Brianna's death certificate or the certifier is stating that those who previously were infected with covid would be risking their very lives by taking a covid vaccine. Either way, the covid vaccine is the proximate and actual cause of Brianna's death.

Cassidy's death certificate (Chapter 1) also stated that covid was the immediate cause of death without any other UCODs, thereby making the immediate cause also the UCOD. Again, if Cassidy is the 7-year-old girl in the VAERS report, ID 2038120, then she reacted in five minutes to the first dose, reacted within one to two days of the second dose, and died within five days of the injection. The medical examiner in Cassidy's case is Michele Matthews. That phrase "complications of ..." seems different from the work of all other medical examiners. Dr. Matthews did not list any UCODs. How can that be?

Dr. Drew Pinsky brought me up to speak from a Twitter Space onto his live show a couple of times. One time, I told Dr. Drew that I observed behavioral habits of certain doctors and medical examiners reflected in the way they filled out death certificates. A good example of this is the certifier of Cassidy's death certificate.

In a search of Massachusetts death certificates from the year 2022, Cause A was filtered for all death certificates that contain the strings, "*COMPLICATIONS*" and "*CORONAVIRUS*." From a total of nearly sixty-four thousand death certificates in the Massachusetts 2022 database, this search returned six death records. All six were certified by Medical Examiner Michele Matthews. Five of the six stated in Cause A, "*COMPLICATIONS OF CORONAVIRUS-19 VIRAL INFECTION*" and one stated, "*COMPLICATIONS OF CORONAVIRUS-19 INFECTION*." None of the six had any UCODs in Cause B, C, or D, which is unusual.

Deaths can be certified by attending physicians, physician's assistants, or medical examiners. Professional medical examiners seem not to practice as physicians, but rather they each certify around four hundred deaths per year as noted in later chapters.

Michele Matthews is a professional medical examiner. The ages of the six people Dr. Matthews certified as having died from "complications" from covid and had no other UCODs in Part I are 58, 53, 7 (Cassidy), 35, 45, and 59. None of these are elderly. Some of the death certificates specified a few Conditions Contributing: "*ASTHMA*" on three records, "*MORBID OBESITY*" on one, "*CHRONIC ALCOHOL ABUSE*" on one, and HIV on one.

What did these people die from, and why is Dr. Matthews not fulfilling her duty to The People?

If Cassidy did die from the covid vaccine and covid was not causal in her death, then her death certificate is doubly fraudulent. We then have to wonder about these other five that have no UCODs. If they died from covid pneumonia, then pneumonia should be the immediate or underlying cause. Neither is there cardiopulmonary arrest in Part I, nor COPD, nor ARDS, nor anything that documents the true cause of death.

And if Dr. Matthews was in the habit of labeling deaths with covid that had no causal relationship to covid, then how many other medical examiners and physicians behaved the same way?

The world enacted policies in 2020 based on data from the locations with the highest death tolls from covid. New Jersey, New York, and Massachusetts were the top three jurisdictions in the world for more than a year in reported covid deaths per population. If Massachusetts is rife with the commission of covid reporting fraud, then the basis for the entire pandemic must be questioned.

The 2021 database contains exactly three records returned by a search using identical search criteria. All three were certified by Michele Mathews. There are no underlying causes listed. Only one of the three has any Conditions Contributing: "*HYPERTENSIVE AND ATHEROSCLEROTIC CARDIOVASCULAR DISEASE, CHRONIC OBSTRUCTIVE PULMONARY DISEASE.*" The reported ages are 37, 62, and 67. What did these people really die from?

The 2020 database contains exactly three records returned by a search using identical search criteria. All three were certified by Michele Mathews. There are no UCODs listed. Two of the three have Conditions Contributing: "*ALZHEIMER'S DISEASE*" for a 94 year old decedent, and "*DIABETES MELLITUS*" for a 74 year old decedent. The third decedent was 28 years old. What did these people really die from, particularly the 28-year-old man? A 28-year-old man died and there is no record of any symptoms on his death certificate except covid. How can this be anything but fraud?

Medical examiners know, or should know, that they have a duty to certify deaths listing only causes in Part I and Conditions Contributing in Part II. It is fraudulent to apply the cause "covid" for accidental deaths resulting from poisoning, such as drug overdoses, or resulting from blunt force trauma, such as from car accidents or falls by elderly people. The results from search criteria such as these yield compelling suggestions of criminal fraud of commission.

A search was made for Massachusetts death certificates recorded in 2020, 2021, and 2022 that specify ICD-10 codes X42 "Accidental poisoning by and exposure to narcotics and psychodysleptics (hallucinogens), not elsewhere classified" and U07.1 "COVID-19."

For 2020, there are eight death certificates that specify both X42 and U07.1. All involve drug overdoses as the immediate or underlying cause. All eight are labeled "*Accident*" deaths.

In 2021, there are five death certificates that specify U07.1 and also specify X42 as the immediate or underlying cause and one death certificate that specifies U07.1 and also X42 as a Contributing Condition, though it is written as "*ACUTE COCAINE INTOXICATION*," which means, in the moment of death, there was enough substance in the blood to cause death. All six are labeled "*Accident*" deaths and the injuries are labeled "*SUBSTANCE ABUSE*."

In 2022, there are twelve Deaths Certificates that specify both U07.1 and X42. All specify drug overdose as the immediate cause, and some specify drug overdoses as the underlying cause. In other words, some died from combined effects of multiple recreational drugs taken at the same time. All twelve are labeled "*Accident*" deaths and the injuries are labeled "*SUBSTANCE ABUSE*."

Multiple medical examiners and physicians certified these deaths, indicating a pattern of fraud across the enterprise of the medical community. Medical examiners are employed by the Commonwealth of Massachusetts, while physicians are employed by private entities such as hospitals, firms, or self-employed.

Another search was done for death certificates that include U07.1 in ICD-10 codes and "*BLUNT FORCE TRAUMA*" in Cause A. In 2020, there are twelve such records. In 2021, there are five. In 2022, there are twelve. All were labeled "*Accident*."

In Massachusetts, for the year 2020, there is a total of 73 deaths in a Manner of "*Accident*" that also carry the ICD-10 code U07.1. In 2021, a search for those same criteria yields 45 records. In 2022, a search for those same criteria yields 76. The total across three years is 194 Massachusetts "*Accident*" deaths assigned the ICD-10 code for death from covid.

Given the willingness of the enterprise of health professionals to commit such blatant fraud in adding covid to accidental deaths, a reasonable citizen will likely doubt all counts of covid deaths. Even the CDC does not claim that the covid shots are effective against accidental death. Imagine how many heart attacks in elderly people may have been misrepresented as covid deaths.

In fact, Medical Examiner Marie Elizabeth Cannon certified one (1) "*Suicide*" death in 2020 with covid in Part II.

Although investigation of these issues could fill a series of books, one additional look at potential fraud of commission follows.

Janice Grivetti is a professional medical examiner who certified totals 327, 479, and 393 deaths in years 2020–2022, respectively.

In 2020, Dr. Grivetti certified ten covid deaths. Three were labeled "*Accident,*" one from acute fentanyl overdose, one from right hip fracture, and one from rib fractures. Seven have covid in Cause A and no underlying causes listed. Among these seven, Part II does list symptoms such as obesity, COPD, and fractures.

In 2021, Dr. Grivetti certified nine covid deaths. Two were labeled "*Accident,*" one from blunt force trauma of torso and one from acute cocaine overdose. Six have covid in Cause A and no underlying causes of death. Among these six, Part II lists symptoms such as obesity, hypertensive cardiovascular disease, alcoholism, cirrhosis, asthma, and pulmonary embolism.

In 2022, Dr. Grivetti certified four covid deaths. Two were labeled "*Accident,*" one acute fentanyl overdose and one blunt force trauma of the neck. Two have covid in Cause A and no underlying causes of death. Among these, Part II lists hypertensive cardiovascular disease, multiple sclerosis, and leukemia.

In ICD-10 codes, those that begin with "J" are "Diseases of the respiratory system." These include pneumonia, COPD, influenza, and upper and lower respiratory issues. Covid is often referred to as a seasonal respiratory virus. If you believe that, then you may expect "J" codes to accompany a covid death.

Dr. Grivetti certified 23 total deaths involving covid spanning the years 2020 and 2021. Of those 23, "J" codes only appeared in two records. One in 2021 was deemed "*RECENT COVID-19 PNEUMONIA*" in Cause B. One in 2020 was deemed COPD in Part II.

Dr. Grivetti did not certify a U07.1 covid death in 2022 after July 11, 2022. Grivetti is a defendant in a lawsuit in the U.S. District Court, District of Massachusetts, for allegedly fraudulently certifying covid deaths.[2] She was notified of this lawsuit on or before September 9, 2022.

These examples of death certificates certified by many medical examiners and doctors seem to indicate large scale fraud of commission in counting covid deaths that had no causal relationship to covid. If someone died from drug overdose or blunt force trauma in the past, the dead bodies were not tested for influenza and labeled influenza deaths. The health records of the decedents were not scanned for positive influenza tests in the past year or more and then labeled influenza deaths. Yet that did happen in years 2020–2022, but with the label of "covid."

Further consider that if the participants in the healthcare enterprise are willing to blatantly label accidents and a suicide with "covid," then they likely would not hesitate to place the label "covid" on deaths involving heart attacks, Alzheimer's, dementia, liver failure, cancers, and other causes in elderly or otherwise terminal people.

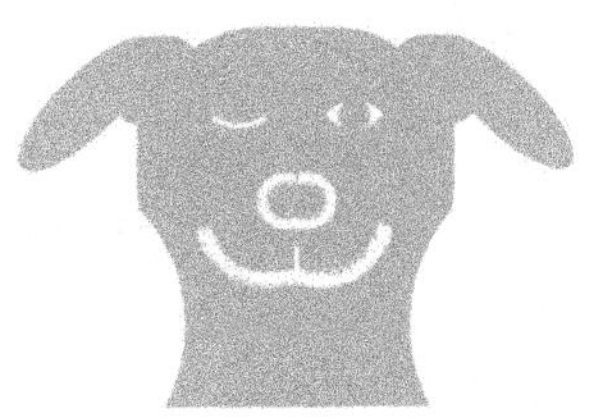

Chapter 6
Fraud of Omission

People have duties. Some are contractual duties entered into under one's own volition. And some are legal duties, the violation of which carries penalties in tort or criminal penalties. Law schools often use the example of a drowning child. The child's parents, someone with lifeguard experience, policemen and firemen, and specific others have a legal duty to save a drowning child when they come across him. However, the average person has no such legal duty. One can watch the child go under water, do nothing, and then walk away without criminal liability. Specific people have a *legal duty to act* based upon their agency, experience, and profession.

Regarding death certificates, physicians and medical examiners attest that the information is true and accurate when they sign the death certificate. They have a duty to ensure a death certificate is true and accurate, to the best of their knowledge, and in conformance with express written standards and expected behavior and practice. This also means that they have a duty not to certify a death certificate if they know the death certificate does not represent the true and accurate cause of death.

A crime of omission is the failure to perform an act that is required as a matter of legal duty. If someone died from blunt force trauma in an automobile crash, then the medical examiner has a legal duty to write "blunt force trauma" or an equivalent phrase as a cause of death. And if the medical examiner found, through medical imaging, that the same crash victim had massive bilateral pulmonary emboli that caused unconsciousness while driving, then the medical examiner has a legal duty to add "pulmonary embolism" as a cause of death. Omission of "pulmonary embolism" while knowing of the bilateral pulmonary emboli is a criminal violation of a legal duty.

Seven-year-old Cassidy's death certificate (Chapter 1) did not mention a covid vaccine or any immunization as a possible cause of death or condition contributing to her death. If Cassidy is the girl in the VAERS report and she did react severely and immediately to both doses, and if the medical examiner knew this information upon certifying her death certificate, then the medical examiner committed a fraud of omission on a public document.

Brianna's death certificate (Chapter 2) is an express fraud of omission beyond reasonable doubt because doctors from the same medical firm where Brianna died wrote a *Brief Report* detailing their knowledge that the vaccine caused her stroke death. Dr. Steven Schwartz, the medical examiner who certified Brianna's death certificate, knew or should have known the root cause of Brianna's stroke death and had a legal duty to include the covid vaccine as a cause of her death.

Some death certificates did mention the vaccine as a cause of death, but the ICD-10 codes, which were assigned by CDC's automated parser and are supposed to represent all causes listed in Parts I and II of the death certificates, included no codes for vaccine or immunization. Some examples of these deficiencies are included in Chapter 8. Clearly, the CDC parser, possibly in conjunction with manual intervention, is inappropriately omitting ICD-10 codes related to immunization or vaccination. If it is incompetence, it rises to malfeasance. If manual intervention is involved, it would be prima facie criminal fraud.

I have listened to doctors and lawyers from all over the United States publicly declare that ICD-10 codes for covid vaccine death are not listed because there are no ICD-10 codes for covid vaccines. This is absurdly false and misleading. The CDC cannot claim they omitted vaccines as a cause of death "because there are no codes."

First, the death certifiers have a legal duty to list a covid vaccine in Parts I or II if there is any hint of contribution in the causal chain of events leading to death. Second, there are plenty of possible codes for the CDC to apply using their parser or manual intervention.

ICD-10 code Y59.0 represents, "Viral vaccines." Y59.8 represents, "Other specified vaccines and biological substances." Y59.9 represents, "Vaccine or biological substance, unspecified." T88.0 represents, "Infection following immunization." T88.1 represents, "Other complications following immunization, not elsewhere classified."

If you hold a McIntosh apple in your hand and a barrel is in front of you labeled, "Apples," would you be acting correctly if you tossed your apple into the barrel? There need not be an ICD-10 code specific to a Moderna or a Pfizer mRNA covid vaccine. The CDC has plenty of appropriate codes to use.

The omission of "vaccine" in Parts I or II on death certificates of people who had onset of symptoms in minutes and death within a day of covid vaccination is a criminally fraudulent act if the medical examiner knew of the injection. This has been happening en masse across the enterprise. Covid vaccine as a cause of death only appears on nine of the nearly 500,000 Massachusetts death certificates certified between 2015 and 2022. Of these, there is but one and only one death certificate which was assigned Y59.0 or T88.1 by the CDC parser; and it listed both. Medical Examiner Rebecca Dedrick certified the death of Solomon A. Kizitoh, who died on January 16, 2021, at the age of 60. Cause A states, "*ACUTE BRONCHOPNEUMONIA AND IDIOPATHIC.*" Cause B states, "*THROMBOCYTOPENIA FOLLOWING COVID-19 VACCINATION*" in "*DAYS.*"

Dr. Dedrick is telling us that the covid vaccine was causal in Solomon's death. And we know from the *Brief Report* about Brianna's stroke death that "*thrombocytopenia is frequent*" in CVST types of stroke death. I often joke that an intern must have been working that day in the medical coding department. Y59.0 and T88.1 appear nowhere else in 2015–2022 despite there being many obvious covid vaccine deaths among the Massachusetts death certificates.

If covid vaccine deaths are not coded, then no one, including the CDC, can possibly know how many deaths were caused by the covid vaccines. It is a criminal act of fraud of omission for the entire health enterprise to systematically omit covid vaccines as a cause of death and/or fail to apply ICD-10 codes for vaccines on death certificates.

Evidence of fraud is plentiful throughout the database of Massachusetts death certificates. A search for death certificates containing ICD-10 codes that begin with Y59 or T88 was performed; and the following examples appeared.

The death certificate for a woman, age 82, who died in 2021, contains the following information. Cause A states, "*ANAPHYLAXIS FOLLOWING IRON INFUSION FOR THE TREATMENT OF.*" Cause B states, "*CHRONIC ANEMIA.*" The ICD-10 codes listed are Y57.9, "Drug or medicament, unspecified," and T88.6, "Anaphylactic shock due to adverse effect of correct drug or medicament properly administered." The ICD-10 codes that the CDC applied to this certificate match the written Causes A and B.

The death certificate for a woman, age 62, who died in 2021, contains the following information. Cause A states, "*PROBABLE ALLERGIC REACTION IN THE SETTING OF RECENT UMECLIDINIUM USE*" in "*MIN.*" The ICD-10 codes listed are Y42.7, "Androgens and anabolic congeners," and T88.7, "Unspecified adverse effect of drug or medicament." The codes match the words in Cause A.

Two more similar death certificates for deaths that occurred in 2021 related to "*COMPLICATIONS OF CANCER THERAPY*" and "*DRUG ADVERSE EFFECT-ASPIRIN*."

In the 2022 database, a search of the same criteria, ICD-10 codes beginning with Y59 or T88, yielded five records. These death certificates expressing ICD-10 codes that begin with Y59 or T88 are evidence that medical examiners and physicians actually do include various oral and intravenous products as causes of death in Parts I and II. Accordingly, they must be aware of these types of causes in order to document them on death certificates. Thus, the CDC does apply the appropriate Y59 and T88 prefix codes as evinced here.

This begs the question, "Why does the CDC fail to apply the appropriate codes to death certificates that document covid vaccines as a cause of death?" The death certificates presented immediately above are prima facie evidence that the family of classification headers appropriate when death is caused by covid vaccine are applied when death is caused by other injectable or orally administered substances.

In other words, there are no legally acceptable excuses for omitting covid vaccines in Parts I or II when they are a cause of death, and no legally acceptable excuses for failing to apply appropriate ICD-10 codes to those death certificates, which specify covid vaccine as a cause of death. There is compelling evidence that, for some reason, the enterprise of healthcare professionals criminally avoids listing covid vaccines in Parts I and II and the CDC also criminally avoids applying the ICD-10 codes available to represent deaths caused by covid vaccines.

PRIMA PARS - CONCLUSION

PRIMA PARS details Massachusetts covid vaccine-caused deaths, likely covid vaccine-caused deaths, a string of stroke deaths from vaccines, likely Vermont covid vaccine-caused deaths, frauds of commission by specifying causes of death as covid when there was no causal relationship to covid, and frauds of omission by omitting covid vaccine as a cause of death when the facts demand its express inclusion.

PRIMA PARS is about people. All of these deaths are people who had families and friends. They were as young as six or seven years old. They deserve the truth to be known. The living deserve to hear the truth to have a chance at informed consent.

Please also know that I spent more than three and a half hours reviewing several hundred death certificates with a medical examiner who worked in Boston during the first covid wave. He wishes to remain anonymous, and I cannot use certain information from him in this book. I do know some of the reasons for criminal conduct by medical examiners and physicians, but that is not the focus of *PRIMA PARS*.

The goal of this book is to communicate the truth as revealed by a compilation of factual information. *PRIMA PARS* explains the breadth and depth of the compiled factual information.

SECUNDA PARS presents correlations of death certificates with VAERS reports and obituaries, but on a larger scale and without the detail in *PRIMA PARS*.

TERTIA PARS presents the results of extensive analysis of all these data.

QUARTA PARS proposes some solutions to correct a corrupt and badly broken system. Thank you for reading *PRIMA PARS*.

SECUNDA PARS

Correlation

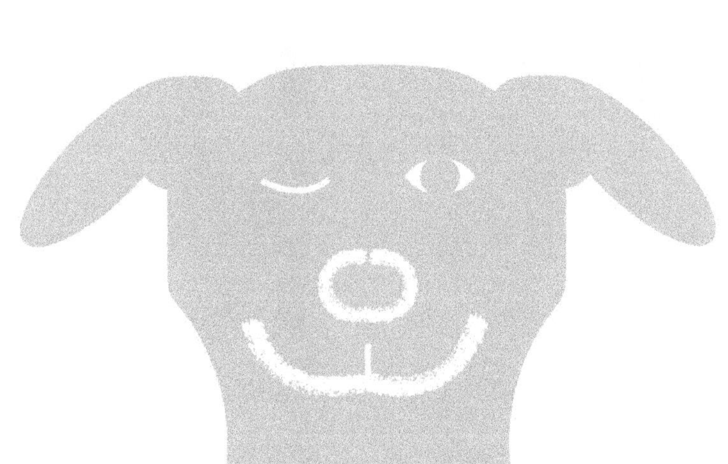

BEYOND REASONABLE DOUBT

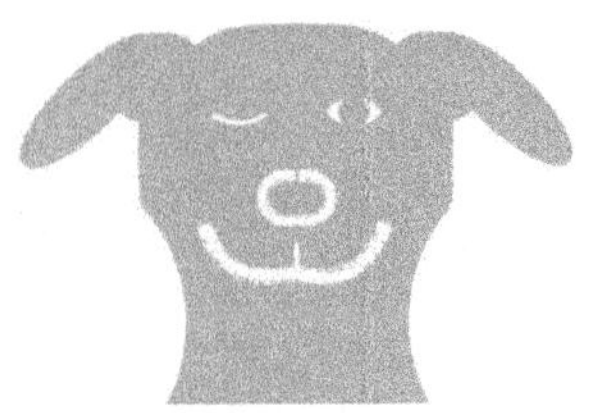

Chapter 7
VAERS

The Vaccine Adverse Event Reporting System (VAERS) was established in 1990 under the U.S. Department of Health and Human Services as an early warning system to detect safety signals in vaccines. As of August 2023, the World Health Organization's website defines "vaccine safety signal" as "information that indicates a potential link between a vaccine and an event previously unknown or incompletely documented, that could affect health. The signal, which may come from one or multiple sources, will suggest a new potentially causal association (or a new aspect of a known association) between a vaccine and an event (or a set of related events), which could be either adverse or beneficial." [1]

As of August 2023, the CDC's website explains, "The information collected by VAERS can quickly provide an early warning of a potential safety problem with a vaccine. Patterns of adverse events, or an unusually high number of adverse events reported after a particular vaccine, are called 'signals.' If a signal is identified through VAERS, scientist[s] may conduct further studies to find out if the signal represents an actual risk." [2]

Of course, detection of early warnings of potential safety problems with a vaccine requires the CDC to diligently monitor the VAERS reports, timely investigate reports which raise concerns, and timely act when indicated. Unfortunately, as shocking as it may seem, there is a complete lack of evidence that the CDC diligently monitored VAERS for safety signals.

VAERS is co-managed by the CDC and the Food and Drug Administration (FDA). The VAERS website states that anyone can report an adverse event to VAERS, that healthcare professionals are required to report certain adverse events, and that vaccine manufacturers are required to report all adverse events that come to their attention.[3,4]

However, the FDA's website states that VAERS is, "... an outgrowth of the National Childhood Vaccine Injury Act of 1986 (NCVIA)." This Act required the creation of a national registry to receive and archive reports of adverse vaccine events. The Act established the reporting mandates for healthcare providers and vaccine manufacturers.[5]

Accordingly, there exists a legal duty for healthcare professionals to report adverse events in VAERS. Reporting to VAERS is not happening as required. Ask an emergency room doctor at any hospital emergency room if they ever filed a VAERS report. We know that no doctor in Brianna's case filed a VAERS report even though six doctors affiliated with Harvard Medical School and Beth Israel Deaconess Medical Center wrote in Brianna's *Brief Report* that they monitor VAERS for similar cases. "*Review of the medical literature and vaccine adverse event reporting system (VAERS) produced no similar cases* ..." [6]

VAERS became a battlefield between factions. Covid vaccine enthusiasts say that VAERS cannot be trusted because anyone can enter a report. As shown in *EXHIBIT H* of *BEAUDOIN v BAKER et al (2022)* [7], the CDC conspired to derogate their own pharmacovigilance system (VAERS) on social media. *EXHIBIT H* is built from FOIA responses to the requests of America First Legal, a 501(C)(3) foundation.[8]

Among the America First Legal FOIA documents is an internal advisory issued by the CDC on May 12, 2021, after Diane died from a stroke and after Brianna died from a stroke. The CDC internal advisory stated, "*Be On the Lookout [BOLO] for: Statements, pictures, posts, or messages containing misinformation about the eligibility of 12- to 15-year-olds for the Pfizer/BioNTech COVID-19 vaccine.*" It also states, "*Potential Impact - Reduced vaccine acceptance.*"

The advisory noted above, part of a CDC slide presentation, was sent by Carol Crawford at the CDC to individuals at Facebook. The presentation included examples of posts that the CDC wanted removed from Facebook. The body of the e-mail coaches the e-mail recipients on how to derogate VAERS.

Why is the federal agency responsible for the early warning vigilance system e-mailing instructions to Facebook management specifying what messages to remove and how to respond to various posts about VAERS and the safety of the covid vaccines?

I first heard of VAERS in February 2021 and began looking at the VAERS data shortly thereafter. I first loaded VAERS files onto my computer on April 4, 2021, in order to document and analyze data, which became the subject of a video I was assigned to produce for a Torts Class I was taking in law school. The video can be found on YouTube under the title *The Hand*

Formula; Economics of Torts; Importance of Torts; Vax tort immunity.[9] I continued to load VAERS data monthly through July 2021 after which my computer could no longer manage the file size of VAERS reports, which were rapidly accumulating in 2021. There were simply too many reports of adverse events.

On June 23, 2021, I created and posted graphics on social media detailing some of the VAERS information of young people who reportedly died shortly after vaccination. It continually surprises me that people dismiss VAERS reports so readily without ever having read them. For example, VAERS_ID 1080840-1 details the death of a 16-year-old girl who is reported to have been vaccinated on March 3, 2021, and died on March 4, 2021. The report was received by VAERS March 8, 2021. The vaccine is listed as "*PFIZER\WYETH MENINGOCOCCAL B (TRUMENBA)*." Adverse Event Description states, "*The day after vaccination, father states that child returned from track practice feeling tired. She went to lay down and he found her face down on her bed, unresponsive and cyanotic.*" [10]

Other accounts include a 15-year-old girl who died from cardiac arrest three to four days after her second Moderna dose, a 17-year-old girl who experienced chest pain and died from cardiac arrest eight days after vaccination, a 16-year-old girl who died from "bilateral large pulmonary embolism" eleven days after vaccination, a 15-year-old boy who died two days after vaccination, an 18-year-old young man who died three days after vaccination, an 18-year-old young man who died fourteen days after vaccination, a 19-year-old woman who died seven days after vaccination, and a 19-year-old young man who died one day after vaccination. This is only a small sample of the VAERS reports of young people who died shortly after vaccination.

On July 23, 2021, I downloaded the 2021 VAERS file and performed text searches to see how often various key character strings appeared. I was searching for potential safety signals, or patterns, related to the large number of reported deaths I was finding. The number of times each key character string was found in the VAERS reports follows:

- "clot" 15,148
- "thrombo" 5,900
- "stroke" 9,714
- "embolism" 3,317
- "aneurysm" 1,247
- "aneurism" 74
- "carditis" 4,656

- "vertigo" 8,970
- "tinnitus" 8,798
- "vomit" 27,682
- "headache" 133,988
- "nausea" 64,567
- "palsy" 6,170
- "guillain" 888

In addition, through July 18, 2021, the 2021 VAERS database contained 5,189 reports of people believed to have died from adverse events connected with a vaccine.

Having had a personal experience with a deep vein thrombosis which was treated with the drug, Xarelto, my growing horror over the human carnage documented in the VAERS reports became even more intense when I discovered the following report:

VAERS ID 1243791:[11]

- *Date Report Received 04/22/2021*
- *Date Vaccinated 04/10/2021*
- *Date of Onset 04/12/2021*
- *Date Died 04/12/2021*
- *Age "21.00"*
- *Sex "Male"*
- *Symptom "DEATH"*
- *Adverse Event Description "Per the father, the deceased received his first shot of Moderna vaccine on Saturday, 4/10/2021 at a local church. He did not work on 4/11/2021. Worked on 4/12/2021. The deceased was found dead at 6:43 p.m. at his home."*
- *History "History of clotting disorder at age 16 with Xarelto treatment and hospitalization"*

I first read the report of the death of this young man in 2021. He had died in mid-April. How was this possible? By February 2021, there were more than enough reports of clotting deaths of young people to qualify as a safety signal. If the CDC and FDA were monitoring the reports and paying proper attention, that safety signal should have triggered an urgent halt on all covid vaccines. This young man's death was completely avoidable.

Despite the torrent of reports of adverse events, our government officials who are trusted to protect the public's health continued to recommend covid vaccines for pregnant women, cancer patients, diabetics, the obese, and other people at high risk for blood clots.

As mandated by the 1986 NCVIA, VAERS is supposed to serve as the "early warning system" which protects the public's health by revealing safety signals. Totaling the VAERS hits for key words related to blood clots ("clot," "thrombo," "embolism") yields more than 24,000 of these serious adverse events through mid-July 2021. Who, in the CDC or FDA, was monitoring the vigilance system to keep us safe?

Not only is it evident that the CDC failed to diligently monitor VAERS for safety signals, they also actively ignored researchers who publicly called out signals in VAERS reports. Dr. Jessica Rose raised a red flag by publishing reports and research papers.[12] However, instead of following up on these serious safety signals, the CDC continued to derogate VAERS. In secret complicity with social media and the press, the CDC endeavored to viciously demean, censor, and de-platform courageous independent researchers. Medical and scientific journals refused to publish research papers that called the government's narrative into question and even engaged in baseless, unethical retraction of papers, which were published after extensive peer review.[13] This blatant government malfeasance together with the unethical and unlawful actions of media and other purportedly independent actors is responsible for an uncountable number of completely avoidable deaths.

By late 2020, I had put aside All-Cause data analyses because the available CDC data was collated in overly large groups which causes important signals to be obscured by Simpson's paradoxes.

By mid-2021, my work with the VAERS records had achieved as much as could be expected. The value of the VAERS records is the clinical experience they contain in the form of case history abstracts. Case histories once served as the essential basis of the medical progress forged by skilled medical clinicians. Now, under the misnomer of "evidence based medicine" (EBM), medical progress has been superseded by medical profits in service of which the government perniciously ignores the lessons and safety signals in the VAERS data. The predictable result is the avoidable deaths of innocent people who were victimized by their misplaced trust in a government, which has shown that it places pharmaceutical industry profits ahead of citizens' lives.

In August 2022, I began to match death certificates to VAERS reports to assemble the smoking gun, which completely exposes the criminal conduct responsible for the deaths of so many innocent people. The resulting matches culminated in *EXHIBIT F*, the foundational evidentiary document in case *Beaudoin v Baker et al (2022)* Docket No. 1:22-cv-11356-NMG pending in U.S. District Court, District of Massachusetts.

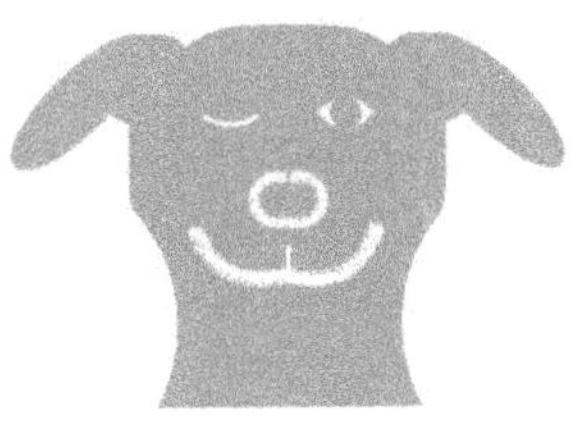

Chapter 8
EXHIBIT F

Record-level source data (RLSD) enables investigation across variables and to detailed levels that cannot be performed using bundled CDC data. In a healthcare context, record-level data means that a medical record contains unique and non-aggregated data elements that relate to a single identifiable individual. Knowing that people were dying from covid or covid vaccines, or both, I felt compelled, in defense of others, to use RLSD, in this case the Massachusetts death certificate data, to document covid vaccine-caused deaths beyond reasonable doubt.

Cassidy, age 7, Brianna, age 30, Eden, age 17, and Karyn, age 45, are but a few examples of deaths caused by covid vaccines. The true cause of these deaths was covered up and fraudulently omitted from their death certificates.

EXHIBIT F of the *Beaudoin v Baker et al (2022)* Complaint, filed in the United States District Court for the District of Massachusetts, comprises 123 pages of hard evidence which document frauds of omission and commission on Massachusetts death certificates. The frauds of omission listed in *EXHIBIT F* fall into two categories: 1) death certificates that mention the covid vaccine as a cause in Parts I or II, and yet have no ICD-10 codes such as Y59.0 or T88.1 listed, and 2) death certificates without mention of a vaccine in Parts I or II correlated to VAERS reports that do mention a vaccine as a cause of death.

The full details included in *EXHIBIT F* are too extensive to permit a quick, comprehensive understanding. For that reason, pages 3–11 of *EXHIBIT F* summarize the exhibit. This chapter presents a review of the summary.

The State File Number (SFN) is a unique number representing each Massachusetts decedent in a given year. The SFN numbers begin again at "1" for each year.

SFN_NUMBER 11199 Solomon Kizitoh died on January 16, 2021, at the age of 60. As previously noted in Chapter 6, Solomon's Massachusetts death certificate is the only one assigned ICD-10 codes for covid vaccine death. Part I states, "*ACUTE BRONCHOPNEUMONIA AND IDIOPATHIC THROMBOCYTOPENIA FOLLOWING COVID-19 VACCINATION*" in "*DAYS*." The assigned ICD-10 codes pertaining to "... *FOLLOWING COVID-19 VACCINATION*" are Y59.0, "Viral vaccines," and T88.1, "Other complications following immunization, not elsewhere classified."

Medical Examiner Rebecca Dedrick fulfilled her duty on Solomon's death certificate. However, the following death certificates refer to a covid vaccine in Part I as a cause of death, but the CDC omitted vaccine or immunization ICD-10 codes from the death certificates. Defendants in *Beaudoin v Baker et al (2022)* may have been able to avail themselves of the defense of "ignorance of fact" before September 9, 2022, when the defendants were served with summonses. However, the notice they received through service of those summonses destroyed the ignorance and, thus, the defense.

After a reasonable time, the governor, Commissioner of the Department of Public Health, Chief Medical Examiner, and four named medical examiners (the defendants) of the Commonwealth of Massachusetts were guilty of fraud because they were given notice of the egregious omissions of vaccine-related ICD-10 codes, yet chose to not act to correct the CDC's omissions and notwithstanding their legal duty.

Martha, SFN_NUM 9150 of 2021, died on February 13, 2021, at the age of 84. Part II of Martha's death certificate states, "*SECOND COVID VACCINATION WAS GIVEN 5 DAYS BEFORE DEATH AND SHE DEVELOPED FEVER AND MENTAL STATUS CHANGES SHORTLY AFTER GETTING IT*." Clearly, the death certifier wanted it understood that a covid vaccine was a likely cause of Martha's decline and eventual death. Vaccine-associated codes are omitted from Martha's death certificate.

Doris, SFN_NUMBER 12117 of 2021, died on February 19, 2021, at the age of 85. Part II of Doris's death certificate states, "*RECEIVED SECOND COVID-19 VACCINE THE PRIOR WEEK*." Again, the certifier of death makes it known that a covid vaccine likely contributed to Doris's death. Vaccine-associated codes are omitted from Doris's death certificate.

Diane, SFN_NUMBER 15403 of 2021, died on March 18, 2021, at the age of 62. Diane is also mentioned in Chapter 2. Part I states, "*ACUTE INTRACRANIAL HEMORRHAGE IN THE SETTING OF THROMBOCYTOPENIA IN A PERSON TREATED WITH COVID 19*

VACCINATION 11 DAYS PRIOR TO PRESENTATION." Medical Examiner Julie Hull clearly wanted it known that Diane's stroke was likely caused by a covid vaccine. Vaccine-associated codes are omitted from Diane's death certificate.

Donna, SFN_NUMBER 16835 of 2021, died on March 19, 2021, at the age of 67. The last underlying cause noted in Cause D of Part I states, "*IN THE SETTING OF RECENT ... COVID-19 VACCINATION.*" Medical Examiner Andrew Elin clearly wanted Part I to include a covid vaccine as the underlying cause of death (UCOD). Vaccine-associated codes are omitted from Donna's death certificate.

Pearl, SFN_NUMBER 17541 of 2021, died on April 4, 2021, at the age of 97. Part II of Pearl's death certificate states, "*COVID 19 VACCINATION.*" Nurse Practitioner Sheryl Derderian purposely and expressly placed those words in Part II. Vaccine-associated codes are omitted from Pearl's death certificate.

Catherine, SFN_NUMBER 20283 of 2021, died on April 16, 2021, at the age of 59. Cause A states, "*CARDIAC ARRHYTHMIA*" in "*SEC.*" Cause B states, "*COVID VACCINATION*" in "*2 DAYS.*" Physician Nada Kerouz clearly and expressly stated that she believed a covid vaccine to have been a cause of Catherine's death. Vaccine-associated codes are omitted from Catherine's death certificate.

Richard, SFN_NUMBER 25261 of 2021, died on May 18, 2021, at the age of 60. Part II states, "*RECENT COVID-19 VACCINE ON DATE OF DEATH.*" To assuage curiosity, Richard died of Cause A, "*CARDIO PULMONARY ARREST*" in "*5 MIN.*" and Cause B, "*SUDDEN DEATH CARDIAC ARRHYTHMIA*" in "*15 MIN.*" Physician Martin Gelman must be credited with honestly certifying Richard's death and making it known that Richard was killed by a covid vaccine in minutes. However, vaccine-associated codes are omitted from Richard's death certificate.

Remember that the defendants in *Beaudoin v Baker et al (2022)* continue to omit vaccine codes from Richard's death certificate more than ten months after being notified of the omission. Accordingly, harm from covid vaccines continues to be hidden from public view. Children and adults died in Massachusetts as a result of booster shots over the ten months (at the time of this writing); the last defendant was notified by summons on September 9, 2022. These deaths are a consequence of criminal omission of conduct concurrent with a legal duty to act.

Laurence, SFN_NUMBER 14456 of 2022, died on March 14, 2022, at the age of 85. Cause A states, "*CEREBRAL VASCULAR DEMENTIA*" in "*5 MOS.*" Cause B states, "*GUILLAIN-BARRE SYNDROME AFTER VACCINATION*" in "*5 MOS.*" Five months before his death, Laurence received a covid vaccine. Soon after vaccination, he developed the Underlying Cause Of Death, Guillain-Barre Syndrome (GBS), which caused the dementia and eventual death five months later. GBS is a known side effect of many vaccines, especially covid vaccines. Physician Charles Rosenbaum certified an honest and seemingly complete death certificate. The CDC failed in its responsibility to apply the missing vaccine codes. This omission was brought to the attention of the defendants, who have not acted to cure the omission in more than ten months. Laurence's death certificate is also now a fraudulent document because of the omission by CDC and the failure of any defendant to correct the fraud.

Daydan, SFN_NUMBER 6554 of 2022, died on January 30, 2022, at the age of 10. Part I states, "*COMPLICATIONS OF BRONCHOPULMONARY DYSPLASIA IN A CHILD WITH A HISTORY OF PREMATURE/PRETERM DELIVERY AT 23 WEEKS GESTATION*" in "*YRS.*" Part II states, "*CEREBRAL PALSY, BILATERAL SUPERIOR VENA CAVA, RECURRENT ASPIRATION, ATELECTASIS, SHORT GUT SYNDROME, GALLSTONE PANCREATITIS, HYPOTHYROIDISM, SARS-COV-2 POSITIVE STATUS POST COVID-19 VACCINATION.*" Daydan is added here not to showcase him as an obvious vaccine-caused death, but rather to ponder the overall death certificate.

Interestingly, the numerous ICD-10 codes applied by the CDC on Daydan's death certificate do not include U07.1 "COVID-19." In the many SARS-COV-2 POSITIVE death certificates I came across, U07.1 was always listed. Why not on Daydan's? Is it because he was vaccinated and, thus, it would have been listed as a "vaccine breakthrough" death? Early in 2021, "breakthrough" infections were a popular topic. The government denied they frequently occurred for many months early in the covid vaccination campaigns.[1] That dam broke later in 2021, and the government stopped saying that the covid vaccine prevents one from getting covid. That the covid vaccines prevented one from contracting covid was a myth created somewhere in the realm of media or politicians. Now, in 2023, people who were vaccinated multiple times for covid are becoming infected by covid multiple times per year, severely and symptomatically.

If Daydan was vaccinated for covid, and the vaccine worked the way vaccines are supposed to work, then why did he test positive for covid? If the vaccine is supposed to reduce symptoms, then why did Daydan die shortly after vaccination? Daydan survived and struggled many years through serious health issues from birth, but died shortly after vaccination.

Why are those with health issues from congenital defects, morbid obesity, and extreme elderly, who were said to be the most susceptible to succumb to covid *per se*, also the most likely to be culled by covid vaccines? In this observation, I have not yet presented the complete picture of the hard evidence. This observation is based on my thousands of hours of research into Massachusetts death certificates. I believe that by the time you finish reading this book, you will also be persuaded by the accumulated mass of hard facts.

If the people, said to have needed the covid vaccine the most, are dying disproportionately more from the covid vaccine, then why do we offer a covid vaccine? Moreover, healthy children are documented herein to die from the covid vaccine in greater numbers than from covid infection, making covid vaccines a vain Death Lottery.

Alfred, SFN_NUMBER 23982 of 2022, died on May 10, 2022, at the age of 88. Cause A, "*DEMENTIA*" in "*YRS.*" Part II stated, "*ADULT FAILURE TO THRIVE, COVID VACCINE.*" Physician Charles Wolff purposely and expressly certified Alfred's death certificate noting a covid vaccine as a contributing condition. Vaccine-associated codes are omitted from Alfred's death certificate.

The bulk of *EXHIBIT F* comprises death certificates matched to VAERS reports. Sometimes three death certificates matched a single VAERS report. Some of these are listed in the exhibit, but most of the exhibit comprises one-to-one comparisons matched beyond reasonable doubt.

Page 4 of *EXHIBIT F* is a list of Massachusetts death certificates matched to VAERS reports. Age, sex, state, date of death, and sometimes symptoms were matched. Often, there was only one person with the same age and sex who died in Massachusetts on a given date. Sometimes, it required attention to Parts I and II to further ensure the correct match was made.

Craig, on Page 20 of *EXHIBIT F*, is an example of correlation.

SFN_NUMBER 68777 Craig died on December 31, 2020, at age 72. Cause A, "*BILATERAL VENTRICULAR FAILURE*" in "*DAYS.*" Cause B, "*MYOCARDIAL INFARCTION*" in "*DAYS.*" Cause C, "*SEPSIS*" in "*DAYS.*"

There is no mention of covid vaccination on Craig's death certificate.

VAERS_ID 0953922 – A man died on December 31, 2020 in Massachusetts at the age of 72. Here is the record of VAERS_ID 0953922:[2]

- *Date Report Received 01/18/2021*
- *Date Vaccinated 12/26/2020*
- *Date of Onset 12/27/2020*
- *Date Died 12/31/2020*
- *Age "72.00"*
- *Sex "Male"*
- *Adverse Event Description "... That evening he reported difficulty breathing and was placed on oxygen; a COVID test was performed and was negative. On 12/30/2020, patient complained of sternal pressure and was transferred to the hospital. The patient died 12/31/2020 and records obtained from the hospital indicated the patient died from a massive myocardial infarction."*

Three other men aged 72 died on December 31, 2020 in Massachusetts.

SFN_NUMBER 68256 William's Cause A is "*COVID 19 PNEUMONIA*" in "*WKS.*" Cause B is "*ACUTE RESPIRATORY FAILURE*" in "*DAYS.*" Cause C is "*MULTI ORGAN DYSFUNCTION*" in "*DAYS.*"

Clearly William is not the 72-year-old male in the VAERS report 0953922. There is no mention of a Myocardial Infarction (MI), heart attack, on William's death certificate.

SFN_NUMBER 68771 Lael's Cause A is "*MULTISYSTEM ORGAN FAILURE*" in "*DAYS.*" Cause B is "*ISCHEMIC CARDIOMYOPATHY*" in "*YRS.*" Cause C is "*CORONARY ARTERY DISEASE*" in "*YRS.*"

Clearly Lael is not the 72-year-old male in the VAERS report 0953922. There is no mention of an MI on Lael's death certificate.

Important to note on the VAERS report is the interval between VAX_DATE and ONSET_DATE—one day. The causes of death will be analyzed in the third part of this book (*TERTIA PARS*). However, the main cause of death will be listed for each record here for the reader to see if these people are dying from respiratory issues such as pneumonia, or circulatory issues such as heart, stroke, and other clotting- or bleeding-related issues. Craig is the first on the list followed by other strongly correlated death certificates and VAERS records. Page 4 of *EXHIBIT F* lists the following:

Fields delineated by semicolons are as follows:

DeathDate; SFN_NUMBER; AGE; SEX; Vax to Onset - Cause

- 12/31/2020; 68777; 72; M; ONE DAY - Heart Attack
- 03/06/2021; 13110; 60; F; ONE DAY - Cardiac Arrest

- 03/08/2021; 13132; 67; M; 2 DAYS - Brain Bleed
- 03/15/2021; 14781; 70; F; SAME DAY - Resp. Failure
- 04/09/2021; 18499; 52; M; ONE DAY - Hemorrhage
- 04/12/2021; 19179; 54; M; 3 DAYS - Arrhythmia
- 04/12/2021; 20085; 67; M; SAME DAY - CP Arrest
- 04/25/2021; 21056; 47; M; ONE DAY - Heart Attack
- 05/08/2021; 23618; 69; M; 5 MINUTES - Card. Arrest
- 05/11/2021; 25223; 59; F; 2 DAYS - Card.Resp.Arrest
- 05/25/2021; 26053; 53; M; HOURS - CLOTS
- 06/21/2021; 30156; 63; F; 3 WEEKS - PE CLOT
- 10/23/2021; 50161; 70; F; ONE DAY - Card. Arrest
- 11/19/2021; 55707; 69; M; ONE DAY - Card. Arrest
- 01/12/2022; 2551; 86; F - JUST AFTER BOOSTER
- 02/24/2022; 12822; 59; M; 2 WKS - PERICARDITIS

Clearly, these people should have ICD-10 codes for immunization or vaccination listed on their death certificates. Clearly, the death certifier should have mentioned covid vaccines as causal in Part I of these death certificates.

One of these death certificates reports an interval of five minutes between covid vaccination and death, yet there is no vaccine associated ICD-10 code applied by the CDC.

Most interesting are the causes of death for these covid vaccine-caused deaths. Most of them are circulatory or blood related, including the heart, which is at the center of the circulatory system.

SUMMARY

EXHIBIT F includes death certificates and VAERS reports detailing Cassidy age 7, Diane age 62, Brianna age 30, Eden age 17, Holly age 42, Charles age 48, and Abigail age 20.

In addition to the evidence put forth in this Chapter 8 regarding correlation of death certificates to VAERS reports in *EXHIBIT F*, the *EXHIBIT F* document filed in the case *Beaudoin v Baker et al (2022)* details accidental deaths from drug overdose fraudulently labeled covid deaths, accidental deaths from blunt force trauma fraudulently labeled covid deaths, vaccine deaths fraudulently labeled covid deaths, and vaccine deaths in which a covid vaccine was fraudulently omitted as a cause of death.

EXHIBIT F is filed as part of *Beaudoin v Baker et al (2022)* and will forever be available to the public through the U.S. District Court system.

EXHIBIT F is one of the most damning documents of hard evidence against covid vaccines and false covid pandemic narratives sworn to under penalties of perjury.

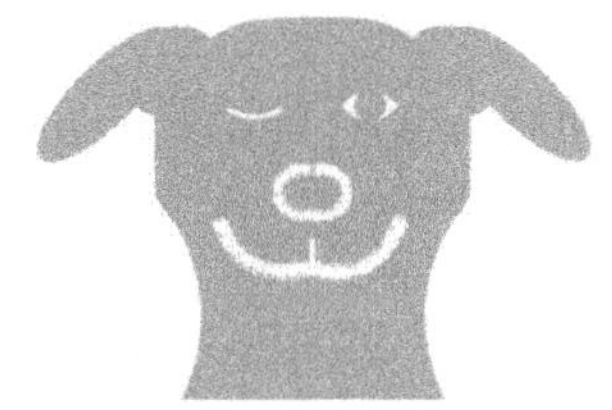

Chapter 9
EBM & Dr. Backer

Around 1990, I moved to a town north of Boston, Massachusetts. Every winter throughout my twenties, I would endure multiple episodes of strep throat, bronchitis, sinus infections, pneumonia, and head and chest colds. I only visited a doctor when I needed a prescription for antibiotics to knock down the bacteria, which were assailing my head, throat, or chest.

I found a doctor who had recently opened his own practice—just a one-man business. Dr. Ronald Backer was probably in his late 50s then, had a pony tail, and was learning his sixth language (Japanese, as I recall). The office was in the bottom unit of a two-family house.

The following winter, when I wanted a prescription, Dr. Backer's schedule was full, but he had taken on a younger partner, Dr. Solomon. The two of them operated as a duo for a few years.

After I got married and moved about an hour away, I maintained Dr. Backer as my primary care physician. Dr. Backer was affiliated with Winchester Hospital in Massachusetts. He and Dr. Solomon moved into office space in downtown Winchester, a short walk from the previous location. They brought in other doctors and the practice grew over the years.

One time, when I was really sick again, I drove an hour to Winchester. Drs. Backer and Solomon were not available, so I had my appointment with Dr. Nada Kerouz, who, you may recall, certified the death certificate for Catherine (Chapter 8, SFN_NUMBER 20283).

I'm sure Dr. Backer is long retired, if he's still with us. I searched on the web for Dr. Solomon and Dr. Kerouz. They are part of Winchester Physician Associates, which is associated with Beth Israel Lahey Health. There are 84 physicians in the practice now. How times have changed.

From the time I was born and into my thirties, physician practices generally had one to ten physicians. In the past two decades, there has been a consolidation of medical practices and of hospital networks to the extent that the personal doctor-patient relationship is now a thing of the past.

I no longer regard the physician I went to each year for about six years before covid as my personal care doctor. When I saw him at the gym during the purported covid pandemic, he told me I have a 1 in 400 chance of dying from covid. He knew I had a DVT, I'm deaf in one ear, I had weird severe vertigo symptoms, and I have tinnitus. He knew that I was physically fit and worked out all the time. Based on the official statistics at that time, my actual chances of dying from covid, without correcting for the fraudulent way covid deaths were counted, was 1 in 55,000. The "1 in 400" number he mentioned was applicable to all ages and across the entire health spectrum, including those with diabetes, morbid obesity, and every other serious co-morbidity. I do not know if he was ignorant of the facts or if he misinformed me on purpose to try to scare me into a covid vaccine.

When I went to an appointment with that physician in the past, he consulted a laptop on a wheeled pedestal table to review my records. It seemed efficient. I trusted him because he was in his sixties. However, when I was seen at that practice by a younger physician and a younger nurse practitioner for symptoms of a spinal injury I suffered, the injury was undiagnosed and misdiagnosed over the course of multiple visits. Eventually, one of my soccer teammates diagnosed me correctly during a short conversation while walking off the soccer pitch. I was experiencing a loss of feeling across my shoulder following a mountain biking accident in which I fractured two vertebrae. My teammate just casually said that my C4 dermatome was affected by a spinal impingement. I never was diagnosed properly by the big office where my physician worked. The shoulder area lacked feeling for years after that accident. Because the nurse practitioner did not properly diagnose the spinal injury, the insurance company offered to pay for an MRI of my thoracic vertebrae that were fractured, but refused to pay for imaging of my cervical vertebrae and disc, which was herniated and causing the loss of shoulder area feeling. Thus, the system left me without care despite my threat of lawsuit.

The point of this soliloquy is to illustrate the gradual deterioration of our healthcare systems and the resulting extinction of personalized, caring medical practice. Traditionally, when a younger doctor in a practice encountered something in a patient that he'd never seen before, he did not defer to the laptop for CDC or NIH recommendations, or for the official, one-size-fits-all Standard of Care. He would bring in a senior doctor in the practice, who'd independently examine the patient. Perhaps the senior doctor would enlighten his junior colleague about the local water supply, or about a genetic propensity of the local ethnicity to react to some local flora. The elder clinician could draw on his wealth of knowledge, accumulated over decades of experience.

The laptop can only mandate the Standard of Care authorized by some distant executive with no medical training whose principle responsibility is to optimize the organization's financial bottom line. This may be an efficient way to maximize profit by facilitating the completion of the patient consultation within the allotted 15-minute time slot, which is now standard in most practices, but it is also very unlikely to deliver any sort of appropriate care to the patients. I want to be diagnosed by a thinking doctor who spends as much time as the diagnosis may require. I want to be treated by a caring physician who sees me as a unique individual, with a unique physiology and unique life circumstances.

Patients at the margins, those with rare issues, used to be able to rely upon the provision of thoughtful physicians and individual care that was appropriate for their unusual circumstances. Nowadays, people are routinely misdiagnosed and mistreated, or completely undiagnosed and untreated, during multiple, stale, and brief appointments. It is now common for a patient, who cannot be correctly diagnosed within the allowed 15 minutes, to be sent out the door after being told that the confusing symptoms are all in the patient's mind.

HOW DID THIS HAPPEN?

Since the 1960s, North American medical schools have been making moves to standardize new methods. Canada reorganized their health care system, medical schools, and public health in 1964. McMaster University introduced "problem-based learning." That system grew into studies of epidemiology and biostatistics directed by David Sackett, who wrote a series of articles on clinical methods in 1981 in the *Canadian Medical Association Journal (CMAJ)*. Gordon Guyatt, also at McMaster, coined the term "evidence-based medicine" (EBM) in 1992.[1.2.3.]

Canadians incubated, fostered, and evangelized EBM throughout the 1990s. From Canada, it spread rapidly into the United States, like a virulent infection. Throughout the U.S., EBM corrupted the traditional flow of learning, turning the concept of clinical medicine, and the scientific method itself, upside down. It soon pervaded every medical school in North America. During the 1990s, it became the sole paradigm that medical school graduates were taught. These recent generations of physicians follow it like automatons follow pre-programmed algorithms.

Whereas clinical experience and the lessons learned from clinical case studies were long acknowledged as the highest form of evidence underlying the practice of medicine, EBM has summarily gouged out that entire sound foundation and relegated it to the trash heap. Clinical experience is now denigrated as merely "anecdotal." Instead of medical wisdom gained through ages of experience, EBM is based on purportedly "peer reviewed studies" which all too often are conducted by researchers with serious conflicts of interest and funded by the very pharmaceutical manufacturers who have financial interests, measured in $billions, in the outcomes of those studies. These studies ignore wide variations in individual patients and distill findings into one-size-fits-all "guidance," which doctors are expected to blindly follow. God help those patients who do not share a physiology with the theoretically average patient.

As a result, doctors are now programmed to follow a central authority (the laptop god on the wheelie table) in diagnosis and treatment. If the CDC says to prescribe remdesivir, they prescribe remdesivir. Even if some doctors have multiple patients die from Acute Renal Failure (ARF), and read medical literature that remdesivir causes kidney failure, those doctors will still err on the side of caution and prescribe remdesivir. But whose side of caution is that? It's the side that says they'd better follow the central authority, else the medical licensing board or certification board may call them to account for failing to follow the central authority laptop god. A renegade "thinking" physician puts himself in a position to be fired, or have his medical license revoked if he should rely on clinical experience to prescribe what he believes to be in the patient's best interest rather than comply with central authority dictates.

It is vitally important for people to understand that the overall system of health care has been hijacked to benefit the providers at the expense of the patients. The executive decision-makers responsible for this criminal perversion exhibit no concern whatsoever for the health and well-being of the people they are supposed to serve. If you find this hard to accept, ask yourself how the system devolved to the point where Medicare pays hospitals a bonus on a patient's entire hospital bill if the hospital administers a drug like remdesivir, which has been shown by evidence to harm the kidneys of a major fraction of patients who receive it.

The recent massive increase in deaths and reduction in fertility and live births are not the result of covid. The evidence in *TERTIA PARS* proves that. There is something else that caused and is causing excess deaths. That something is a new culture among physicians that was instilled over the past thirty years by EBM. The culture enabled a corrupt system to exploit covid to put The People under siege. That culture enabled the authoritarian disruption of the sacred doctor-patient relationship. Without that change in healthcare culture, there would have been neither covid, not the covid vaccine.

One physician in California was asked a question by a Silicon Valley executive on an open social media audio forum. Thousands were listening. The executive asked the physician a question based on the following hypothetical situation. If you vaccinated twenty patients and ten were dead in a week, would you stop using that vaccine? I was shocked that the question was even asked. I found it insulting to the physician. But then, my shock was overtaken by the physician's answer. The physician stated that he would have to consult the most recently available literature before making that decision. The conversation continued and the physician stood his ground. He would not deviate from EBM dictate—not even if ten of his own patients die in a week. Do you want to be a patient of that physician?

This is the evil which has destroyed the field of medicine. People outside the medical industry cannot fathom how a system can go so awry. Lives are lost and destroyed by "the system" as few speak up or speak out. The system has become powerful enough to personally and professionally destroy those with the courage to speak up.

The paradigm of EBM became the mantra of EBM. Patient-centric medical practice from caring and insightful physicians has been stifled by the automation of the hive mind. EBM may sound good to a hospital executive with no medical training. EBM may function well as a system for indoctrination on a large scale. But EBM is unsafe for children and other living creatures.

Canada's socialized and centralized healthcare system was not preferred by patients. That's why many Canadians gave up on their system and came to the United States. Much to the misery of U.S. citizens, centralized healthcare is now here in USA.[4]

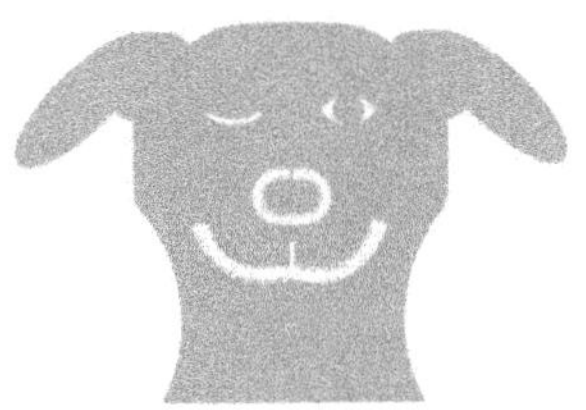

Chapter 10
The Minnesota Memorandum

Near the end of Chapter 9 were mentioned Acute renal failure (ARF) and remdesivir. It is asserted that, if remdesivir is prescribed and administered for COVID-19 patients, then the hospital and doctors can make a windfall from federal incentive programs such as the *New COVID-19 Treatments Add-On Payment (NCTAP)*.[1] That program along with a *Federal Register* entry dated April 25, 2022[2] explains the complex schema of compensation for administering the drug remdesivir, also known as "Veklury." This chapter continues that vein of subject matter, bringing more COVID facts to the reader.

Although this book mainly covers Massachusetts and Vermont death certificate records and data, Chapter 10 reviews the *Minnesota Memorandum* sent by John Paul Beaudoin, Sr. to the Governor, Lieutenant Governor, Attorney General, and Health Commissioner of Minnesota. The official title of the document is *MEMORANDUM: NOTICE OF HEALTH EMERGENCY REQUIRING IMMEDIATE INVESTIGATION OF DEATHS BY ACUTE RENAL FAILURE IN MINNESOTA*.[3]

The *Minnesota Memorandum* is narrowly tailored to alert the listed Minnesota state officials of an epidemic of Acute renal failure involved *excess* deaths totaling approximately one thousand six hundred in 2021 and 2022. The evidence in the memorandum depicts *excess* ARF deaths beyond what is normal and *expected* from years 2015–2019. The opening paragraph and *INTRODUCTION* of the memorandum explain the purpose and raise alarm about ARF.

> *This Memorandum is legal notice to the above-named Minnesota officials jointly and severally, hereinafter known as "the agents." The intent in providing this Memorandum is to protect the health and safety of Minnesotans, who are dying at alarming rates from*

a specific cause of death, not covid. The best solution [is] *to act on the recommendations in the § "RECOMMENDATIONS."*

INTRODUCTION

Minnesotans are in the throes of an epidemic of Acute Renal Failure (hereinafter known as "ARF"). ARF-involved deaths are now arguably greater than the covid pandemic per se. Yet Minnesota state officials seem to be ignorant of this fact. Notice raises ignorance.

Evidence of excess ARF deaths is provided in EXHIBIT A. The excess ARF deaths in 2021 and 2022 totals approximately one thousand six hundred (~1,600) Minnesotan souls. That word "excess" means 'more than expected by trend established from baseline years 2015–2019.'

Each ARF death is multiple life-years-lost compared to an average covid death being one (1) life-year-lost in Minnesota. Much younger people are died [sic] *from ARF. Families who lose a parent or child are devastated far more than if an elderly relative in their eighties or nineties dies.*

Each of the named agents has a legal duty to act upon the information and belief detailed in this Memorandum and in EXHIBIT A. Failure to conduct an investigation, provide public findings, and act to prevent injury or death to Minnesotans will constitute sufficient mens rea to prosecute the agents under federal felonies, including homicide crimes.

Minnesota public officials have access to State vital records, health records, and immunization registry databases. Refusal to investigate and determine the commonality among the thousands (1,000s) of excess ARF deaths will constitute a negative act concurrent with a legal duty to act. Inaction is a crime despite what the CDC or FDA officially or unofficially communicate to the agents. The information necessary for agents of Minnesota to make informed public health decisions regarding the health and safety of Minnesotans lies in the records of

> *Minnesota, not the CDC or FDA; and no CDC recommendation can absolve the agents from the crime of knowingly, willfully, and recklessly ignoring Minnesota's own health, immunization, and death databases in favor of mere and threadbare CDC recommendations.*[3]

The *Minnesota Memorandum* further explains the meaning of legal "notice," the awesome responsibility that state officials have manifest in a "legal duty to act," the officials' lack of "qualified" or "sovereign immunity" for criminal conduct including inaction concurrent with a "legal duty to act," and the fact that there is no "statute of limitations" for most homicide crimes.

The factual allegations laid out in the memorandum document the incredible levels of *excess* ARF deaths in Minnesota.

Figures 10.1–10.4 depict two sample age groups from *EXHIBIT A* of the *Minnesota Memorandum*. The years of anomaly and the numbers of excess deaths in such young people speak for themselves. ARF-involved deaths is a health emergency of immense proportion not seen since the Spanish flu of 1918 and 1919; yet it seems that there is not a single mention of it by any agent of the Minnesota state health department or the CDC.

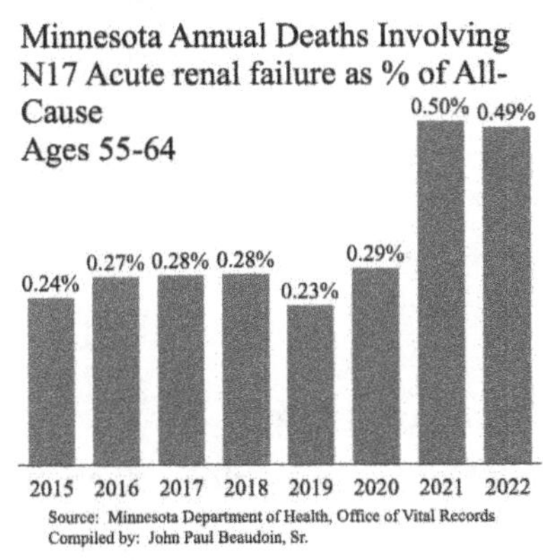

Figure 10.1

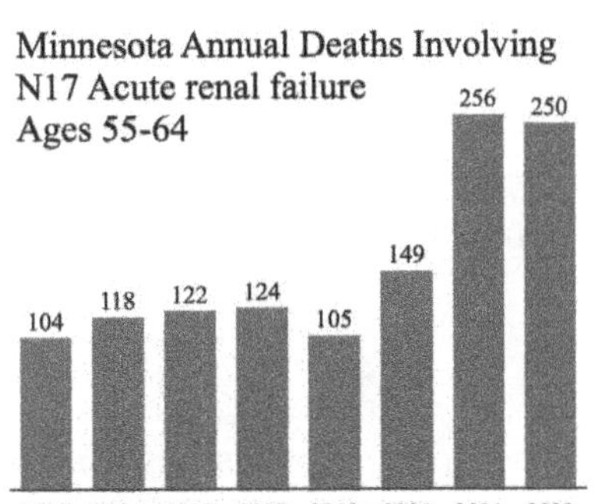

Year	Excess	Excess % over Expected
2020	32	27.4%
2021	138	117.3%
2022	131	110.8%

Figure 10.2

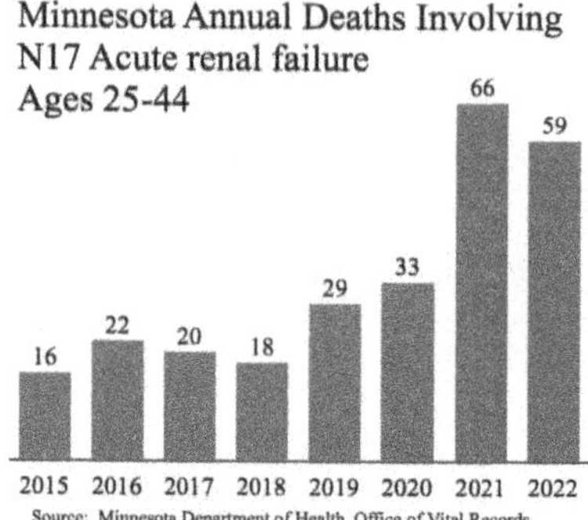

Year	Excess	Excess % over Expected
2020	5	19.6%
2021	36	121.5%
2022	27	84.4%

Figure 10.3

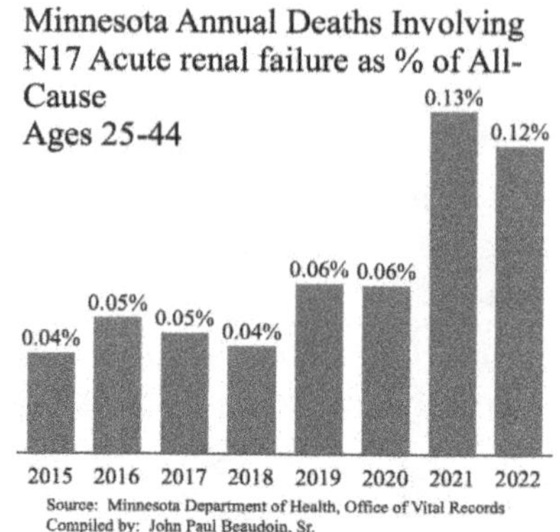

Figure 10.4

THESIS

Once notified of the health emergency factually described in the *Minnesota Memorandum*, the government officials have a legal duty to act by investigating the evidence presented to them; and inaction resulting in further injury to Minnesotans constitutes the requisite criminal negligence and deliberate indifference to convict them for various homicide crimes in both state and federal jurisdictions.

The *All Ages* totals for *Minnesota Annual Death Involving N17 Acute renal failure* shown in Figure 10.5 is a succinct representation of the magnitude of this epidemic of sudden kidney failure. After adjusting for total All-Cause deaths in a year, Figure 10.6 *Minnesota Annual Deaths Involving N17 Acute renal failure as % of All-Cause* shows that ARF in the first year of covid was within normal bounds.

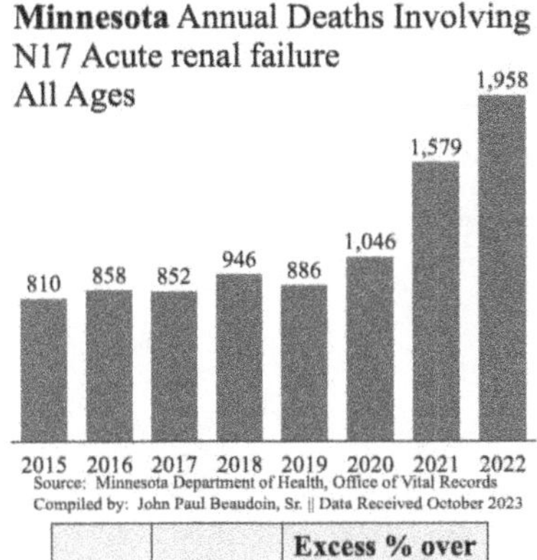

Year	Excess	Excess % over Expected
2020	104	11.0%
2021	613	63.4%
2022	968	97.7%

Figure 10.5

Minnesota Annual Deaths Involving
N17 Acute renal failure as a percent
of All causes
All Ages

1.90% 1.99% 1.92% 2.11% 1.95% 2.00% 3.07% 3.83%

2015 2016 2017 2018 2019 2020 2021 2022

Source: Minnesota Department of Health, Office of Vital Records
Compiled by: John Paul Beaudoin, Sr. || Data Received October 2023

Figure 10.6

The *Minnesota Memorandum* recommends to the Minnesota state officials that they first verify the information expressed in the memorandum, then correlate the individual health case records with the Minnesota Immunization Information Connection (MIIC) system to determine covid vaccination status of the decedents, then correlate or investigate the use of remdesivir (Veklury), baricitinib, and other medicaments that may have caused the premature death by ARF. The *RECOMMENDATIONS - RELIEF* section closes with a call for immediate development of a root-cause analysis and action plan. Anything less is a violation of their legal duty.

The *CONCLUSION* of the Minnesota Memorandum reiterates the *THESIS* in enumerated form: A) officials named have legal duties, B) the memorandum is legal notice that razes ignorance, C) inaction concurrent with a legal duty to act and after being notified constitutes the requisite *mens rea* (guilty mind) to convict, D) subsequent deaths after a reasonable time after notice is an injury that completes the crime, E) homicide crimes have no statutes of limitations, F) Grand Jury investigations will happen some day and it's easier to cure the failings now than face a Grand Jury later, and G) investigate now, publish the results, otherwise, failure to act is criminal negligence.

One three-word line quoted from the Minnesota Memorandum sums up the entire memorandum to the state officials.

Do your job.

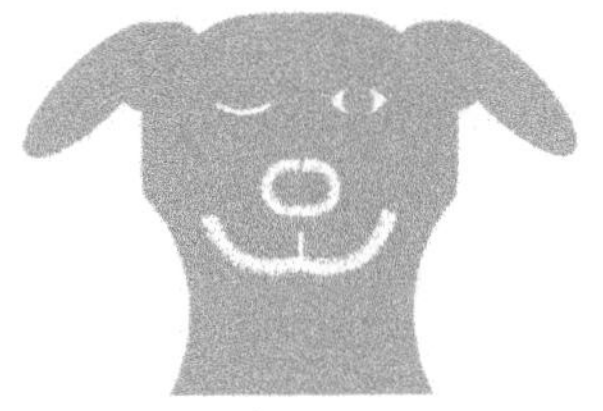

Chapter 11
The Vermont Memorandum

The *Vermont Memorandum and EXHIBITS* (*VM&E*)[1,2] comprise a formal legal notice, delivery of which was completed by May 25, 2023, to 21 officials of the State of Vermont.[3] This 18-page memorandum is entitled, "*NOTICE OF MISREPRESENTATION REQUIRING PUBLIC ADMISSION AND CORRECTION OF VITAL RECORDS.*"

The *VM&E*, sent by John Paul Beaudoin, Sr., is legal notice that apprises top Vermont (VT) officials in all three branches of government of misrepresentations on VT death certificates. Some VT death certificates make no mention of a covid vaccine where the vaccine is the likely cause of death. The same correlation technique employed on Massachusetts records was performed on VAERS reports and VT death certificates.

The *Vermont Memorandum* begins with the following text:

> *This Memorandum is legal notice to the above-named Vermont officials jointly and severally, hereinafter known as "the agents." The intent in providing this Memorandum is not to scold, blame, or accuse, but rather to offer opportunity to the agents to cure misrepresentations in official state documents. Failure to cure the misrepresentations after receiving notice rises to criminal liability where intent of inaction and a legal duty to act are concurrent. After notice imparts knowledge, further injury that flows from inaction can be causally traced to the agents, thus resulting in additional criminal violations. The misrepresentations are being used as a basis to enact public health and safety policies that are injuring Vermonters. The best solution for the agents, and in the public interest, is to fulfill the simple, economical, and righteous recommended actions in the section below named "RECOMMENDATIONS."*

The third (3rd) paragraph from the *Introduction* of the *Vermont Memorandum* states:

> *Vaccine Adverse Event Reporting System ("VAERS") reports and Vermont Death Certificates comprise evidence of proximate and actual causation, which leads to and creates reasonable belief that the C19 vaccines caused numerous Vermont deaths.*

EXHIBIT A of the VM&E

The *VM&E* includes 44 pages of supporting exhibits. *Exhibit A* details death certificate misrepresentations exposed by correlating the certificates with corresponding VAERS records.

Dorothy died on January 5, 2021, at the age of 87 in the State of Vermont. On her death certificate, Cause A states, "*complications of Dementia with psychosis*" in "*1-2 weeks*." Cause B states, "*dementia*" in "*1-2 years*." Part II states, "*chronic kidney disease, hypothyroid, venous stasis*."

VAERS_ID 0942072 is the report of an 87-year-old woman from Vermont who died on January 5, 2021. VAX_DATE states, "*01/02/2021*." Adverse Event Description states, "*Death occurred 3 days after vaccine receipt; attributed to complications of her chronic advanced dementia with aspiration at age 87. No evidence of acute vaccine reaction*." [4]

There is no reasonable doubt that Dorothy is the woman in the VAERS report. Dorothy died three days after vaccination, which apparently isn't acute enough in time for death to be an acute reaction. Let the reader decide, especially in the context of all the other deaths.

Here is a comment I made on Page 2 of *EXHIBIT A* of the *VM&E* with regard to Dorothy's death. Read this in the context that I am not a doctor, but rather a concerned citizen. Dorothy had become violent in her dementia as noted in the VAERS report under HISTORY.

> *In a person with dementia, the already leaky vessels in the brain can become immediately and further damaged from the C19 vaccine, known to cause endothelial damage. Why would anyone vaccinate a person with a "venous stasis" condition knowing the thrombotic and platelet dysregulation issues that occur from the C19 vaccine? Violence is a normal result of leakage.*[2]

John died on February 21, 2021, at the age of 82 in the State of Vermont. Death certificate Cause A states, "*Non ST Elevation Myocardial Infarction*" in "*days*." Part II states, "*Pulmonary fibrosis possibly linked to prior radiation therapy for late b cell lymphoma which was in remission*."

VAERS_ID 1072218 is of an 82-year-old man from Vermont who died on February 21, 2021. VAX_DATE states, "*02/13/2021*." Adverse Event Description states, "*Patient hospitalized for NSTEMI (from 2/18/2021 to 2/20/2021) and discharged on hospice/comfort care. Patient died 2/21/2021*." [5]

There is no reasonable doubt that John is the man represented in the VAERS report. The NSTEMI heart attack occurred at least as early as 2/18/2021 per the VAERS report. That is a maximum of five days after vaccination. There are widespread reports of NSTEMI shortly after covid vaccination. For example, Martin, mentioned in Chapter 4, who died from NSTEMI heart attack within three days after his covid vaccination. Martin was 52 years old. The VAERS_ID associated with Martin's report is 1247687.

Someone reported John's death to VAERS on March 4, 2021. There is no mention of a vaccine on John's death certificate. This misrepresentation by omission must be corrected. Once Vermont officials received the *VM&E*, they had a reasonable time to cure the misrepresentation. After a reasonable time after legal notice, failure to cure the misrepresentation will constitute criminal fraud.

Stanley died on March 16, 2021, at the age of 79 in the State of Vermont. Death certificate Cause A states, "*Neuromuscular disorder (type unspecified)*" in "*54 years*." Part II states, "*Atherosclerotic cardiac and cerebral vascular disease (presumed)*."

VAERS_ID 1169181 is of a 79-year-old man from Vermont who died on March 16, 2021. VAX_DATE states, "*03/13/2021*." Adverse Event Description states:[6]

> *Wife reported that no side effects from vaccine noted until 3/16/2021 when patient had arm and back pain and wanted to go back to bed and she noted he was extremely sweaty at that time.*

> *He was lifted back to bed and was reportioned [sic] several times because he could not get comfortable. She went to get him a drink from the kitchen and heard a guttural sound and rushed back to find him unresponsive and blue in color. She called ""911"" and patient was dead upon arrival (and a DNR) so the Medical examiner arrived and pronounced him dead. She states sx [sic] started at about 4pm and he was pronounced dead at about 5pm. Medical examiner determined a heart attack cause of death. The family not sure that the vaccination had anything to do with death but wanted it to be reported.*

There is no reasonable doubt that Stanley is the man represented in the VAERS report. Stanley died only three days after vaccination from what the medical examiner determined to be a heart attack. There are widespread reports of NSTEMI shortly after covid vaccination. Again, for example, Martin, mentioned in Chapter 4, who died from NSTEMI heart attack within three days after his covid vaccination. Martin was age 52. The VAERS_ID associated with Martin's report is 1247687.[7]

Someone reported Stanley's death to VAERS on April 5, 2021. There is no mention of a vaccine on Stanley's death certificate. This misrepresentation of omission must be corrected. Vermont officials had a legal duty to cure Stanley's death certificate after they were notified of the misrepresentation.

Ethel died on April 23, 2021, at the age of 98 in the State of Vermont. Death certificate Cause A states, "*Congestive Heart Failure*" in "*24 hours.*" Cause B states, "*Myocardial Infarction*" in "*24 hours.*" Cause C states, "*Hypertensive cardiovascular disease*" in "*years.*"

VAERS_ID 1267587 is of a 98 woman from Vermont who died on April 23, 2021. VAX_DATE states, "*04/21/2021*" Adverse Event Description states, "*patient woke up on 04/22/2021 with shortness of breath and weakness. On exam, she was hypotensive, tachycardic and edematous.*" Lab Data states, "*4/22/2021 EKG: A fib, RVR, 145 bpm, q wave abnormalities showing ischemia inferiorly and anterolaterally.*" [8]

There is no reasonable doubt that Ethel is the woman represented in the VAERS report. Ethel died only two days after vaccination from a heart attack.

The most interesting part of the VAERS report is the tachycardia noted in the Lab Data field. "*145bpm*" is a super-fast heartbeat for a teenager, let alone a 98-year-old woman. 4/22/2021 is when they noticed Ethel's heartbeat was racing. It was likely racing shortly after vaccination the day before.

Some may say that she was age 98, so she could have died from old age. But the fast heartbeat (tachycardia) is known to occur from covid vaccines. Regardless of her age, Ethel's case contributes important evidence of damage to the heart from covid vaccines. And she lost her life from it within two days. A covid vaccine ran her heart out of beats.

Someone reported Ethel's death to VAERS on April 28, 2021. There is no mention of a vaccine on Ethel's death certificate. This misrepresentation of omission must be corrected. Vermont officials had a legal duty to cure Ethel's death certificate after they were notified of the misrepresentation.

Rebecca was 23 years old and died on May 24, 2021 in Vermont. Death certificate Cause A mentions liver cancer that metastasized to her lungs and abdomen in only "*3 months*." There is nothing else mentioned beyond Cause A.

VAERS_ID 1343614 is of a 23 woman who died on May 24, 2021. Her VAX_DATE is May 18, 2021. Her ONSET_DATE is May 20, 2021, only two days after her vaccination date. There is no reasonable doubt Rebecca is the woman in the VAERS report. The SYMPTOM_TEXT states, "*presented to ED dept confused, incr n/v, weakness. Received palliative carex4 days. deceased 05/24.*" [9]

Rebecca was dying anyway. Why did they give her a covid vaccine? She presented to the Emergency Department confused with nausea and vomiting. That sounds like she was having a stroke. Rebecca's life and death should not be for naught.

Entering a VAERS report takes a significant amount of time, and someone spent the time to enter a VAERS report for Rebecca. Given the medical notation and lab data, someone privy to Rebecca's hospital file entered her VAERS report.

EXHIBITs B, C, D, E, and F of the VM&E

Exhibit B of the *VM&E* details *Death Certificates Stating that C19 Vaccine is Causally Related to Death.*

At least four Vermont death certificates mention a vaccine in Parts I or II. These four are detailed below.

- Barbara died at the age of 96 in the State of Vermont on May 29, 2021. Cause A states, "*Generalized medical deconditioning, multifactorial: see part 2*" in "*months.*" Part II states, "*Hypertensive and atherosclerotic cardiovascular disease; Old age; Clinical impression of generalized decline following Covid-19 Johnson & Johnson Vaccine 5/7/2021.*" Clearly, Steven Shapiro, who certified Barbara's death, wanted it to be known that the J&J covid vaccine was causal in Barbara's death.
- Marion died at the age of 102 in the State of Vermont on September 11, 2021. Cause A states, "*Probable Acute Myocardial Infarction*" in "*1-2 weeks.*" Cause B states, "*Coronary Artery Disease*" in "*>5 years.*" Cause C states, "*Congestive Heart Failure*" in "*>5 years.*" Cause D states, "*Hypertension*" in "*>10 years.*" Part II states, "*Covid Positive Test Result in Asymptomatic Vaccinated Person.*" The question here is not whether a vaccine killed Marion. She was 102 years old. She survived the second year of the Spanish flu as a newborn in 1919 and every other disease since then. The real question is – why would someone inject an experimental vaccine into a 102-year-old woman? Were they trying to save her? Marion may have been killed by a covid vaccine, but no one was interested in exploring this. An autopsy would have been needed to look for endothelial inflammation and the types of WBCs (white blood cells) present at time of death.
- Leland died at the age of 86 in the State of Vermont on September 16, 2021. Cause A states, "*Inanition*" in "*weeks.*" Cause B states, "*COVID 19 breakthrough infection after fully vaccinated*" in "*1 month.*" Part II states, "*Rheumatoid Arthritis, Depression, personal history of squamous cell cancer metastatic to parotid gland.*" Inanition generally means exhaustion from lack of food or water, or both. It could be from mental or physical reasons. The timing in the year is important. What actually killed Leland? Did covid

vaccine injury to Leland's immune system, a known side effect of covid vaccines, precipitate the breakthrough covid infection listed as a cause of death? Or was the inanition the result of the commonly employed hospital covid protocol involving withholding of hydration and nutrition?

- Karyn died at the age of 45 in the State of Vermont on November 21, 2021. Karyn's case is reviewed extensively in Chapter 4.[10]

Regarding the timing of Leland's "*breakthrough*" case, remember the first half of 2021 when the CDC and news media tried to make "*breakthrough*" infections seem rare to support the fallacious official narrative that covid vaccines precluded any and all infection. The "experts" stated on news broadcasts and government press conferences that covid vaccines prevent infection, "If you get vaccinated, you will not get covid." [11]

Then, in the autumn of 2021, when evidence was overwhelming that covid vaccines did not prevent infection, the media and CDC went quiet on the "*breakthrough*" concept and shifted to saying that covid vaccines were never meant to prevent covid infection, but rather only to reduce symptoms, hospitalization, and death. The latter was stated despite the complete lack of supporting evidence. They fabricated the cover story to replace the previous cover story, and only after-the-fact did they attempt to buttress the deception with weak, under-powered studies.

One can assume that everything reported in the media that was attributed to the CDC and FDA was not based on evidence, but instead originated as focus-group-tested marketing propaganda. The coup de grâce being the completely unsupported three-word slogan, "*safe and effective*." Indeed, we now have conclusive evidence that the covid vaccines are neither.

And if covid vaccines do not prevent infection, do not prevent transmission, and there is no reasonably believable evidence that a covid vaccine reduces symptoms, hospitalizations, or death, then why is, or was, it mandated? How was the power of government invoked to solicit and coerce an experimental treatment upon The People; an exercise of Russian Roulette wherein some will die, some will be maimed for life, and the lucky ones will not react, at least not over the short term? How many victims of this dangerous 'game' still believe that they've protected themselves from a terrifying disease portrayed by government to be extremely deadly? As the actual RLSD in the reports presented in this book reveal, any feeling of safety was purely illusory.

EXHIBIT C of the *VM&E* lists some one hundred fifteen VAERS reports of people from Vermont that contain the character strings: *carditis*, *tachycard*, *ischemi*, *clot*, *embol*, *rhythmi*, and *thromb*. The header text in *EXHIBIT C* states, "*VAERS records to be investigated.*"[2]

EXHIBIT D of the *VM&E* comprises eight pages detailing 29 Vermont death certificates.[2] These death certificates contain words or character strings that are suggestive of covid vaccine harm and should, therefore, be investigated. The investigation could start with a simple one-minute look-up of each vaccination record. Collating vaccination records with these death certificates could quickly confirm or refute covid vaccination as a cause of death in the respective cases.

Examples in *EXHIBIT D* include Erik, a 16-year-old boy who died on January 2, 2022, from death certificate Cause A "*pancytopenia*" in "*weeks*" and Cause B "*lymphoblastic lymphoma*" in "*months*." This was a fast-acting cancer that killed this boy in months. Perhaps few would immediately regard Erik as a potential covid vaccine victim. However, I have been immersed in the data for more than a year. *TERTIA PARS* of this book presents evidence of a causal association of covid vaccines with lymph node cancers, bone marrow cancers, and other blood cancers, which are at three hundred percent of normal in some ICD-10 codes since covid vaccines were introduced. Unlike 2020 when such cases were appearing only in the elderly, lymph node cancer and bone marrow cancer have increased sharply in much younger people. Erik's death should be investigated.

Jeremiah died on January 7, 2022 at age 37. Jeremiah's death certificate Cause A states, "*Cardiac arrest*" in "*hours*."

Aiden died on February 18, 2022 at age 16. Aiden's death certificate Cause A states, "*Hypoxic-ischemic encephalopathy*" in "*15 hours*." Cause B states, "*Presumed seizure*" in "*15 hours*." Cause C states, "*Epilepsy and neurocognitive disorder due to STXBP1 mutation*" in "*16 years*."

While Aiden had issues his entire life, encephalopathy is revealed in *TERTIA PARS* to be much more common in 2021 and 2022. If there is a connection between neurological damage and covid vaccines, then Aiden would be a good example to study. Just as someone with a clotting issue should not be vaccinated for covid, perhaps people with Aiden's issues of epilepsy and neurocognitive disorders should not be vaccinated for covid either.

The particularly notable issue is not the possible connection, but rather the absolute refusal of the medical community to study what is right in front of them. The content of this book details a massive amount of information readily available to medical researchers, yet the conspicuous avoidance of this trove of real data is obvious to anyone who follows the research.

There are too many to include here. I'll conclude this section on *EXHIBIT D* of the *VM&E* with Capri who died on February 18, 2022 at the age of 37. Capri's death certificate Cause A states, "*Pulmonary thromboembolism*" in "*minutes*" and a DVT in her leg, and with history of coagulopathy in years. If this young woman had clotting issues, why did she take a covid vaccine? Did the covid vaccine kill her?

The *VM&E* recommends querying the Vermont vaccination records for each of the decedents listed in *EXHIBIT D* for any temporal relationships between covid vaccination and death. Surely, it is the dutiful thing to do in the public interest. Empty claims of "*no evidence to implicate covid vaccines in ...*" are meaningless absent a reasonable effort to uncover evidence. Collating vaccination records with these death certificates could quickly confirm or refute covid vaccination as a cause of death in the respective cases. The interests of public health and safety demand this simple investigation.

EXHIBIT E of the *VM&E* details five Vermont death certificates involving *myocarditis* for decedents aged 44, 51, 64, 77, and 96.[2]

EXHIBIT F of the *VM&E* details four Vermont death certificates involving *pericarditis* for decedents aged 47, 59, 82, and 83.[2]

EXHIBIT G OF VM&E

EXHIBIT G comprises twenty Vermont VAERS reports. Not all of these involve deaths. Many are reports of serious conditions that left patients permanently maimed or injured for a period of time. Many injuries are life-threatening.

A man, age 41, VAERS_ID 1505017, experienced clots in his legs that traveled to his lungs, threatening his life. This occurred a month and a half after vaccination for covid.[12]

A woman, age 25, VAERS_ID 1999297, experienced a "*myocardial injury*" and chest pain within three days of vaccination; diagnostic tests were inconclusive.[13]

A woman, age 67, VAERS_ID 1150385, experienced blood clots in her arm three days after vaccination. The clots were at the site of a catheter placed for surgery seven weeks earlier. She had had clots there before the vaccination. The following question must be asked. Given a patient, known to have recently developed blood clots, and, given that covid vaccines are known to cause clots, why would health care professionals endanger the life of that person by administering a covid vaccine?[14]

A girl, age 9, VAERS_ID 2540777, was injected on December 29, 2021. The onset date listed is January 6, 2021, eight days later. The symptoms include "*dizzy spells*," "*headaches*," and "*body pain*." The symptoms worsened after a second dose was administered. The little girl, only 9 years old, was later diagnosed by the pediatrician with POTS (postural orthostatic tachycardia syndrome). As will be detailed in *TERTIA PARS*, tachycardia diagnoses have increased substantially since 2021, when covid vaccines were introduced. Dysautonomia, associated with tachycardia, has also exploded since early 2021; and not only in the elderly like Ethel, age 98. Younger people like this unfortunate 9-year-old girl are also suffering.[15]

EXHIBIT G concludes with a VAERS report similar to that of Cassidy (Chapter 1), but without ending in death. I cannot help wondering if the parents of this boy understand the seriousness of his condition. It is not likely that they would be aware that Cassidy may have died from the same kind of injury.

A boy, age 8, VAERS_ID 2122755, was vaccinated on December 4, 2021 with his second Pfizer dose at around 1:15 PM. His first dose was administered on November 12, 2021 at 4:30PM, when he was still 7 years old. Symptoms included "*severe stomach pain*" on December 5, one day after the second dose. "*Fever*" and "*nausea and vomiting*" also followed within two days of the injection.[16] These are the exact same symptoms, in the same timeline that were detailed in the report with VAERS_ID 2038120, believed to be associated with 7-year-old Cassidy. May God bless and protect this boy from further harm.

CONCLUSION B in the *Vermont Memorandum* states, "*This Memorandum and the EXHIBITS A through G serve as legal notice, providing knowledge of misrepresentations by omission on state records, specifically Death Certificates*."[1]

CONCLUSION G in the *Vermont Memorandum* states, "*The agents should take their opportunity to simply publish the full truth using information from Vermont state records, despite the truth being in conflict with CDC and FDA criminally reckless recommendations.*[1]

The *Vermont Memorandum* with a page noting a web link to the *EXHIBIT*s was sent via certified mail on May 22, 2023, to the following Vermont officials: Governor PHIL SCOTT, Lieutenant Governor DAVID

ZUCKERMAN, State Attorney General CHARITY CLARK, State Treasurer MIKE PIECIAK, Secretary of State SARAH COPELAND HANZAS, State Auditor DOUG HOFFER, Health Commissioner MARK LEVINE, Deputy Health Commissioner KELLY DOUGHERTY, Deputy Health Commissioner JULIE AREL, Chief Medical Examiner ELIZABETH A. BUNDOCK, Sergeant at Arms JANET MILLER, Senate President Pro Tempore PHIL BARUTH, Speaker of the House JILL KROWINSKI, Chief Justice PAUL L. REIBER, Associate Justice HAROLD E. EATON, JR., Associate Justice KAREN R. CARROLL, Associate Justice WILLIAM D. COHEN, Associate Justice NANCY J. WAPLES, U.S. Senator BERNIE SANDERS, U.S. Senator PETER WELCH, U.S. House Representative BECCA BALINT.[3]

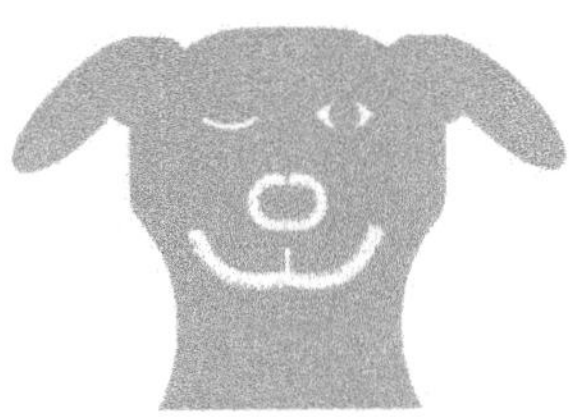

Chapter 12
Obituaries

Last names will not be used in this chapter because this chapter is not about correlated death certificates to VAERS records.

These are Massachusetts pulmonary embolism deaths in people under age 23, who are not described as obese or diabetic, and who do not appear to have had chronic health issues. The families of these decedents were likely told that these deaths were from covid or were accidental. I don't know if any of these deaths were caused by a covid vaccine, but any prudent Massachusetts official sharing responsibility for the public's health and well-being would certainly be expected to devote the minimal amount of time it takes to query the immunization records available in the Massachusetts Department of Public Health. The People of the Commonwealth should demand this simple investigation in the public interest.

Emily died in Massachusetts at the young age of 21 on January 7, 2022. The obituary states that Emily died "*after suffering cardiac arrest due to Covid-19.*" Emily's death certificate SFN_NUMBER 1115 Cause A states, "*PULMONARY EMBOLI.*" There are no other causes mentioned in Parts I or II. "*Covid*" is not mentioned on this death certificate. I do not know why it is mentioned in the obituary online. Could it be related to the Federal Emergency Management Authority's (FEMA) requirements to qualify for up to $9,000 of assistance in covid-related funeral expenses?[1]

From personal experience, I can understand why families may not wish to be contacted about the loss of a child. When my son John died, I withdrew and did not talk to many people. I just sat at home for two years until covid hit. I did go to a group once a month for fathers who lost children. We sat in a circle and told our stories of our sons and daughters, how we are coping, and how we plan to continue living without our children. For me, that ended when the group sent an e-mail early in 2021, "**Vaccinated Only**," written in boldface type. I waited about a year and then finally sent one of them a message about how I felt. Many of us don't want to continue life without our children. Some of us wake up every day disappointed that we woke up. To be in the presence of other men who've experienced such loss was calming. Then it was gone ... callously.

For those who wonder how parents of children can remain silent upon learning that their child died from a covid vaccination, I have no answer for you. Everyone is different. I only tried to contact two families about their children's deaths. In each case, I abandoned the effort after two attempts received no reply. It's done. It's over. And nothing is going to bring their children back. If years had not already passed since my son died, I don't know if I'd be doing this research. I only want to save the children whose parents still don't know the perils and who may risk their children under the needle again.

I cannot un-know what I have learned from my research. The numbers in *TERTIA PARS* are neither statistical nor complex. They are stark. And they plainly depict the carnage for all to understand.

Emily is said to have had a stellar high school record and was a senior at a local university. God bless Emily and her family. What caused a pulmonary embolism in a healthy 21-year-old woman? The death certificate omits covid as a cause though Massachusetts medical examiners often write covid as a cause from a simple positive test. An explanation of the true cause may arise from a look at her vaccination record. Maybe she was never vaccinated for covid. Or maybe a covid shot killed her. Massachusetts owes The People an answer.

Meghan died in Massachusetts at the age of 22 on November 6, 2022. Her obituary makes no mention of a cause of death for Meghan. Meghan's death certificate SFN_NUMBER 53585 Cause A states, "*CARDIAC ARREST*" in "*HRS*," Cause B states, "*RIGHT VENTRICULAR FAILURE*" in "HRS," and Cause C states, "*PULMONARY EMBOLISM*" in "*HRS.*" There are no other causes listed in Parts I and II. The last UCOD, the root cause, is a pulmonary embolism.

Meghan was an accomplished young lady with two degrees from college and a new career in a profession using both her college degrees. Meghan's and Emily's deaths leave great big gaping holes in the hearts of their parents and families. What caused Meghan's PE? Was she vaccinated for covid? Her profession and employer suggest she would have been required to take the covid vaccinations. Hold-outs were fired and did sue their employer. May God bless Meghan and her family. Let peace and justice enter among us.

Alicha M. St. Croix died in Massachusetts at the age of 22 on November 13, 2022. Her obituary states that Alicha, "*passed away ... following complications from giving birth.*" Alicha's death certificate Cause A states, "*PULMONARY EMBOLISM*" in "*DAYS,*" and Part II states, "*CARDIOMEGALY.*"

There is no mention of pregnancy on Alicha's death certificate in Part I or Part II. Yet her death record contains the ICD-10 code O99.4, "Diseases of the circulatory system complicating pregnancy, childbirth and the puerperium." How did the CDC know to do that? This is evidence that the pulmonary embolism complicated the pregnancy. Still, we do not know what caused the pulmonary embolism, which is a common effect from covid immunizations.

Alicha's daughter will never know her, and her family will certainly miss her every time they see Alicha's daughter. Alicha was predeceased by her mother. Some families have an unfair amount of loss. Was Alicha covid vaccinated, and when? The Commonwealth of Massachusetts owes The People answers to these questions.

This brief chapter is a departure from the hard evidence, which is the book's foundation. It is not meant as an element of debate. It is meant to convey the simple fact that every one of these inadequately explained deaths of young people could be clarified with a simple immunization record look-up, which requires barely one minute of clerical time to perform.

TERTIA PARS

Data Analyses

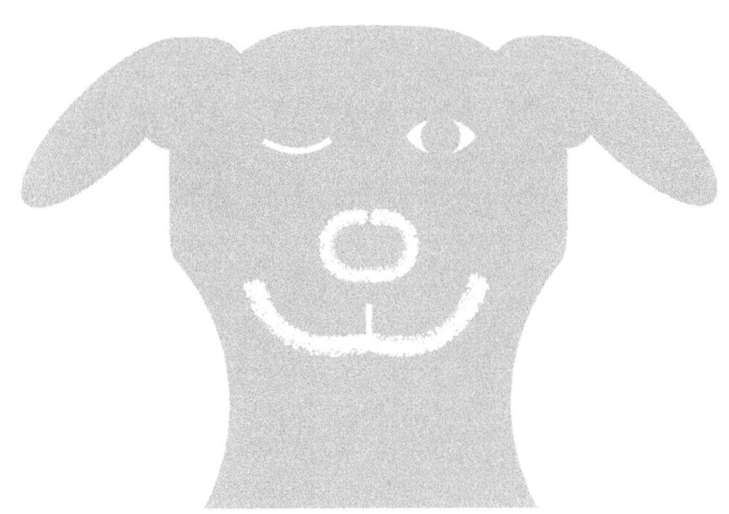

RES IPSA LOQUITUR

"The thing speaks for itself"

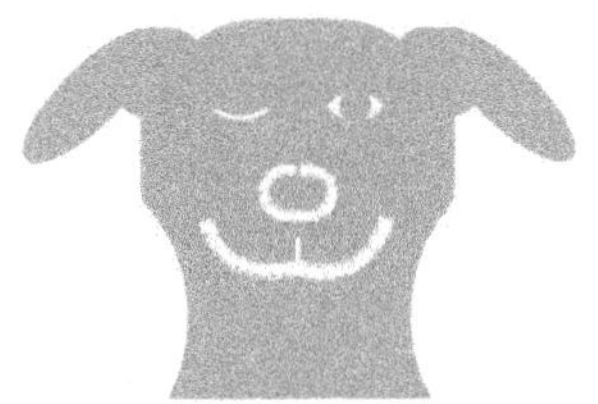

Chapter 13
All-Cause & Simpson's Paradoxes

Apples can be separated by variety (McIntosh, Gala, Red Delicious). Applesauce cannot be.

The CDC gives the world applesauce. Data from the CDC has been de-identified and bundled into sets of variables. Thus, no researchers have been able to tease out the individual signals well enough to learn what is happening, to whom, and when within the span of 2020–2023.

This analysis, based on Massachusetts death certificates, is likely more robust than anything else published thus far. Individual causes of death, as well as combinations of causes of death, can be correlated by age, sex, town, or any other variable available on a death certificate.

The CDC employs about 11,800 people[1] and the Massachusetts State Department of Public Health employs about 3,500 people.[2] Both of them hoard data and bundle it in ways which diminish its utility. They use these data bundles to generate and publish nearly useless statistics that become the basis for endless arguments among various factions over what is true. Is data bundling intended to obscure safety signals of pharmaceutical products? The fact that this data bundling obscures safety signals is clear and indisputable.

Upon receiving the Massachusetts Death Certificate database in February 2022, I wanted to get this valuable information into the hands of experts in statistical analysis. I offered it to several professors and people holding PhDs, as well as a British data hound. Joel Smalley immediately produced a good piece of work in his Substack article.[3]

About two weeks after Joel's article was published, the Commonwealth of Massachusetts coincidentally removed more than four thousand covid deaths from the count, but added about four hundred at the same time, citing a change to how they count covid deaths. This occurred around March 10, 2022.[4]

Massachusetts had put the population through fear and panic for two years and then it just dropped 4,000 purported covid deaths from the rolls–some sixteen percent–and no one blinked.

Massachusetts, New York, and New Jersey led the world in purported covid deaths per population for the first year of covid. These three states were used to scare the world. People should care about such a drastic reduction.

After Joel's article, professors who downloaded the database apparently did not see enough value in it to engage in analyzing death certificates. Frustrated at the lack of activity, I started experimenting with searches and filters using a spreadsheet utility. Soon after that, as more frustration set in, I re-learned spreadsheet functions. Before long, my workbook comprised about thirty spreadsheets with cells calling sheet to sheet. Now, all I have to do is type in one ICD-10 code and the computer operates for ten to fifteen minutes until all my graphs and tables are generated for that one ICD-10 code.

Using those spreadsheets, the first thing I wanted to look at was All-Cause deaths. Was the CDC data consistent with the Massachusetts data online and consistent with the death certificate database I newly possessed?

I graphed daily deaths for all years 2015–2021. I used years 2015–2019 as the baseline for comparison. Solid lines represent 2015–2019, dashed lines represent 2020, and dotted lines represent 2021.

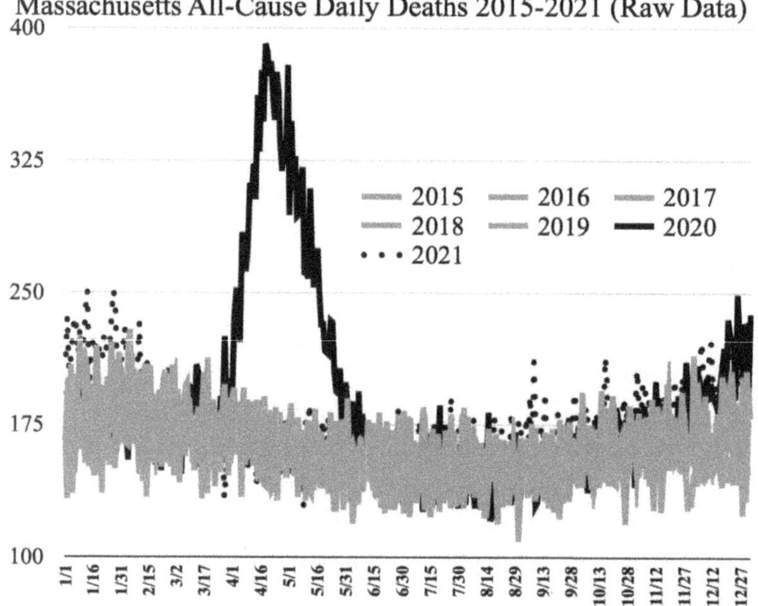

Figure 13.1

The gray lines, representing daily deaths each year for 2015–2019, make a nice gray band that one can consider 'normal.' No curve smoothing was used in making this graph.

The black line is 2020. The obvious first wave depicts an epidemic from mid-March to mid-June. The black line also pops up above the gray band at about the end of November or the beginning of December. This appears to be a seasonal respiratory virus second wave, which is much smaller than the first wave, as would be expected.

The dotted line plot is 2021, which begins on the left where the black line plot left off on the right. The winter wave ends around February as the dotted line plot disappears into the normal gray band until mid-July. That caught my attention. Why would the 2021 dotted line plot rise above the normal black band unseasonably in July? And why would it stay there for the rest of the year?

The next figure shows the pattern more clearly.

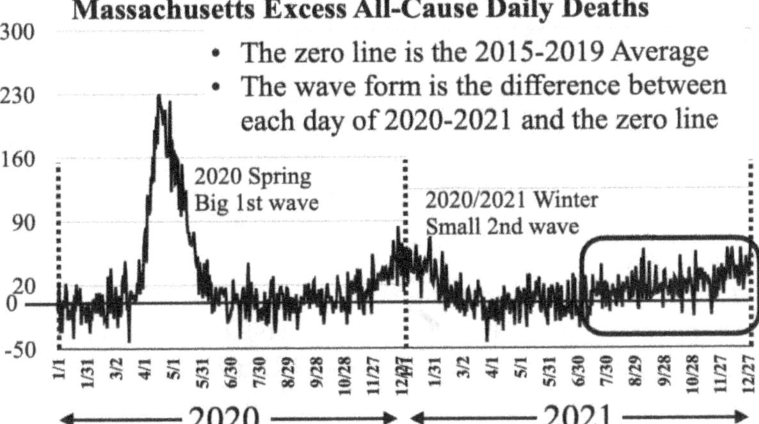

Figure 13.2

The graph above is a continuous plot for 2020 on the left and 2021 on the right. The zero-line is the average of 2015–2019 for each day. The plot depicts the differences for each day between the actual number of daily deaths during 2020–2021, and the 2015–2019 average. *Id est*, it is simply a plot of excess All-Cause deaths for both years. Until mid-2021, the peaks behave like a seasonal respiratory virus behaves.

The first big wave is the 2020 Massachusetts epidemic which lasted only eight to nine weeks. There is a return to zero excess deaths with the arrival of warmer weather in June, exactly the behavior a seasonal respiratory virus normally displays.

By the end of November or beginning of December 2020, the second wave begins and continues until around February 2021, where it returns to zero. This again is normal behavior for a seasonal respiratory virus.

Some will say that the introduction of the covid vaccine caused the 2nd wave to drop in early 2021, but that cannot be true. The plot reverses from an increasing slope to a decreasing slope on the front-side of the wave. It's the Gompertz second derivative for those who understand calculus.

The important fact is that the change in curve from increasing slope to decreasing slope happened long before any reasonable number of people were covid-vaccinated, if any at all.

One thing for sure is that the 2021 plot returns to zero around February 2021 and stays there until July. My initial thought was that covid was gone or seasonally in its "off" state.

We'll next consider Simpson's paradox. First, please notice the rectangle with rounded corners surrounding the second half of 2021. The rectangle highlights the anomaly which bothered me. Excess deaths are continuously above zero unseasonably, from July through the end of the year; some ten to twenty excess deaths every day for half a year. That amounts to two to four thousand excess deaths over six months. What caused thousands of excess deaths unseasonably?

Professional, well-known epidemiologist professors state that SARS-CoV-2 is not a seasonal virus. They do not have record-level source data. They base that conclusion on bundled CDC data, which are compromised by Simpson's paradoxes. I assure you that covid, as it was in 2020 and has been since, exhibits the textbook behavior of a seasonal respiratory virus when the confounding signals from negative externalities (vaccines, deadly hospital protocols, etc.) are filtered out.

A Simpson's paradox occurs when two or more visible and independent signals interact to partially or fully cancel their individual visible behaviors. This can result in erroneous conclusions about the magnitude or existence of the independent effects. The routine practice by CDC and other government agencies of combining large amounts of raw data into a small number of groups virtually guarantees that Simpson's paradox will be operating. For example, combining the data from countries with different climates and situated on opposite sides of the equator is guaranteed to obscure any seasonality in the data.

Simpson's paradox can explain why, if covid vaccines are truly deadly to some people, and mass vaccination began in January 2021, there appear to be no excess deaths from February 2021 through July 2021, inclusive. Some vaccine vigilance pun- dits postulated that there is a five month delay between administration of a covid vaccine and a subsequent resulting death. However, the fundamental medical understanding of pulmonary embolism, stroke, heart attack, and other acute conditions completely refutes the five month delay theory. The theory simply does not make sense.

Regardless of whether the covid virus or covid vaccines were responsible for excess death, the evidence of what is happening must be embedded in the RLSD death certificate data. I decided to explore the 2020 death certificate data to see what evidence might emerge. In order to reduce the possibility that underlying signals could be masked by Simpson's paradox, I did not combine data across diverse categories. I began by looking at what was happening over time by age at time of death. I already had all of the RLSD data loaded into spreadsheets. As one might imagine, these spreadsheets are very large, comprising several million individual cells, each of which contains a number. The human eye-brain system, as miraculous as it may be, is not well suited to finding meaningful patterns by examining immense arrays of numbers. I decided to produce a "heat map" of the data. Readers, no doubt, are already familiar with many forms of heat maps. For example, weather radar maps are a form of heat map where the colors plotted on the map indicate the intensity of the rain at each point. In this case, I produced a heat map indicating the intensity of excess deaths for each cell included in the map.

On a weather radar map, each point on the map corresponds to an actual geographical location. On my heat map, each cell corresponds to an actual period of time and an actual age group. For example, one cell in my heat map corresponds to the deaths of people aged 65 through 74 during the first two weeks of March 2020. On a weather radar map, intensity is a measure of how hard it is raining at each point on the map. In my heat map, intensity is a measure of the difference in the number of deaths for each time period and age group compared to the baseline number of deaths for that time period and age group as calculated from the average of the death certificate data for 2015 through 2019.

General readers may skip over the following section, which explains how the intensity for each cell is calculated. This is for the benefit of readers who are familiar with simple statistics.

The intensity, I, of excess deaths for each cell is calculated as

$I = (N - M) / SD$ where,

N = Number of Deaths in a 2020 or 2021 cell

M = Mean of deaths in corresponding cell for years 2015–2019

SD = Standard Dev. of deaths in the corresponding cell for 2015–2019, and

where, in the heat map,

light gray indicates $I \geq 2$ sigma, $I < 8$ sigma EXCESS

medium gray indicates $I \geq 8$ sigma, $I < 16$ sigma EXCESS

dark gray indicates $I \geq 16$ sigma EXCESS

nnn indicates $I \geq 2$ sigma DEFICIT

NNN indicates $I \geq 8$ sigma DEFICIT

Each row of the heat maps in Figures 13.3 and 13.4 represents a semi-monthly period. "1H" includes the 1st through 15th of each month, except February, which includes the 1st through the 14th. "2H" includes the 16th through the last day of each month, except February, which includes the 15th through the last day of February.

Each column of the heat map represents the indicated age group.

If the excess deaths in a cell do not differ significantly from the corresponding mean during the 2015–2019 baseline years, the cell is left unshaded.

If the excess deaths in a cell are moderately greater, the cell is shaded light gray.

If the excess deaths in a cell are much greater, the cell is shaded dark gray.

If the excess deaths in a cell are eminently greater, the cell is shaded black.

If there are moderately fewer deaths in a cell than in the corresponding baseline data, that deficit is indicated by placing "nnn" in that cell; and if the deficit is larger, that is indicated by placing "NNN" in the cell.

Massachusetts All-Cause Deaths Heat Map

2020 Standard Deviations from 2015-2019 Mean for each Age group and Semi-Monthly Period

	25-44	45-54	55-59	60-64	65-74	75-79	80-84	85+
January 1H								
January 2H								
February 1H		nnn						
February 2H								
March 1H								
March 2H								
April 1H								
April 2H								
May 1H								
May 2H								
June 1H								
June 2H								NNNNN
July 1H								
July 2H							nnn	nnn
August 1H								nnn
August 2H								
September 1H							nnn	nnn
September 2H								
October 1H								
October 2H								
November 1H								
November 2H								
December 1H								
December 2H								

HUGE WAVE
EXCESS DEATH

No Signal in this box
80-84 & 85+ DEFICIT
NO EPIDEMIC Jun-Dec

SMALL WINTER WAVE

Source: Vital Records of The Commonwealth of Massachusetts dated April 2023
Compiled by: John Paul Beaudoin, Sr.

Figure 13.3

That large first wave shown in the waveform graphs, Figures 13.1 and 13.2, is quite evident in the 2020 Heat Map, Figure 13.3. The first covid wave of deaths in Massachusetts lasted only 8 to 9 weeks. Moreover, it mainly affected those aged 65 and older quite badly. It did impact those aged 25–59 to a much lesser degree, and those aged 60–64 to a medium degree.

All summer and most of the autumn of 2020, there was no signal. In fact, there was a deficit of deaths among those aged 80 and above. A deficit in the deaths of elderly immediately following a wave of excess deaths during an epidemic is the result of the "dry tinder effect." The "dry tinder effect" occurs when those, such as the elderly and infirm, who were likely to die in the coming months anyway, instead succumbed to the stresses of an infectious disease. Succumbing earlier clears the forest of "dry tinder." Once the forest floor is cleared of dry tinder, the likelihood of another forest fire is low until more dry tinder accumulates. Since people cannot die twice, a deficit of deaths manifests after such a first wave of disease. In viewing Figure 13.3, it is useful to keep in mind that the average age of death in Massachusetts from 2015 to 2019 is 75.6.

The scarcity of excess deaths from June through October of 2020 in Figure 13.3 is compelling evidence that covid is a seasonal disease. This heat map reveals that during 2020 covid behaved exactly like acknowledged seasonal diseases such as flu and the common cold.

Some claim that masks, social distancing, and other measures made covid disappear all summer in 2020. However, it is clear in Figure 13.1 that the first wave deaths had already declined close to the historic baseline by the time the Massachusetts governor mandated masking on May 6, 2020.[5]

As mentioned above, the decline in "rate of change" in daily deaths occurred before the peak of the first wave of deaths in Figure 13.1. Thus, the evidence is clear that these masking and distancing mandates had nothing to do with the shape or triggered changes of the covid All-Cause deaths curve representing Massachusetts. Moreover, the data for the subsequent two years confirm the seasonality of covid disease.

Figure 13.4 is the heat map for the 2021 death certificate data. Considered together with the plot of aggregate All-Cause mortality in Figure 13.2, the 2021 heat map depicts Simpson's paradox in operation.

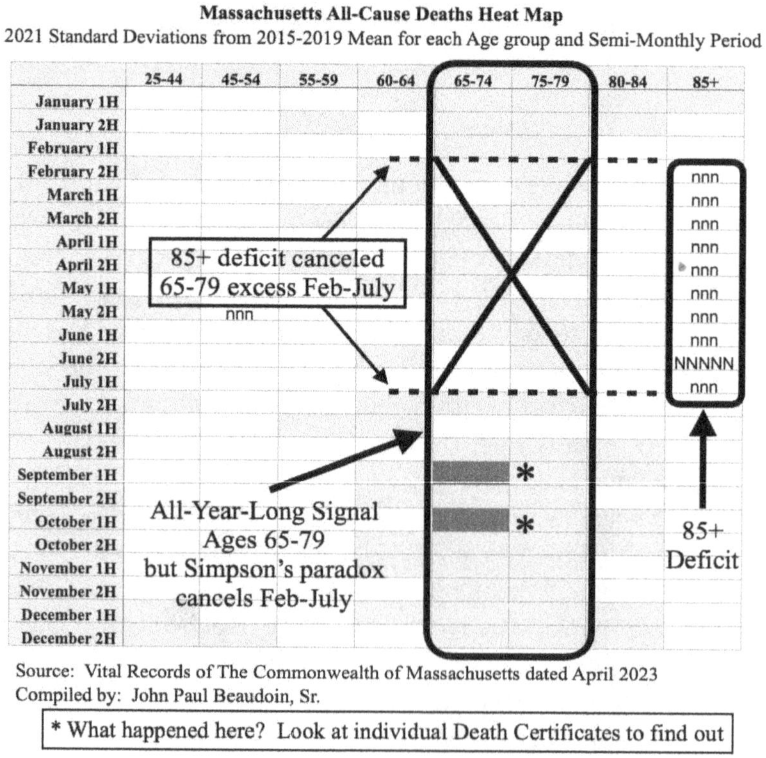

Massachusetts All-Cause Deaths Heat Map

2021 Standard Deviations from 2015-2019 Mean for each Age group and Semi-Monthly Period

25-44
45-54
55-59
60-64
65-74
75-79
80-84
85+

January 1H
January 2H
February 1H
February 2H
March 1H
March 2H
April 1H
April 2H
May 1H
May 2H
June 1H
June 2H
July 1H
July 2H
August 1H
August 2H
September 1H
September 2H
October 1H
October 2H
November 1H
November 2H
December 1H
December 2H

85+ deficit canceled
65-79 excess Feb-July

nnn

nnn
nnn
nnn
nnn
nnn
nnn
nnn
nnn
NNNNN
nnn

All-Year-Long Signal
Ages 65-79
but Simpson's paradox
cancels Feb-July

*
*

85+
Deficit

Source: Vital Records of The Commonwealth of Massachusetts dated April 2023

Compiled by: John Paul Beaudoin, Sr.

* What happened here? Look at individual Death Certificates to find out

Figure 13.4

Whereas Figure 13.2 shows 2021 All-Cause deaths returning to the historical 2015–2019 over the span from February through July 2021, the heat map in Figure 13.4 reveals the paradox in operation. All-Cause deaths for 65–74 and 75–79 age groups are above normal all year long. Yet, the line plot in Figure 13.2 goes to zero from February through July 2021 because the deficits in 85+ age group cancels out the excess deaths in the two age groups spanning 65–79 over the same period.

The heat map in Figure 13.4 reveals the pronounced lack of seasonality in *excess* deaths during 2021. Compare that to the clear seasonality revealed in the 2020 heat map in Figure 13.3.

Covid seems to have switched from highly seasonal behavior in 2020 to a complete absence of seasonal behavior in 2021. How is this possible? Is the shift in behavior on the calendar boundary between 2020 and 2021 a complete coincidence, or is there a clue there? Is it possible that one or more externalities, manifested in Massachusetts in 2021, impacted the level of excess deaths? Is it possible that the mass administration of covid vaccines, which began at the start of 2021, is adding non-seasonal excess deaths? Could the aggressive inclusion of remdesivir in hospital treatment protocols, beginning at the end of October 2020, be adding non-seasonal excess deaths?

Notice the darker two cells in the 2021 Heat Map (high- lighted by asterisks) in Figure 13.4. I wanted to learn why those were relatively higher than the others around them. I thought that a detailed review of the individual records for the decedents in those two cells might reveal what is responsible for the anomalously high level of deaths in those cells.

I filtered the 2021 Death Certificate spreadsheet for ages 65– 74 and for the first (1st) half of September and the first (1st) half of October. I scanned down the Cause A column and noticed "PULMONARY EMBOLISM" and "CARDIOPULMONARY ARREST" many times in Cause A during those periods and in that age range. This piqued my interest in ICD-10 codes as an easy way to track and analyze specific causes of death. Thus began my work on ICD-10 code analyses.

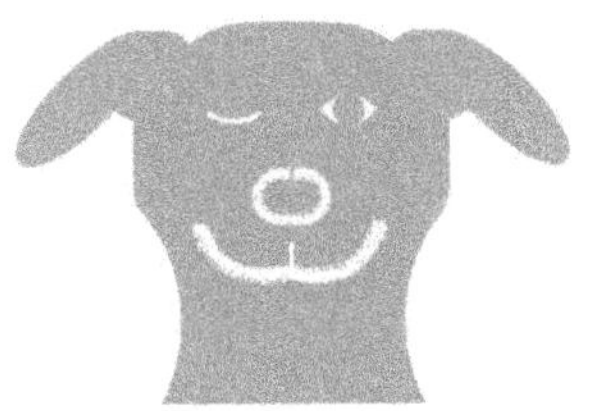

Chapter 14
ACP v Blood

ACP v Blood examines the differences in the causes of death during 2020 as compared to 2021 and 2022.

"*ACP*" means "All-Cause, Covid-19, and Pneumonia." The three individual components exhibit the same pattern going from the first covid year 2020 to the first covid vaccine year 2021. Thus, they are treated as a group. Figure 14.1 shows that *excess* deaths in each of these categories during 2021 declined by roughly 50% from their 2020 levels.

"*Blood*" is used in this chapter as a catchall for the deaths involving abnormalities in blood, blood forming organs, and problems with the blood transport system comprising the heart, veins, arteries, and capillaries. Figure 14.2 shows that in the transition from 2020 to 2021, instead of dropping in concert with the ACP causes, *Blood* causes of death increased substantially.

CHAPTER THESIS

If causes of death that are acute symptoms are patterned inversely to the disease as a cause of death, then it is likely something else besides the disease is causing those acute symptoms leading to death.

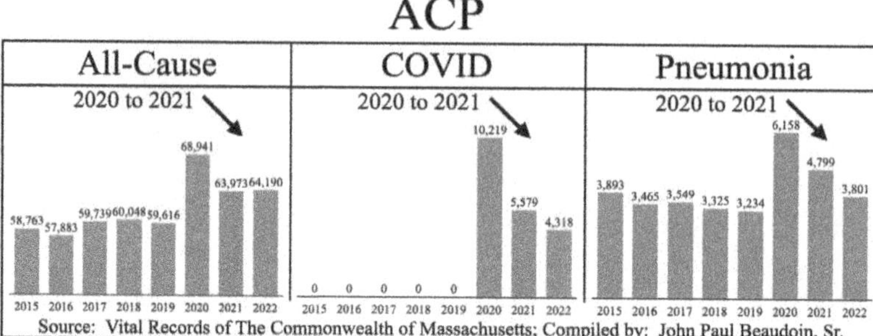

Figure 14.1

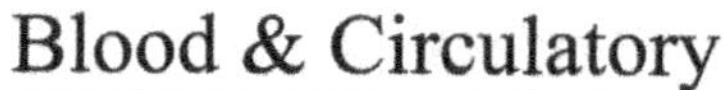

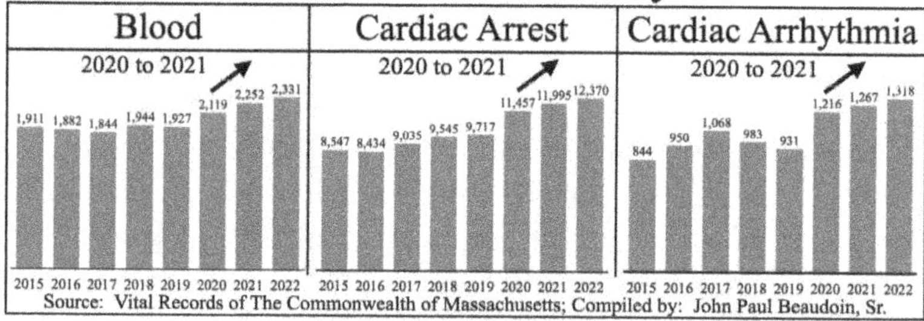

Figure 14.2

CALCULATION OF EXCESS & EXPECTED DEATHS

"*Excess* deaths" is a term that is widely used, but seldom explained in detail. Conceptually, it is simply "the number of deaths more than *normal*" or "the number of deaths more than *expected*." *Normal* and *expected* share a common meaning in this context.

Excess deaths are simply the difference between *actual* deaths and *expected* deaths. In this case, *actual* deaths are counted directly from the death certificates for the given time period. Only God knows the true number of "*normal*" deaths that should have occurred in a given year. Humans can only estimate that number. This estimation is calculated differently by different researchers. *Expected* deaths are estimated from the statistics derived from prior years. In this book, the *actual* numbers for years 2015 through 2019 are used as a basis for what is *normal*.

I'm very conservative in my choice of methods to calculate *expected* deaths because I abhor exaggeration and hyperbole when important issues are involved. Different calculation methods will result in different values for *expected* deaths. I am careful to always choose the method which yields the highest number for *expected* deaths which, in turn, will yield the lowest number for *excess* deaths.

General readers may skip the following section, which explains how *expected* is calculated for the analyses reported in this book. These details are included for the benefit of readers who are familiar with simple statistics.

Expected is estimated based on only five data points from the five baseline years, 2015–2019. Since population is continuously changing over time, total deaths for each year generally trend proportionally to the trend in population. To incorporate any such trends in my estimates for expected deaths, I use my spreadsheet SLOPE and INTERCEPT functions to build a TREND methodology, which calculates the best linear least-squares fit to the five baseline data points. If the TREND method determines that the trend in the baseline years for a particular cause of death has a negative slope, I use the simple average of the five baseline years, 2015–2019 instead of the trend. In such cases, the average will produce a higher estimate of normal deaths than the trend and a correspondingly lower number of *excess* deaths. This conservative approach minimizes the risk of overstating the number of *excess* deaths for that cause of death.

I do not use any outlier detection to exclude any of the base- line years. All five baseline points are always retained for the fit performed by the TREND method. As it happened, 2018 was a bad year for many causes of death. If outlier detection were applied to the baseline data for many of these causes of death, the data for 2018 would be excluded, the estimates for *expected* deaths would be lower, and the numbers for *excess* deaths would be correspondingly higher.

BEHAVIORS & PATTERNS

I began studying ICD-10 codes in order to track causes of death. Each ICD-10 code begins with a letter which corresponds to a general category of causes of death. For example:

- "J" for Respiratory system causes
- "I" for Circulatory system causes
- "D" for Blood and blood forming organs causes

The first codes I looked at represent pulmonary embolism. There are only two main codes for pulmonary embolism:

- I26.0 for "Pulmonary embolism with mention of acute cor pulmonale"
- I26.9 for "Pulmonary embolism without mention of acute cor pulmonale"

Note that "cor pulmonale" refers to enlargement and failure of the right ventricle, which would normally indicate a chronic condition.

2021 deaths involving I26.9 **increased** to 115% of the 2020 level, while 2021 deaths involving covid **decreased** to 55% of the 2020 level. This is an example of an inverse relationship.

Since pneumonia is supposed to accompany covid, I looked up all the pneumonia ICD-10 codes. That is when I noticed that medical examiners and physicians seem to rely on generic words in Parts I and II of death certificates. Generic words, without specificity, are often assigned ".9" codes by the CDC.

Most of the pneumonia-involved deaths were assigned the code J18.9 "Pneumonia, unspecified." Normally, death certifiers should specify if the pneumonia is viral, bacterial, or fungal, each of which has a subcategory ICD-10 code of its own. For example, bacterial pneumonia can be J15.2, "Pneumonia due to staphylococcus" or it can be J15.3, "Pneumonia due to streptococcus, group B" or another specific type. However, during the initial waves of the covid virus, it was recognized that many deaths were caused by an out of control immune reaction known as a cytokine storm. Accordingly, if the death certifier concluded that the pneumonia was caused by a cytokine storm rather than by a pathogen, then he would just write,

"PNEUMONIA," in Parts I or II, which would be assigned the code J18.9 "Pneumonia, unspecified."

While learning all of this, I noticed patterns in respiratory versus circulatory codes. To be exhaustive, I put together a spreadsheet using both AVERAGE and TREND methods. The spreadsheet showed a stark and crucial difference between 2020 and 2021. Each spreadsheet row held the results for a different code. I focused on "I" (circulatory) codes and "J" (respiratory) codes. Figure 14.3 depicts the results. The cells indicating the greater excess death percentages are highlighted.

ICD Code	ICD Description							2020 AVERAGE method Δ	2021 AVERAGE method Δ
Raw Data 2015	Raw Data 2016	Raw Data 2017	Raw Data 2018	Raw Data 2019	Raw Data 2020	Raw Data 2021	Part Yr Raw Data 2022	2020 TREND method Δ	2021 TREND method Δ
J12	Viral pneumonia, not elsewhere classified							3050.9%	890.6%
13	5	7	14	14	334	105	71	2302.9%	600.0%
J15	Bacterial pneumonia, not elsewhere classified							99.1%	98.5%
177	138	171	153	162	319	318	324	104.9%	106.2%
J18	Pneumonia, unspecified							72.4%	34.5%
4,044	3,587	3,665	3,413	3,295	6,209	4,843	3,840	100.3%	65.2%
J22	Unspecified acute lower respiratory infection							282.4%	(70.6%)
8	3	12	4	7	26	2	5	300.0%	(68.8%)
I26	Pulmonary embolism							27.5%	47.1%
709	645	709	688	732	888	1,025	986	22.8%	40.0%
I46	Cardiac arrest							25.9%	31.7%
8,738	8,596	9,200	9,669	9,848	11,593	12,131	12,535	13.7%	15.2%
I49	Other cardiac arrhythmias							24.6%	30.5%
1,169	1,265	1,401	1,329	1,319	1,616	1,692	1,730	15.0%	17.3%
I80	Phlebitis and thrombophlebitis							22.2%	41.0%
212	267	263	219	209	286	330	305	31.3%	55.4%

Figure 14.3

A clear change in the patterns is evident between 2020 and 2021. Respiratory "J" codes dominated 2020 as highlighted by the shaded stripe down through those cells. Circulatory "I" codes dominated the 2021 column as highlighted by the shaded stripe down through the cells.

The significance of the stark change in ***symptom spectrum profile*** cannot be overstated. Viruses do not change how they kill people on a year boundary. After all, they cannot plan to cause pneumonia deaths one year and then abruptly switch to cause pulmonary embolism and stroke deaths the next year. Something other than covid began killing people with circulatory system pathologies in 2021. There is no question about it.

As I created more sheets, formulae, and graphs, and explored for patterns involving additional ICD-10 codes, the ***symptom spectrum profile*** of *excess* death began to take shape.

Beginning in 2021, the causes of *excess* deaths comprised mostly the blood transport system (circulatory system), blood forming organs (marrow and lymph), the blood itself, and blood- related cancers (leukemia, bone marrow cancer, lymph node cancer, acute promyelocytic leukemia).

I created more than 1,000 graphs of causes of death. Only a few examples were selected for this book to illustrate certain theories, patterns, and evidence.

ALL-CAUSE DEATHS

"All-Cause" is the most important data set because it is the one category that is not readily amenable to fraudulent manipulation. Either people died or they did not die.

Death certificates exist for actual people. Their records include family members, the death certifier, the funeral director, and the burial location or cremation. The number cannot be padded with fake deaths unless all the people in each record are in on the scam; and that would be darned near impossible.

Specific causes can be manipulated by changes in policy on short notice. But All-Cause deaths actually happened.

Figure 14.4 depicts the first All-Cause graph.

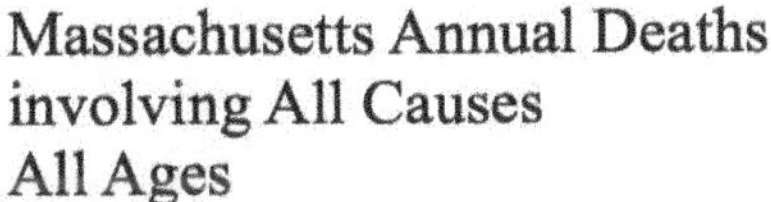

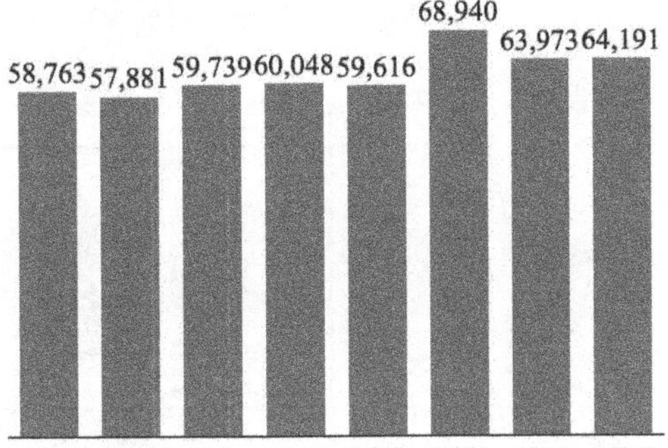

Year	Excess	Excess % over Expected
2020	8,569	14.2%
2021	3,214	5.3%
2022	3,045	5.0%

Figure 14.4

All-Cause deaths were up 14.2% over the *expected* value in 2020, 5.3% in 2021, and 5.0% in 2022.

The boundary between 2020 and 2021 is important because it is also the boundary between the covid year without any covid vaccines and the years when covid vaccines were widely administered.

Governments and covid vaccine proponents claim that the covid vaccine is effective because *excess* deaths declined year over year from 2020 to 2021.

However, if the covid vaccine worked as claimed, All-Cause deaths should have returned to near baseline in 2021, and fully to baseline or below in 2022. Accordingly, *excess* All-Cause deaths should have returned to near zero in 2021, instead of remaining elevated with an excess of 3,214. By 2022, *excess* All-Cause deaths should have returned to zero or below zero instead of remaining high at 3,045.

Examining All-Cause deaths within age groups in Figure 14.5 might provide more insight into the transition from 2020 to 2021.

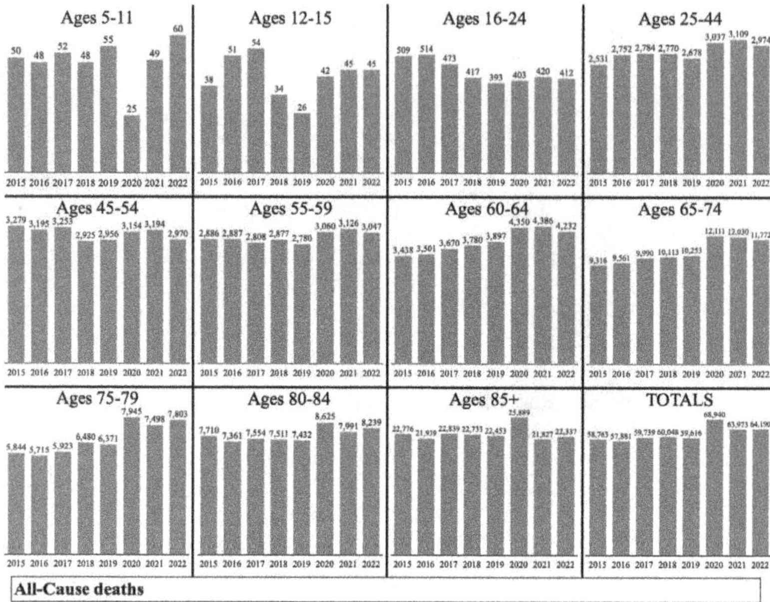

Data Source: VITAL Records of The Commonwealth of Massachusetts dated April 2023
Compiled by: John Paul Beaudoin, Sr.

Figure 14.5

Every age group from ages 5 through 64 shows an increase of All-Cause deaths from 2020 to 2021. *Excess* deaths for ages 65–74 look almost equal in 2020 and 2021. *Excess* deaths for every age group above age 74 decreased from 2020 to 2021.

Those who claim that the covid vaccine is effective cannot explain why everyone under age 65 died in greater numbers in 2021 than in 2020. Those over age 84 who were unhealthy and fragile would be expected to die from covid in higher numbers during 2020. Since those unhealthy and vulnerable elderly could not die twice, it would be expected that that age group would have fewer deaths from all causes in 2021 irrespective of vaccine effectiveness. If covid vaccines worked as claimed, then why did more people under age 65 die in 2021 than in 2020? There is only one thing that changed in 2021, which could be responsible for this significant increase in these deaths—widespread administration of the covid vaccines. This evidence of the lethality of the covid vaccines is unambiguous and irrefutable.

Semi-monthly plots of deaths for the years 2015 through 2022 provide additional insights. Figure 14.6 includes two graphs. The upper graph comprises semi-monthly plots of the cumulative deaths across each year. The lower graph shows running plots of deaths for each semi-monthly period. A mathematician would recognize the lower plots as the first derivatives of the upper plots for the corresponding years.

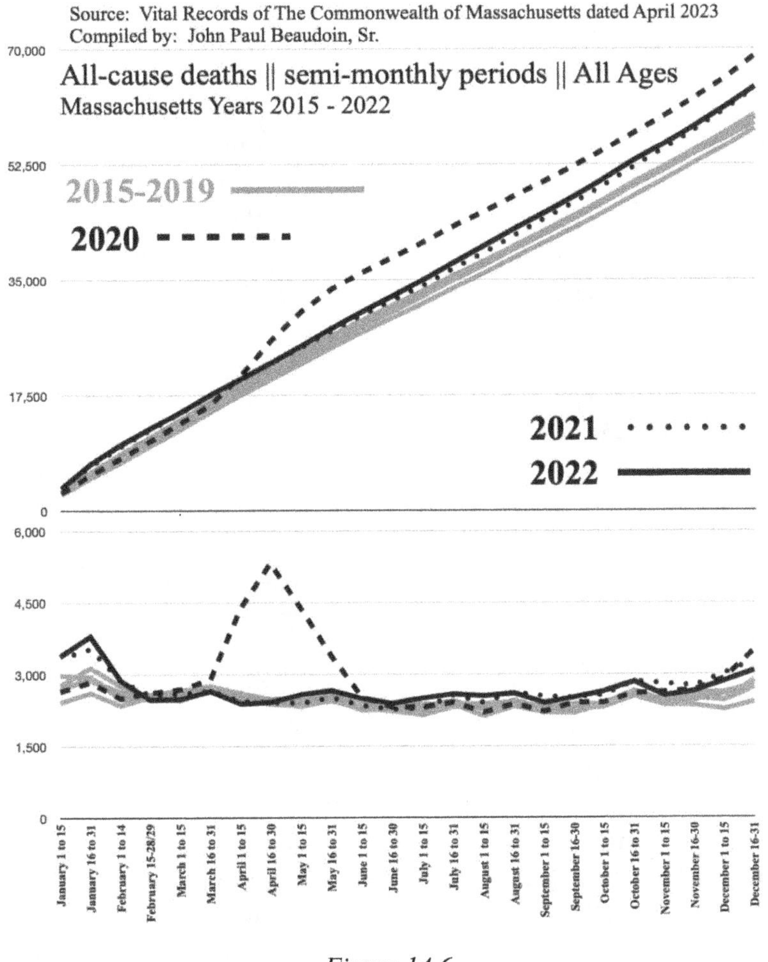

Figure 14.6

Excess deaths for 2020 through 2022 are clearly visible wherever the plots for those years lie above the gray band, which comprises plots for the baseline years 2015 through 2019. The first wave of excess deaths during spring 2020 jumps right off the page. Whether the direct action of the virus, or the extraordinary government policies imposed in response to the emerging epidemic, or a combination of these two factors were responsible for these excess deaths, it is clear that something significant occurred from mid-March to mid-June 2020.

In these line graphs, the slopes of the plots in the upper graph are important. In the upper graph, notice that the slope of the 2020 plot increases during the big spring peak shown in the lower graph. Only during the mid-March to mid-June wave in the lower graph does the gap open between the 2020 plot and the plots for baseline years 2015–2019.

The lower plot clearly shows that after that first wave in 2020 ended, deaths returned to the *expected* level indicated by the gray band comprising the baseline years. The upper graph shows that the 2020 plot and band of plots for the baseline years track in parallel after the peak. In other words, from June through December, the slopes for all the baseline years are about the same as the slope of the 2020 plot. When the slopes are roughly equal, it means that an equal number of people died each day across the respective years. Clearly, there is no sign of a covid epidemic during the summer of 2020. The lower graph's plots confirm that there are no *excess* deaths during that period. This halt to the epidemic cannot be due to effective covid vaccines because they had not yet been deployed for mass administration to the public. Clearly, covid exhibited the classic behavior of a ***seasonal*** respiratory illness. To claim covid is not seasonal would require ignorance of the actual data.

To be clear, after the first wave killed many elderly people during the spring of 2020, the covid epidemic was over. The normal, greatly diminished second wave over the winter of 2020/2021 in no way comports with the concept of an epidemic. The epidemic had ended by June 2020 and general immunity had been established long before the vaccines were administered to anyone in the general population.

The covid vaccines did not save any lives in 2020 because they had not yet been administered. There is no evidence that covid vaccines saved anyone in 2021 since deaths among everyone younger than 65 were higher in 2021 than in 2020 and the elderly who had not succumbed to covid in 2020 continued to die at elevated rates in 2021 compared to the baseline years. The covid vaccines did not protect anyone from the factor or factors that were responsible for the continued excess deaths during 2021. The semi-monthly waveform plots by age group shown in Figure 14.7 provide more insight.

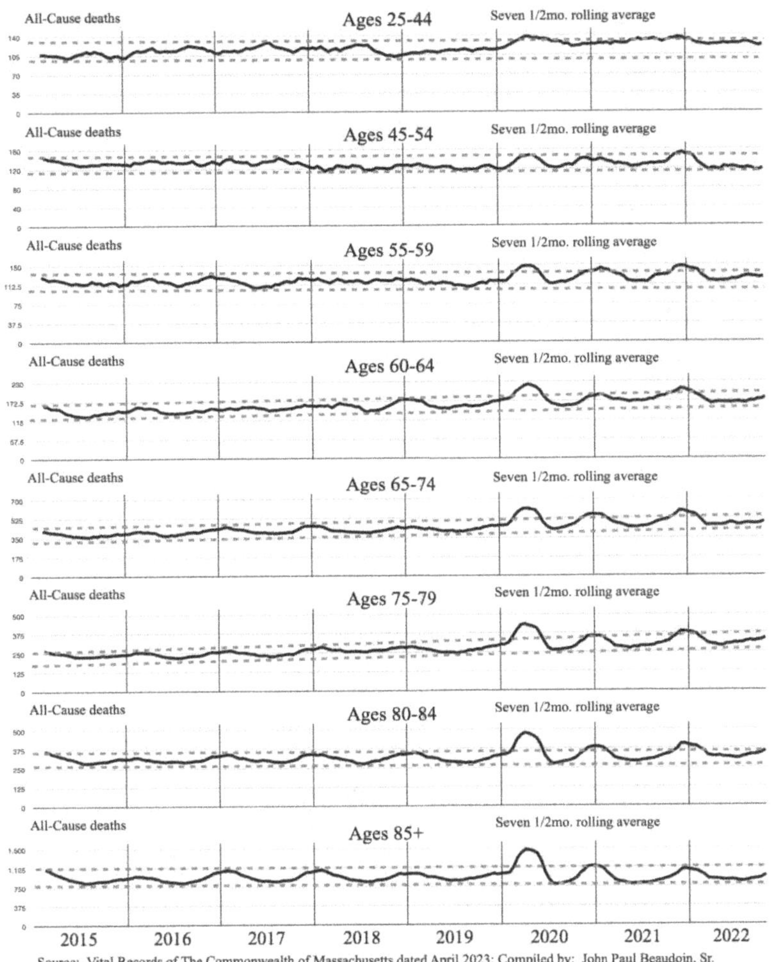

Figure 14.7

The northeast United States' normal seasonal pattern of deaths is clearly evident in the undulating traces for the older age groups in the baseline years 2015–2019. The amplitudes of the seasonal peaks in the baseline years are more pronounced in the plots as age increases.

In 2020, the late season emergence of the March to June seasonal peak is evident. Smaller seasonal peaks return during the subsequent two winters 2020/2021 and 2021/2022. However, in addition to the classical seasonal peaks evident in the younger age groups, the plots exhibit an additional signal which is absent from the baseline years. This additional signal will be discussed in detail later in this book.

Notice the slopes of the "guard rails" indicated by the dashed gray lines. Call them "peak" and "trough" guard rails. The guard rails indicate the maximum and minimum extents of seasonal peaks and troughs during the baseline years. During the summers of 2021 and 2022 the seasonal peaks do not return to the expected values which the guard rails indicate. This means that excess people were dying every day, even in the summer, from something that is not seasonal.

Clearly something did kill many elderly people during the first wave in spring 2020. This first wave followed the nominal behavior of a contagious respiratory epidemic.

COVID-19 DEATHS

Beginning April 1, 2020, two new ICD-10 codes were activated for covid:

- U07.1 COVID-19, virus identified
- U07.2 COVID-19, virus not identified

Essentially 100% of the Massachusetts death certificates received by the CDC after April 1, 2020, which specify covid in Parts I or II, was assigned the U07.1 code by the CDC. This includes certificates for deaths that occurred in March and were received and coded by the CDC after April 1. This chapter does not consider the U07.2 code because it has gone unused and there are effectively zero death certificates that were assigned this code.

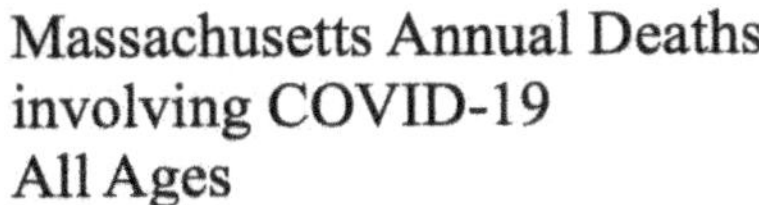

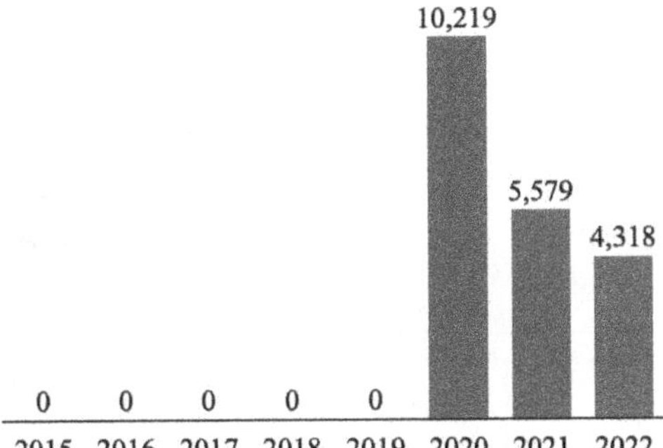

Source: Massachusetts Department of Health, Office of Vital Records
Compiled by: John Paul Beaudoin, Sr. || Data Received April 2023

Year	Excess	Excess % over Expected
2020	10,219	
2021	5,579	
2022	4,318	

Figure 14.8

Figure 14.8 shows the total number of Massachusetts death certificates assigned the U07.1 code by the CDC. Note that the baseline years all show exactly zero deaths since they precede the emergence of the disease. That means that the *expected* deaths for the years 2020 through 2022 is exactly zero. Therefore, all covid deaths are *excess* covid deaths. Also, it is not possible to calculate values for % Δ from *expected.*

In Figure 14.8, first notice that COVID-19 deaths in 2021 dropped to 55% of the 2020 level much like *excess* All-Cause deaths for 2021, which dropped to 18% of the 2020 level. Both categories exhibit the same general pattern.

Figure 14.9a shows that there were 14,794 total *excess* All- cause deaths over years 2020–2022. Yet there are purportedly 20,116 covid deaths over the same period. If covid is a deadly epidemic responsible for an anomalous number of additional deaths of otherwise healthy people, how could there be 5,323 more covid deaths than *excess* deaths?

Figure 14.9b shows a plot of the semi-monthly All-Cause *excess* deaths together with a plot of the semi-monthly covid deaths. This provides some insights about the reason for the discrepancy of covid deaths exceeding All-Cause *excess* deaths.

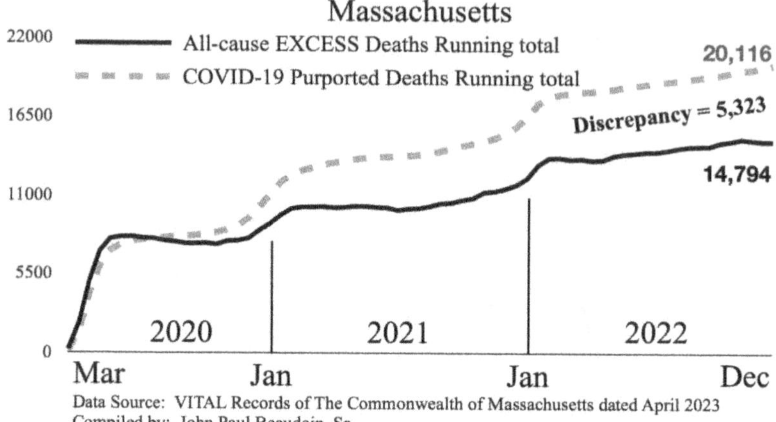

Figure 14.9a

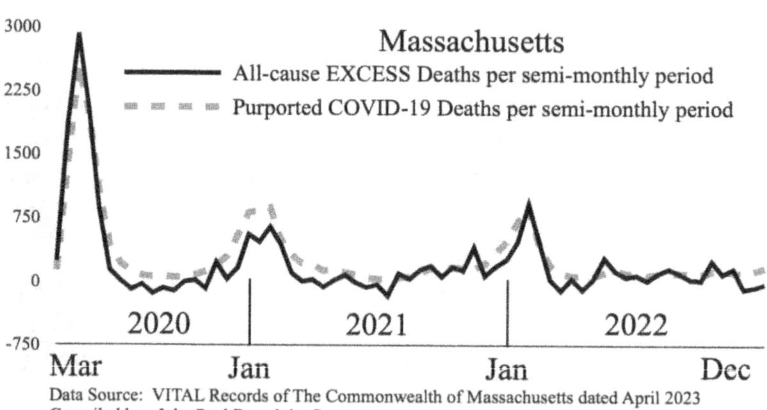

Figure 14.9b

The plots of *excess* deaths (solid lines) in Figures 14.9a and 14.9b clearly show the classic behavior of a seasonal infectious respiratory virus. The first wave emerged in March 2020. All-Cause *excess* deaths rose sharply to a peak in April at which time they declined as sharply, returning to the baseline value (slightly below zero *excess* deaths) by June. By every measure and definition, the covid epidemic was over in June 2020. As would be expected, the plot for covid deaths (dashed gray line) closely tracks *excess* deaths from the onset of covid in March 2020 through early May 2020.

Note that beginning mid-May 2020, the plot of covid deaths begins exceeding the plot of *excess* deaths. This is highly likely the result of two factors: 1) The elderly and infirm, who would contribute to the baseline of *expected* deaths irrespective of covid, were diagnosed with covid at or near the time of their deaths. *Id est*, their deaths are counted as covid deaths, but they do not contribute to the tally of *excess* deaths because they died in the normal course of the human life cycle "with" covid rather than "from" covid; or 2) they get counted as covid deaths due to a false positive covid test or erroneous misinformation on the death certificate, whether intentional or unintentional. Similarly, these deaths are counted as covid deaths, but they do not contribute to the tally of *excess* deaths because they occurred in the normal course of the human life cycle.

As will be explored more in Chapter 18, the average age of covid deaths in Massachusetts in 2020 is 81.3. The average age of deaths in 2015–2019 ranged from 75.3 to 75.8—a tight distribution. Thus, the average age of covid deaths is nearly 6 years higher than the baseline average age of deaths in 2015–2019. Figures 14.9a and 14.9b clearly show that most of the *excess* deaths in 2020 occurred in March through June, which is consistent with the prior explanations of overcounting beginning in that time.

The CARES Act was signed into law on March 27, 2020.[1] The CARES Act incentives began implementation in April and May of 2020. Those incentives include monetary bonuses for hospitals that reported covid deaths. This incentive and others are solicitations and behavior modifications. The greater the monetary incentive to the hospital and doctors, the greater the number of non-covid-caused deaths that will be labeled as covid deaths. It worked as designed. The taxpayers' money was transferred to hospitals, pharmaceutical companies, and doctors, mostly in Massachusetts, New Jersey, and New York during the first year of covid.

A much weaker second wave of covid is evident over the winter of 2020/2021. This is also consistent with the classic behavior of a seasonal infectious respiratory virus. The significant overcounting of covid deaths continues to be evident all the way through mid-2021. Is covid overcounting due to hypersensitivity from covid panic, fueled by the unprecedented declaration of a state of emergency, over a fairly routine viral outbreak, magnified by powerful government financial incentives to attribute deaths to covid? This question begs for speculation.

A third wave of covid is evident over the winter of 2021/2022. However, this wave shows some divergence from the classic behavior of a seasonal infectious respiratory virus. Normally, a third wave is expected to be weaker than a second wave, but in this case, it is approximately equal to the second wave. Note that overcounting of covid deaths reemerges during the third wave.

There is another significant anomalous behavior visible in Figure 14.9b. Note that the plot for All-Cause *excess* deaths does not return to the baseline level of zero after June in 2021 and continues at an elevated level during 2022. This anomalous behavior is also evident in Figure 14.7. It is an alarming and clear indication that something non-seasonal is causing a significant number of *excess* deaths.

Even though the plots of covid deaths and All-Cause *excess* deaths converge during July through November 2021 and through much of 2022, this does not indicate that these additional non-seasonal *excess* deaths are related to some sort of non-seasonal behavior of covid. To the contrary, this would require sudden, discontinuous changes in the rate of overcounting of covid deaths. There is nothing which would account for such a strange, intermittent change in covid overcounting rates. The remainder of this book will present unambiguous evidence that this non-seasonal increase in *excess* deaths is not due to covid, but is instead the result of the fatal effects of covid vaccines.

Figure 14.10 shows the COVID-19 line graphs to be nearly identical in shape to the ideal Gompertz function shown in Figure 14.11. The Gompertz growth function is used in disease and superspreader modeling.[2]

Source: Vital Records of The Commonwealth of Massachusetts dated April 2023
Compiled by: John Paul Beaudoin, Sr.
U07.1 COVID-19 involved deaths || semi-monthly periods || All Ages
Massachusetts Years 2015 - 2022
2015-2019
2020
2021
2022
12,000
9,000
6,000
3,000
0
3,000
2,250
1,500
750
0
January 1 to 15
January 16 to 31
February 1 to 14
February 15-28/29
March 1 to 15
March 16 to 31
April 1 to 15
April 16 to 30
May 1 to 15
May 16 to 31
June 1 to 15
June 16 to 30
July 1 to 15
July 16 to 31
August 1 to 15
August 16 to 31
September 1 to 15
September 16-30
October 1 to 15
October 16 to 31
November 1 to 15
November 16-30
December 1 to 15
December 16-31

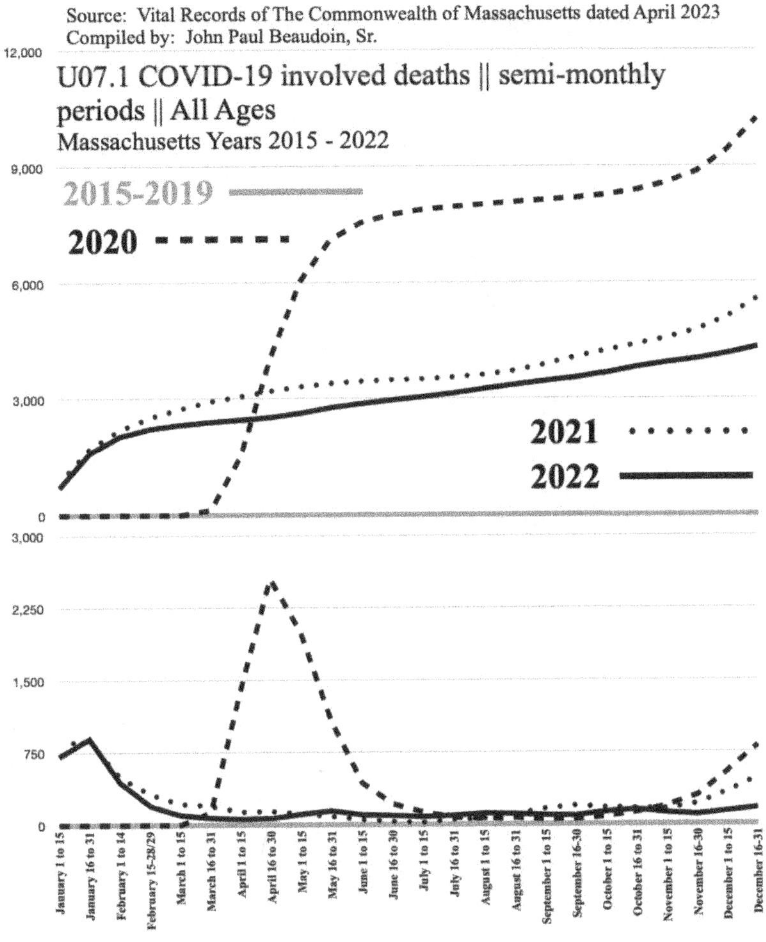

Figure 14.10

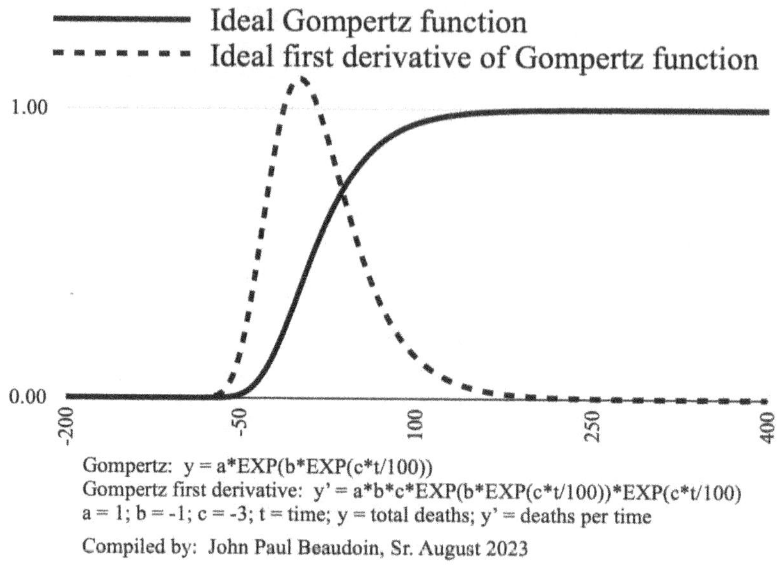

Figure 14.11

COVID-19-involved deaths in 2020 make a nearly ideal Gompertz curve and its first derivative in time. The first wave is stark. The second wave begins at the end of the year and continues until February of 2021. There is a third wave in the winter of 2021/2022.

Notice the slopes of the lines in the upper graph. The 2020 line is nearly flat all summer long, almost ideal, and then begins to bend up again in November.

However, the 2021 and 2022 graphs never flatten out. They remain at a pronounced positive slope all summer long. In fact, 2022, beginning in March, depicts a nearly straight upward line through to the end of the year. That means there is no seasonality and the same number of purported covid-involved deaths are occurring in May and August as in November.

A quick look at age groups in Figure 4.12 will explain who is purportedly dying from covid.

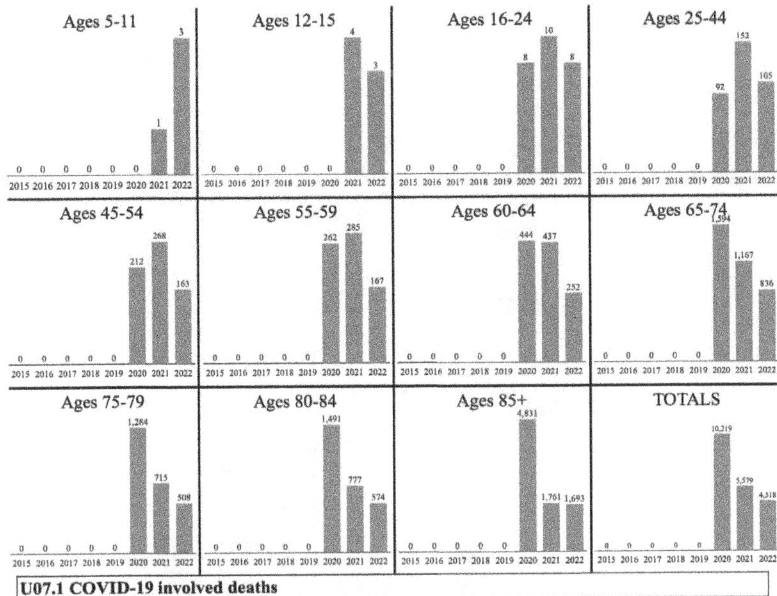

Figure 14.12

From ages 5 through 59, more people died from covid-involved deaths in 2021 than in 2020. Above age 64, fewer people died from covid-involved deaths in 2021 than in 2020.

For All-Cause deaths, the pattern is the same. From ages 5 through 59, more people died from All-Cause deaths in 2021 than in 2020. Above age 64, fewer people died from All-Cause deaths in 2021 than in 2020.

The behavior of the first wave in 2020 is indirect evidence that people did die from covid because the patterns of All-Cause and COVID-19 are similar. One can logically attribute the *excess* deaths in the first wave to a disease, whether the deaths were caused by the disease *per se* or by improper treatment of those who fell ill with the disease. The *excess* thereafter bears scrutiny against disease patterns. Summer deaths in 2021 do not fit the pattern established in 2020.

After the first wave of deaths concludes in June 2020, the pattern of deaths deviates from that of a seasonal respiratory virus. In order to further explore the deviations, consider deaths involving a specific cause related covid.

J18.9 PNEUMONIA DEATHS

The most frequently recorded pneumonia ICD-10 code J18.9, "Pneumonia, unspecified," is examined next. Figure 4.13 presents Massachusetts J18.9 deaths for 2015 through 2022.

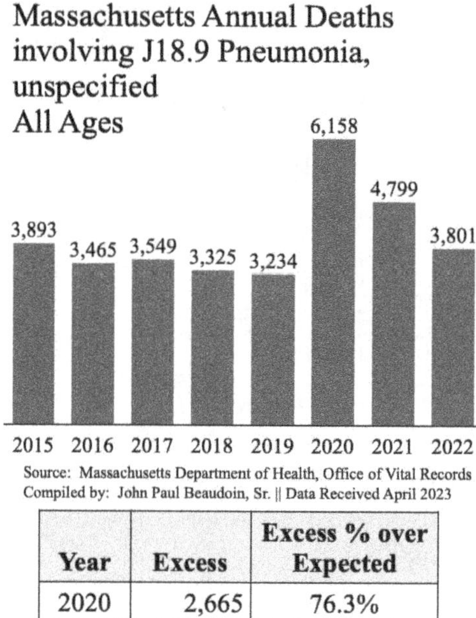

Year	Excess	Excess % over Expected
2020	2,665	76.3%
2021	1,306	37.4%
2022	308	8.8%

Figure 14.13

J18.9 "Pneumonia, unspecified" follows the same pattern as covid deaths. 2021 *excess* deaths involving J18.9 decreased to 49% of the 2020 *excess* level, while 2022 J18.9 *excess* deaths decreased to 11.5% of the 2020 *excess* level. This is similar to covid deaths, but not to All-Cause deaths. This is important to note. Covid and pneumonia are much lower from 2021–2022, but All-Cause is not that much lower.

The semi-monthly plots of *excess* pneumonia deaths shown in Figure 14.14 also exhibit behaviors similar to the corresponding plots for covid deaths and All-Cause deaths.

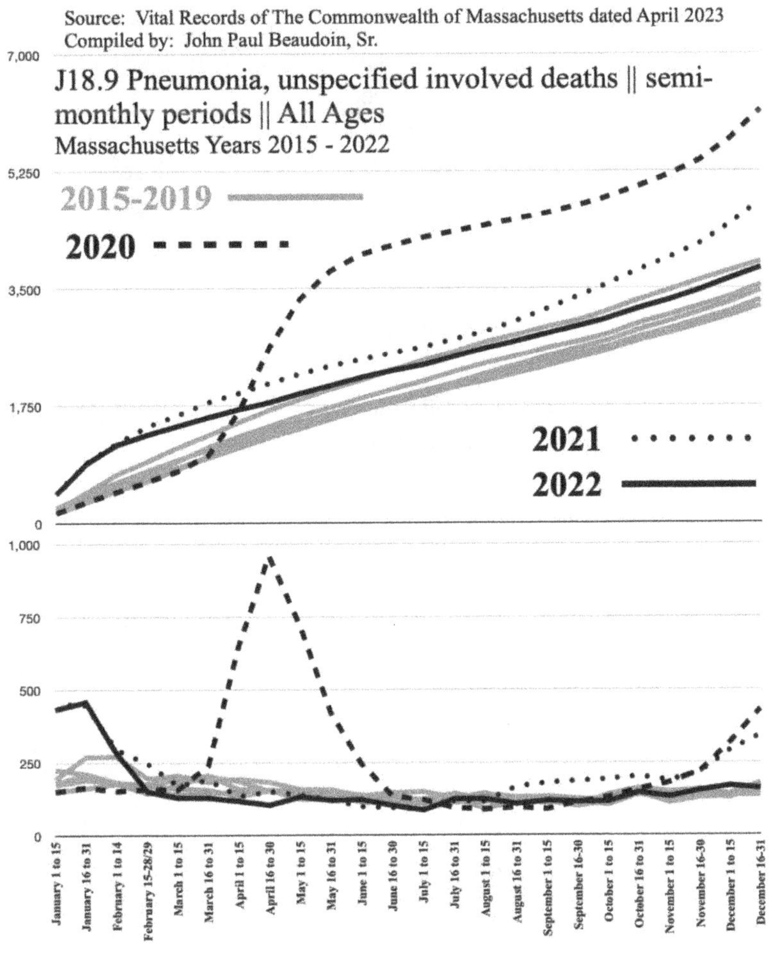

Figure 14.14

The plot for 2021 shown in the lower panel of Figure 14.14 shows a significant anomaly from August through October. There is a significant elevation of pneumonia deaths occurring unseasonably during those months. Even year 2020, with its high covid death counts, does not show the elevation in pneumonia deaths seen in 2021. The death certificates show that pneumonia accompanies kidney failure as well as various respiratory ailments.

The emergence of a third wave of pneumonia deaths in November 2021 is consistent with the expected behavior of a *seasonal* respiratory illness.

There are two main points to understand. 1) The pneumonia graph is similar to both covid and All-Cause graphs in the major rises and falls from

2020 to 2021. 2) A half year into the covid vaccination campaign of 2021, several months after the great majority of people had already received two doses, an increased number of people were dying from pneumonia unseasonably in the summertime and early fall.

Figure 14.15 shows how these deaths were distributed among age groups.

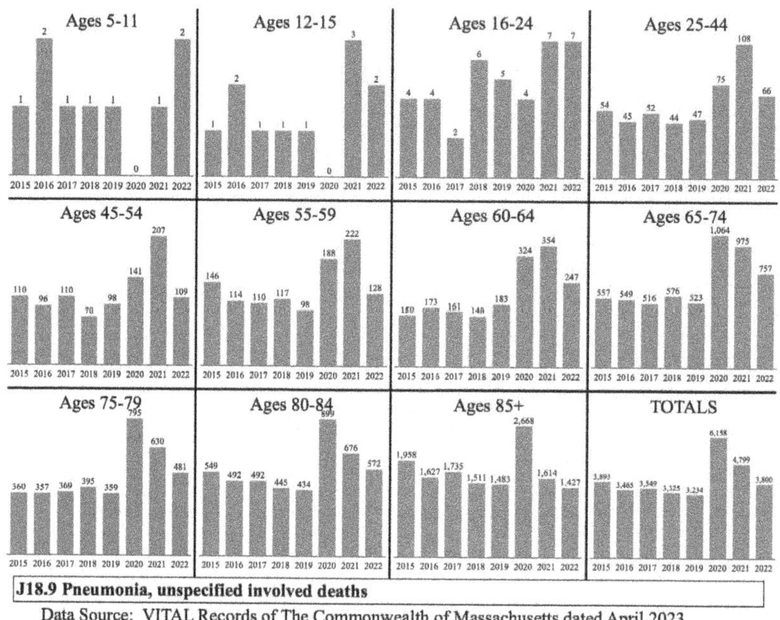

Figure 14.15

Figure 14.15 shows that in ages 5 through 64, more people died from pneumonia-involved deaths in 2021 than in 2020. Above age 64, fewer people died from pneumonia-involved deaths in 2021 than in 2020.

The same behavior is displayed by All-Cause and covid-involved deaths. This makes three death categories which display the same pattern.

If the vaccine is effective, then why did more younger people die from pneumonia in 2021? Fewer deaths among older people were expected because so many fragile elderly were killed during the large first wave in spring 2020. Recall the Heat Map in Figure 14.2 that shows how the first wave culled the elderly population.

Some may assume that a high number of younger people would have died with pneumonia during January and February 2021 because they were not yet eligible to be vaccinated. The line plots in Figure 14.16 for ages 25 through 44 clearly contradict that assumption. Not only is the second wave for that age group much lower than the first wave, the 2021 summer trough also never returned to baseline. There is an unseasonal summer signal of *excess* pneumonia deaths there. This is completely inconsistent with the *seasonal* behavior of an infectious respiratory disease.

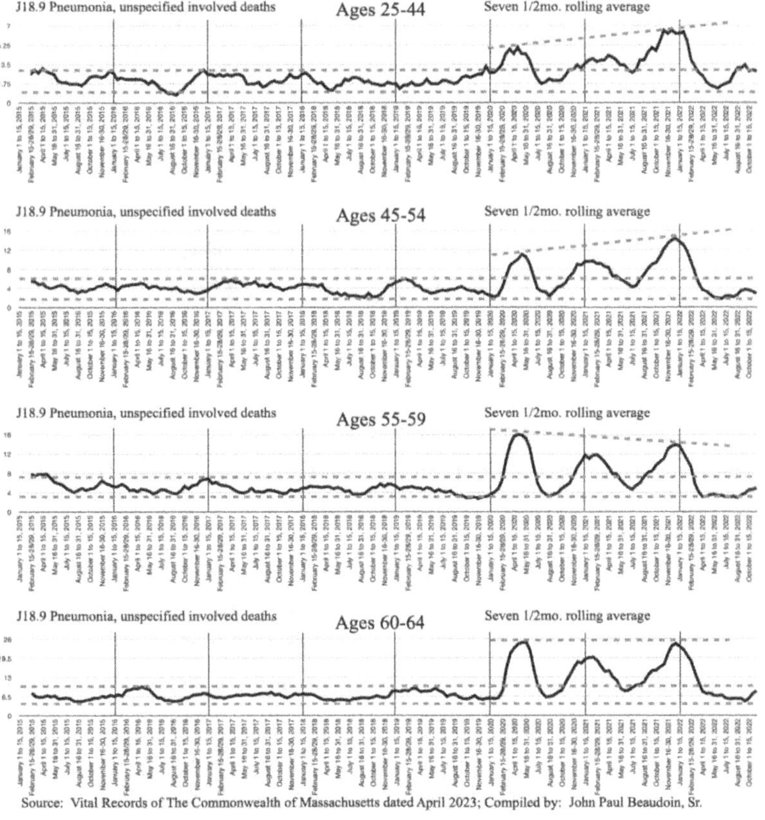

Figure 14.16

Also note that for ages 25 to 54, the covid era third wave of pneumonia is worse than the first wave. Normal *seasonal* behavior of an infectious respiratory disease exhibits a steady decrease in mortality during each subsequent wave. The line plots for ages 55 through 64 exhibit the normal diminishing patterns. In engineering terms, the waves in the line plots for the older ages exhibit damped harmonic behavior. The line plots for ages 25 through 54 indicate an unstable, out-of-control system with an induced externality adding energy to a system of chaos and death.

The *excess* begins in the summer of 2021 where the trough fails to return to the *expected* natural baseline. Thereafter, the waveform takes off even higher during the winter of 2021/2022. Something other than *seasonal* covid is causing a significant *excess* number of unseasonal pneumonia deaths a full year after the first wave of covid at a time when nearly everyone had already encountered the covid virus. In other words, the *excess* unseasonable pneumonia deaths during 2021 were caused by something other than covid.

SIDEBAR - COMBINATIONS

When working with Record Level Source Data (RLSD) such as death certificates, it is possible to explore relationships among combinations of factors. This alone is sufficient reason for researchers to demand RLSD data from governments.

Exploring relationships among factors can reveal additional aspects of the underlying truths embodied in the data. For example, consider how many of the U07.1 COVID-19-involved deaths also involved J18.9 Pneumonia, unspecified. With RLSD, it is an easy calculation. The pattern is very interesting, and very telling.

In 2020, 2021, 2022, there were 10219, 5579, 4318 U07.1 covid-involved deaths, 6158, 4799, 3801 J18.9 pneumonia-involved deaths, and 3176, 2491, 1405 deaths involving both codes, respectively.

The percentages of covid decedents who also had J18.9 pneumonia in 2020–2022 are 31.1%, 44.6%, 32.5%.

The percentages of J18.9 pneumonia decedents who also had covid in 2020–2022 are 51.6%, 51.9%, 37.0%.

Covid deaths as a percentage of All-Cause deaths each year 2020–2022 are 14.82%, 8.72%, 6.73%.

J18.9 pneumonia deaths as a percentage of All-Cause deaths each year 2020–2022 are 8.93%, 7.50%, 5.92%.

Both covid and J18.9 pneumonia-involved deaths as a percentage of All-Cause each year are 4.61%, 3.89%, 2.19%.

Using a computer spreadsheet with RLSD, it is easy to explore any combination or combinations of factors. I created generators that allow me to specify any combinations of codes and see the results in seconds.

Please be aware that one "ordinary" man who is not a professional software engineer created this system in a few weeks and it appears to be far better than anything that any federal or state government agency provides to The People. The CDC and state health departments employ a total of approximately a quarter of a million people in the United States. Why do we fund them if they do not openly provide "We The People" with useful information?

Earlier in this book, it was mentioned that governments hoard data and provide little utility from it. These combinations are an example of what I meant. Scientists and doctors the world over seem to unquestioningly accept the limited bundles of data they are given by governments. Governments tell citizens and researchers that RLSD is private, and the requestors walk away accepting that response from governments. The data belongs to The People, and anything less than transparency of every possible data point is not acceptable. Where appropriate, the legitimate privacy interests of individuals can be respected with routine procedures to de-identify the data. It reeks nefariously when governments improperly hoard and conceal data. It is even more problematic that people accept government malfeasance without complaint.

The most startling pattern in the relationships above is that more than fifty percent of J18.9 deaths also had covid in 2020 and 2021, but then it dropped to 37.0% in 2022. That should be very concerning to anyone who believes that people are actually dying from covid en masse. How can a disease just change how it kills?

I26.9 PULMONARY EMBOLISM DEATHS

Recall that there are two ICD-10 codes for pulmonary embolism (PE):

I26.0 represents "Pulmonary embolism with mention of acute cor pulmonale"

I26.9 represents "Pulmonary embolism without mention of acute cor pulmonale"

The I26.0 dataset for years 2015–2022 is {3, 4, 2, 2, 2, 3, 1, 2}. Since the numbers are so small, there is no point in looking at the I26.0 code.

Those death certificates that do not mention acute cor pulmonale do not mean that acute cor pulmonale did not present. It merely means that it was not mentioned on the death certificate.

Figure 14.17 shows the total number of annual PE deaths for I26.9 for "Pulmonary embolism without mention of acute cor pulmonale" for 2015–2022 together with the *excess* number of PE deaths for 2020–2022.

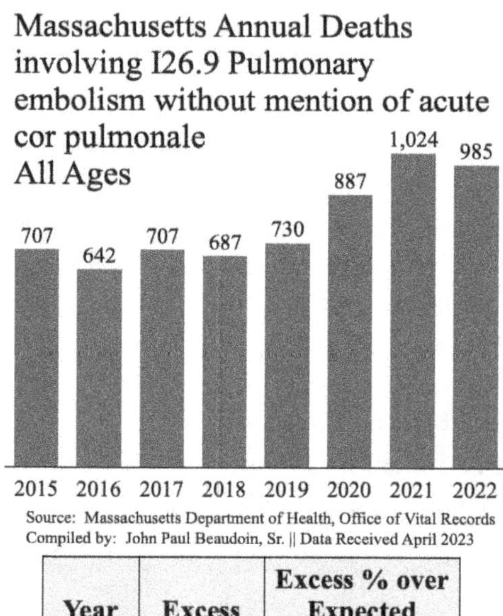

Year	Excess	Excess % over Expected
2020	165	22.9%
2021	293	40.1%
2022	245	33.1%

Figure 14.17

Note that *excess* PE-involved deaths increased significantly, 78%, from 2020 to 2021. In contrast, *excess* All-Cause deaths decreased 63% and covid deaths decreased 45% from 2020 to 2021. Clearly, something killed many more people by clots in their lungs (PEs) in 2021 compared to 2020.

In 2021 and 2022, each of the 538 *excess* PE-involved deaths was a real human being who had families and friends. The percentages of *excess* PE-involved deaths above the expected level are 40.1% in 2021 and 33.1% in 2022. Many more covid vaccines were administered in 2021 than in 2022. PE is known to be a short-term acute response to covid vaccines.

Thus, it is expected that PEs would drop along with covid vaccine uptake from 2021 to 2022.

Data, as of December 31, 2021, from the Massachusetts DPH, shows that "Grand Total Doses Administered" was 12,751,822.[3]

Data, as of December 26, 2022, from the Massachusetts DPH, shows that "Total Doses Administered" was 17,332,868.[4]

Nearly 13 million doses of covid vaccine were administered in Massachusetts in 2021 compared to about 4.6 million covid vaccine doses administered in 2022 in Massachusetts. The general correlation between vaccine administration and PE-involved deaths is not conclusive proof that the vaccinations are causing these deaths, but it is persuasive evidence. Moreover, the fact that the 2022 PE-involved deaths barely declined in proportion to the sharp decline in vaccinations suggests that the risk of PE-involved death may increase cumulatively with each additional booster. Rather than speculate on the potential cause-effect relationship, please simply understand the numbers submitted and the possible causation in acute, mid-term, and long-term adverse effects.

Some will point to 2020 being higher than baseline years 2015–2019. However, the 2020 *excess* PE-involved deaths are only 1.9% of the massive *excess* All-Cause deaths in 2020. In 2021, *excess* PE-involved deaths climb to 9.1% of 2021 *excess* All-Cause deaths. In 2022, *excess* PE-involved deaths remained similar to 2021 at 8.0% of 2022 *excess* All-Cause deaths. If PE were caused by covid, then I26.9 PE should have gone down with ACP in 2021 and 2022. The PE-involved deaths trend is notably inversely related to the ACP trend. Covid cannot have caused the massive increase in PE-involved deaths in 2021 and 2022. Some other factor or factors must be responsible for these excess deaths.

The semi-monthly plots in Figure 14.18 show when the *excess* PE-involved deaths occurred.

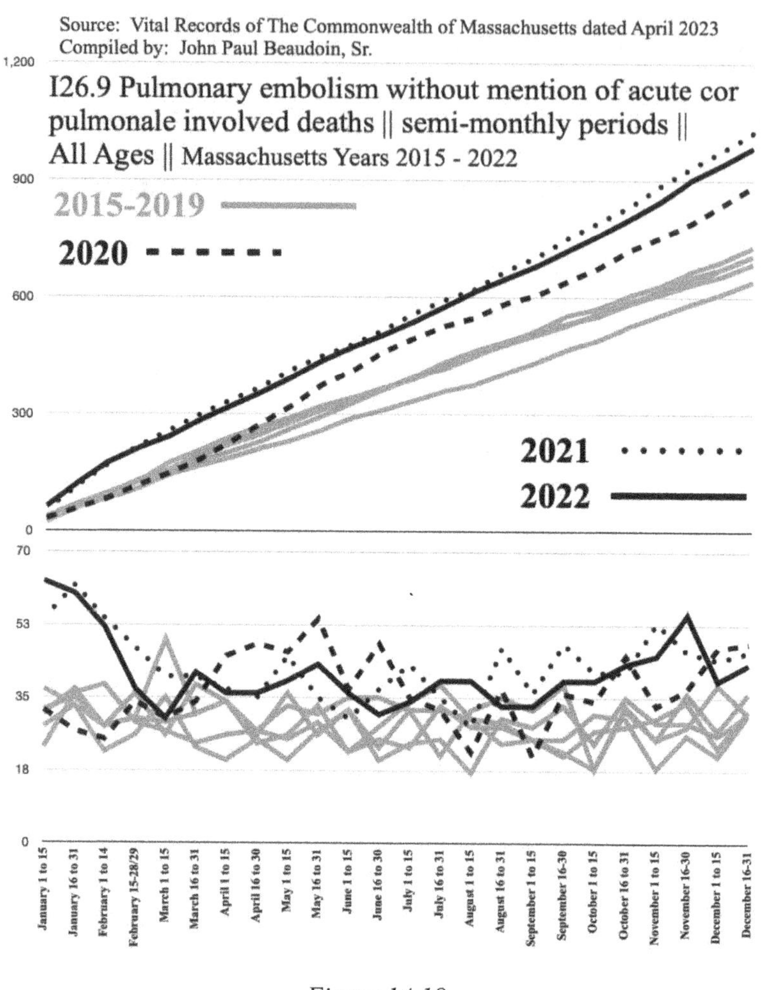

Figure 14.18

Figure 14.18 clearly shows that 2020 *excess* PE deaths began during the 2020 first wave in mid-March but continued to occur for a few weeks after the first wave ended in May. PE-involved deaths returned to the baseline in July and remained there until October, at the beginning of the seasonal second wave. The slope of the 2020 dashed line plot in the upper graph clearly separates from baseline 2015–2019 years during the spring. And then, the 2020 PE-involved deaths slope runs parallel to the baseline years 2015–2019 until beginning to edge up in October. In other words, 2020 PE *excess* generally tracked with ACP. The 2020 PE *excess* is *seasonal* and could be solely related to infection with covid or government protocols in response to covid. The age groupings will give us more insight into who died.

While 2020 PE-involved deaths were *seasonal*, the pattern changed beginning in 2021. In addition to peaking in sync with the second *seasonal* covid wave during winter 2020/2021, PE-involved deaths remained in *excess* during the summer and into the fall when they increased again in sync with the third covid wave during winter 2021/2022. It is clear that there is something unrelated to covid which is contributing additional *excess* PE-involved deaths all year long.

Please consider, in deciphering these graphs, that more than one thing can be contributing to the *excess* PE deaths. Covid could be responsible for triggering some of the PE and government interventions could have caused as many or more deaths as covid did. The public was subjected to extraordinary interventions, including lockdowns, masks, vaccines, remdesivir, early treatment protocols (or suppression of early treatment), withholding of antibiotics, and many more externalities other than covid.

If covid alone were solely responsible for *excess* PE-involved deaths in 2021, then why did PE deaths increase when ACP declined? Viruses do not change how they kill on a year boundary. There is no question that other externalities were in play in Massachusetts during 2021 and 2022.

Figure 14.19 showing age groups adds more clarity. Recall that ACP deaths are patterned 'younger up' and 'older down' from 2020 to 2021 with the switchover at around age 60. This is not the case with PE-involved deaths.

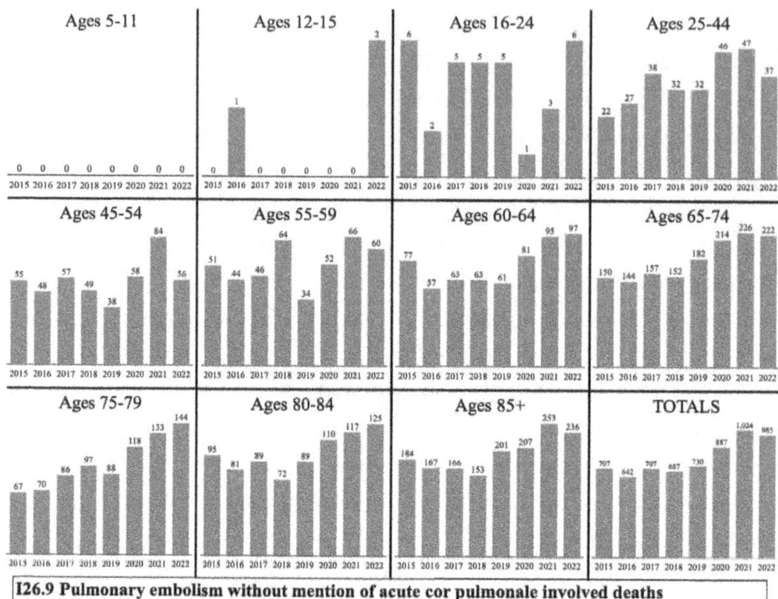

Figure 14.19

Figure 14.19 shows that PE deaths for every age group 45 years old and older increased from 2020 to 2021. The numbers in the groups under age 25 are too small to be useful for analysis. PE deaths in the "Ages 25–44" group remained essentially flat between 2020 and 2021. The "Ages 45–54" group rose substantially from 2020 to 2021. This relatively young age groups rose 45% from 58 to 84 PE-involved deaths. This group's deceased were real people in the prime of life who likely had children who depended on them.

In Massachusetts, mostly elderly people took "boostah" doses of covid vaccines. Note that "Ages 75–79" and "Ages 80–84" groups suffered more PE-involved deaths in 2021 than 2020 and even more in 2022 than 2021. Did these age groups take the most boosters in 2022?

The greatest evidence might be in the "Ages 85+" group, which is nearly normal in PE-involved deaths in 2020, the year of the great "pandemic" [sarcasm]. Those over age 84 started dying involving PEs when the covid immunizations were rolled out. And who would challenge the cause of death of someone over 84 years old? But a signal is a signal. If more older people died from PEs after vaccination and did not die from PEs after having covid, then the correlation is obvious and should be immediately studied. The signal of PE-involved deaths was clear by February 2021 in the VAERS data. This ignorance of VAERS by the government must be willful. Two full years of covid vaccination yielded 500 *excess* PE-involved deaths.

Figure 14.20 next shows I26.9 PE-involved deaths as a percentage of All-Cause deaths.

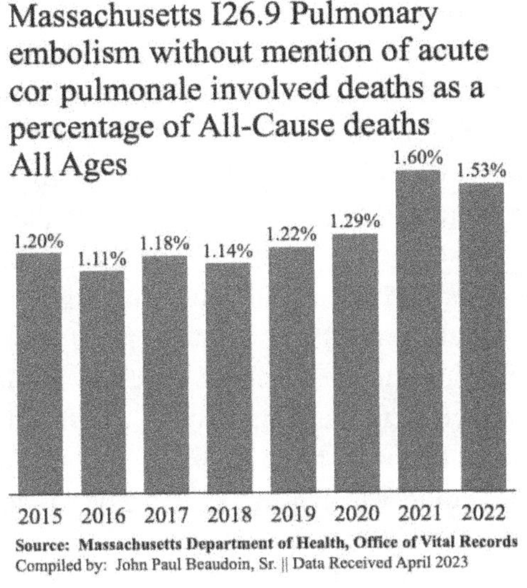

Figure 14.20

PE-involved deaths can be considered in proportion to All-Cause deaths by dividing PE-involved deaths by All-Cause deaths. In 2020 PE-involved deaths are only slightly elevated compared to baseline years 2015–2019. There appear to be few to no *excess* PE-involved deaths in 2020.

The picture changes dramatically coincident with the start of mass covid vaccination in 2021. In 2021, PE-involved deaths as a percentage of All-Cause deaths rose substantially. The increase was sustained in 2022. Years 2021 and 2022 are starkly anomalous and coincide perfectly with the covid “vaccine” rollout.

SUMMARY OF PULMONARY EMBOLISM DEATHS

By the hard evidence in *PRIMA PARS* and *SECUNDA PARS*, we know that PEs are involved in many covid vaccine deaths. **The graphs just presented provide the scale evidence that more than five hundred *excess* people were killed in Massachusetts involving pulmonary emboli very likely caused by covid vaccination.**

By most accounts, when families ask doctors if a covid vaccine possibly caused the PE, the doctors in Massachusetts often say there is no correlation between the two. The evidence from individual record and large data set analyses in this book provides truth; and the truth refutes the prevarications by doctors in Massachusetts. PEs resulting from covid vaccines are a massive loss of life consequence of covid vaccines in Massachusetts.

People of Massachusetts, and the world, are faced with a choice to believe 1) doctors, who have been coerced and solicited to deny any correlation between covid vaccination and PE, or 2) facts and truth from official records herein provided.

I46.9 CARDIAC ARREST DEATHS

Since the introduction of covid vaccines, there has been a continuous stream of news reports of young people and professional athletes collapsing and dying during strenuous training or competition. Others are being discovered dead in their beds. These tragedies usually involve heart issues.

Figure 14.21 depicts deaths associated with ICD-10 code I46.9, “Cardiac arrest, unspecified,” from 2015 through 2022.

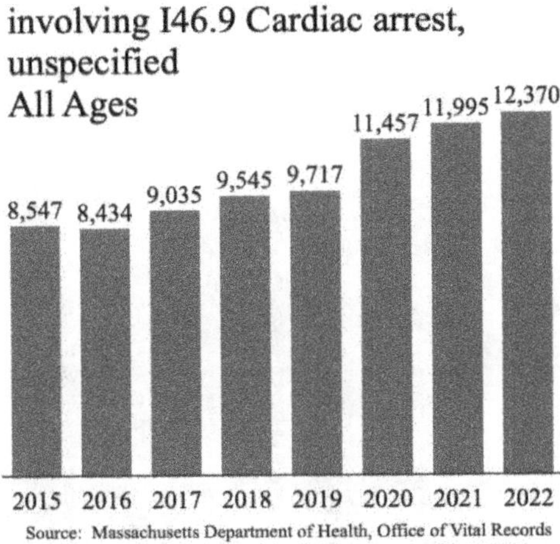

Year	Excess	Excess % over Expected
2020	1,366	13.5%
2021	1,559	14.9%
2022	1,589	14.7%

Figure 14.21

In Figure 14.21, years 2021 and 2022 *excess* cardiac arrest-involved deaths total 3,148 real people with families and friends.

Adjusting for total All-Cause deaths each year yields the following cardiac arrest-involved deaths as percentages of All-Cause deaths graph in Figure 14.22.

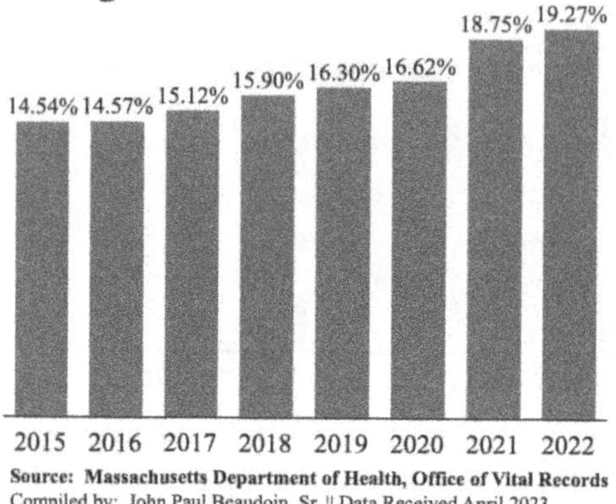

Figure 14.22

In Figure 14.22, the 2020 *excess* Cardiac arrest-involved deaths disappears into the 2015–2019 baseline trend of bars.

2021 and 2022 *excess* Cardiac arrest-involved deaths jump off the page as distinctly greater than the 2015–2020 trend. Note that 2020 is here included in the baseline years as a trend. Why not? In proportion to All-Cause deaths, it's not in *excess*.

If a specific cause of death is in the ***symptom spectrum profile*** of a disease, then it will synchronously rise and fall over time with the disease as a cause of death. Because Cardiac arrest-involved deaths went up from 2020 to 2021 when covid-involved deaths went down, covid and cardiac arrest are inversely related.

Some other externalities must be responsible for this major increase in the number of *excess* Cardiac arrest deaths.

More than three thousand *excess* Cardiac arrest-involved deaths in one state occurred in 2021 and 2022. One would expect the Commonwealth of Massachusetts or CDC to investigate this per their legal duties. Alas, they neither investigated nor have they responded to my lawsuit with action to investigate. With eyes tightly shut, the CDC and FDA and state governments continue to covid vaccinate unabashedly.

These cardiac arrest graphs look nothing like the ACP pattern. The 2020 to 2021 Cardiac arrest and ACP patterns are again inversely correlated.

The semi-monthly plots in Figure 14.23 show when the I46.9 Cardiac arrest-involved deaths occurred.

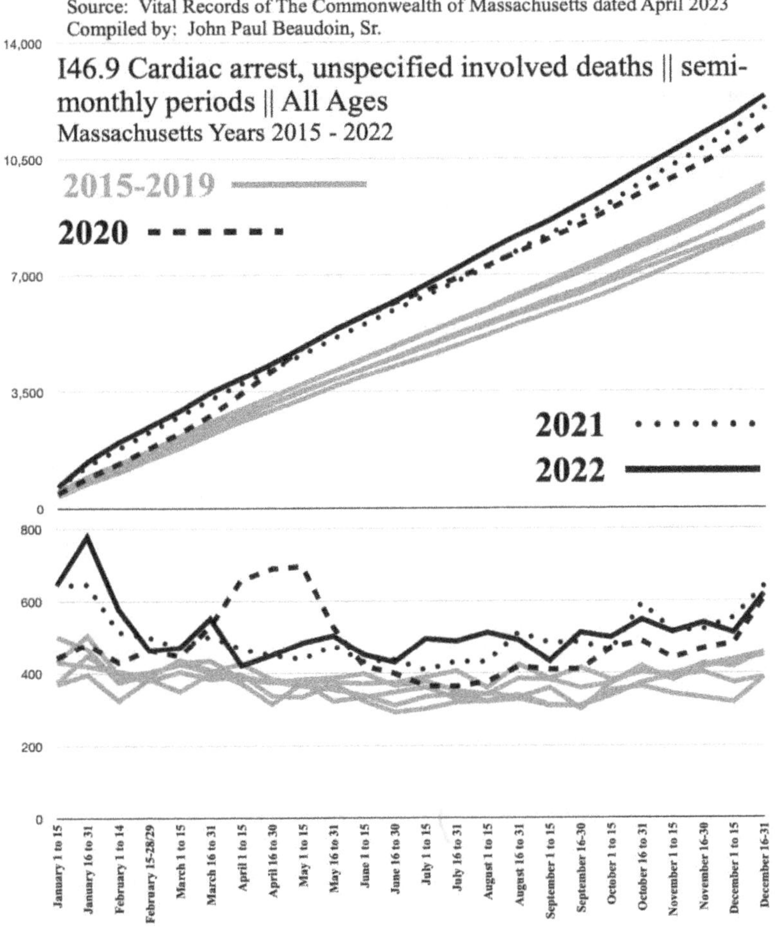

Figure 14.23

In the lower panel of Figure 14.23, it is evident that there are two principle components that contributed to the *excess* deaths from 2020 through 2022. ***Seasonal*** waves riding on a continuously elevated base of non-seasonal *excess* deaths are clearly visible.

The year 2020 Cardiac arrest-involved deaths dashed line plot depicts the obvious ***seasonal*** spring wave mid-March to mid-May. The year 2020 plot also rises at the end of the year in December, the beginning of the second ***seasonal*** wave.

Cardiac arrest-involved death plots also depict normal ***seasonal*** waves at the beginning and end of each of years 2021 and 2022. Note that the second wave during winter 2020/2021 is almost as high as the first wave despite the fact that the second wave of covid deaths is significantly lower that the first wave. Even more surprising is that the third seasonal wave of Cardiac arrest-involved deaths during winter 2021/2022 is even higher than the first wave though the third wave of covid-involved deaths is far lower than the first.

Anomalously, there is also an externality of *steady-state excess* Cardiac arrest-involved deaths all spring, summer, and fall of both 2021 and 2022, but not in 2020. This is a key finding.

The upper Cardiac arrest-involved deaths graph in Figure 14.23 shows ***steady-state*** (straight line positive slope) signal component all-year-long in years 2021 and 2022.

Also in the upper graph, year 2020 Cardiac arrest-involved deaths dashed line plot rose with a steeper slope than 2021 and 2022 only during March through May, corresponding to the first covid wave. Then the slope over the remainder of 2020 decreased to track parallel to the plots for the baseline years, 2015 through 2019. Note that the slopes of Cardiac arrest-involved deaths for 2021 and 2022 June through November are steeper than the slopes of the baseline years and the slope of 2020 June through November. This corresponds to the higher number of Cardiac arrest-involved deaths in 2021 and 2022. This is clear evidence of a huge epidemic of Cardiac arrest-involved deaths, which are unrelated to covid.

Figure 14.24 depicts the age profiles of Cardiac arrest-involved deaths.

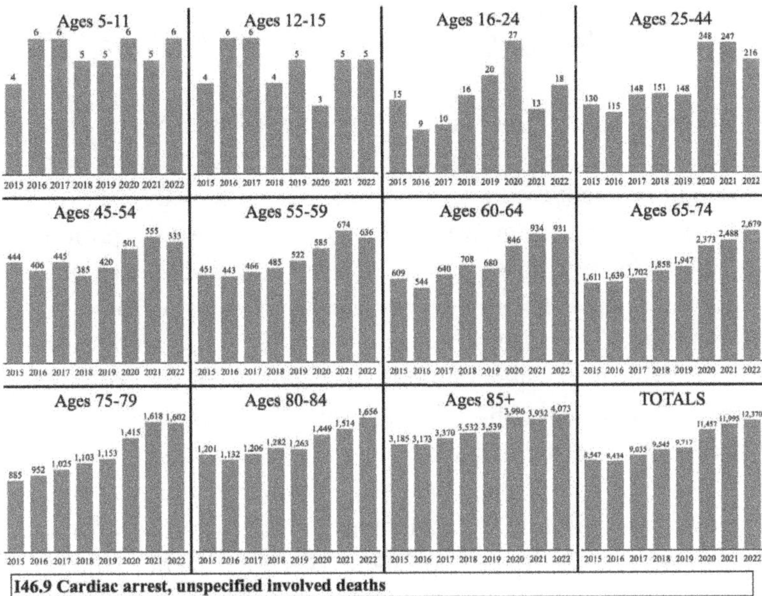

I46.9 Cardiac arrest, unspecified involved deaths

Data Source: VITAL Records of The Commonwealth of Massachusetts dated April 2023
Compiled by: John Paul Beaudoin, Sr.

Figure 14.24

Figure 14.24 shows that Cardiac arrest-involved deaths "Ages 25–44" group are almost equal from 2020 to 2021, thus breaking the ACP pattern of the younger aged going up and the older going down year over year.

Remember that the switchover occurs around age 60 in ACP, whereas Cardiac arrest-involved deaths were greater in 2021 than in 2020 for ages 45 through 84. And the "Age 85+" group is nearly equal from 2020 to 2021.

The ACP pattern of younger "up" and older "down" is completely broken by Cardiac arrest. Nearly all cardiac arrest age groups increased from 2020 to 2021.

Two facts should be considered when viewing the plots for "Ages 85+"; the oldest age groups took the most booster covid "vaccinations" in 2022 in Massachusetts and the oldest age groups died at greater rates from Cardiac arrest-involved deaths in 2022.

A conservative figure of more than three thousand excess Cardiac arrest-involved deaths occurred in 2021 and 2022 in age groups all the way down to 25 years old. This is an inverse signal relative to the ACP pattern. Clearly, covid did not cause these Cardiac arrest-involved deaths. Something else did, and it began in 2021.

I49.9 CARDIAC ARRHYTHMIA DEATHS

Arrhythmia is considered next. Many middle-aged people died in their sleep. Younger athletes died during or just after intense athletic activity and many were also discovered unresponsive or dead in bed.

Many have seen cardiac waveforms displayed on a heart monitor. The heart regulates its own contractions by producing a sequence of electrical potentials which flow through the muscle fibers, causing them to contract in a coordinated way. Inflammation or other cellular disruption can interfere with the proper generation of the sequence of electrical potentials. Inflammation can also result in the creation of scar tissue, which interferes with the orderly flow of the electrical potentials through the heart's muscle fibers.

Any disruptions of this sort can interfere with the orderly beating of the heart. The result is a partial or complete loss of efficient pumping action, which can quickly result in unconsciousness or death.

Figure 14.26 shows Massachusetts deaths involving ICD-10 code I49.9, Cardiac arrhythmia, unspecified, for the years 2015 through 2022.

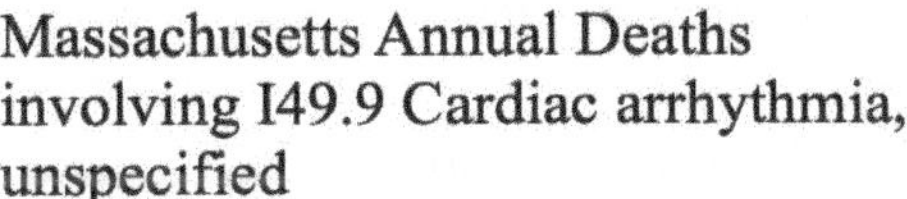

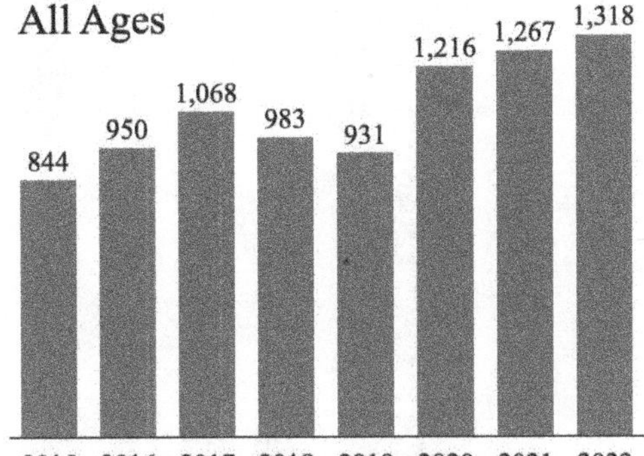

Source: Massachusetts Department of Health, Office of Vital Records
Compiled by: John Paul Beaudoin, Sr. || Data Received April 2023

Year	Excess	Excess % over Expected
2020	199	19.5%
2021	229	22.1%
2022	259	24.5%

Figure 14.26

By now the pattern exhibited by the Cardiac arrhythmia deaths is becoming familiar. The ACP pattern of *excess* is broken again in Cardiac arrhythmia-involved deaths as it is in Cardiac arrest- and Pulmonary embolism-involved deaths.

Years 2021 and 2022 Cardiac arrhythmia-involved deaths are greater than in 2020. ACP all went "down," while arrhythmia deaths went "up" from 2020 to 2021. Accordingly, Cardiac arrhythmia-involved deaths are also related inversely to ACP.

The *excess* Cardiac arrhythmia-involved deaths in 2021 and 2022 total 488 people who had families and friends who cared about them.

Figure 14.27 shows the percentage of total All-Cause deaths for each year involving Cardiac arrhythmia. Again, the patterns are familiar.

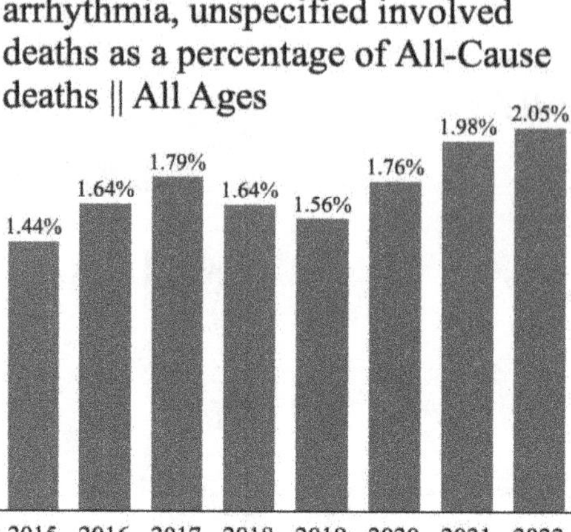

Figure 14.27

Figure 14.27 shows that the increase in the raw number of Cardiac arrhythmia-involved deaths in 2020 disappears when adjusted by the number of All-Cause deaths in 2020. Note that the adjusted value for 2017 even exceeds the 2020 value.

Clearly, something bad happened in 2021 and 2022 that caused an increase in Cardiac arrhythmia-involved deaths.

The semi-monthly plots in Figure 14.28 reveal when Cardiac arrhythmia-involved deaths occurred.

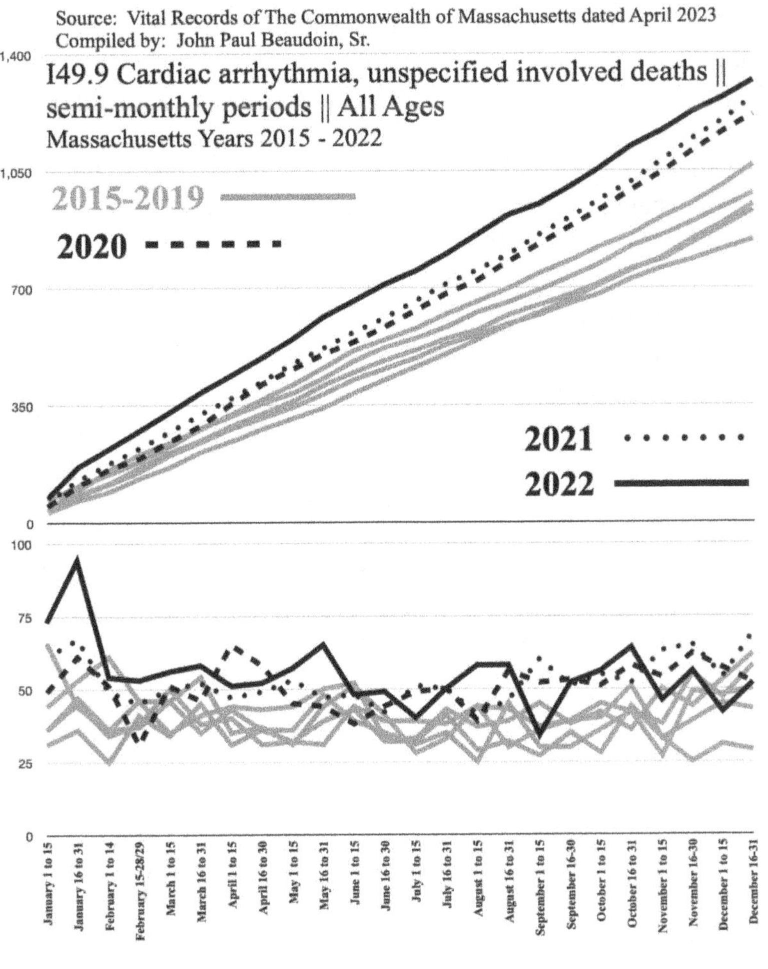

Figure 14.28

In Figure 14.28, the *seasonal* behavior of Cardiac arrhythmia-involved deaths lacks significance, if it exists at all. The first wave in spring of 2020 is barely visible. Again, the second wave during winter 2020/2021 exceeds the first wave, and the third wave during winter 2021/2022 exceeds the second wave, even though covid deaths were successively lower over those two winters.

Find, again, patterns deviant from ACP. Instead of the normal behavior of a *seasonal* disease in which each successive wave is smaller, Figure 14.28 shows each successive wave is greater. Furthermore, the off-season behavior also increased each successive year. Cardiac arrhythmia deaths in 2020 returned to baseline level after the first spring 2020 wave but did not stay at baseline for the entire year. And the elevation above baseline increased in each subsequent year, 2021 and 2022.

Nearly 500 *excess* Cardiac arrhythmia-involved deaths in two years, 2021 and 2022, from one cause of death, is significant. One tenth of that was enough to stop vaccine rollouts nationwide in the past. This data is for just one state and one single cause of death, yet the *excess* is ten times more than nationwide totals that stopped prior vaccines. This is more evidence that nothing was going to stop these covid immunizations from widespread distribution. The Department of Defense maintained full throttle unleashing Operation Warp Speed on The People regardless of the evidence of harm, which was very clear by February 2021. Diane Dubois died in March. Brianna McCarthy died in April. Eden MacDonald died in June 2021. Apparently, willfully unconcerned, our state and national government officials continued to push covid vaccines, while aggressively censoring any questioning voice.

Does the Massachusetts Department of Public Health remain willfully ignorant of the stark increase in Cardiac arrhythmia-involved deaths?

Figure 14.29 depicts Cardiac arrhythmia-involved deaths by age groups.

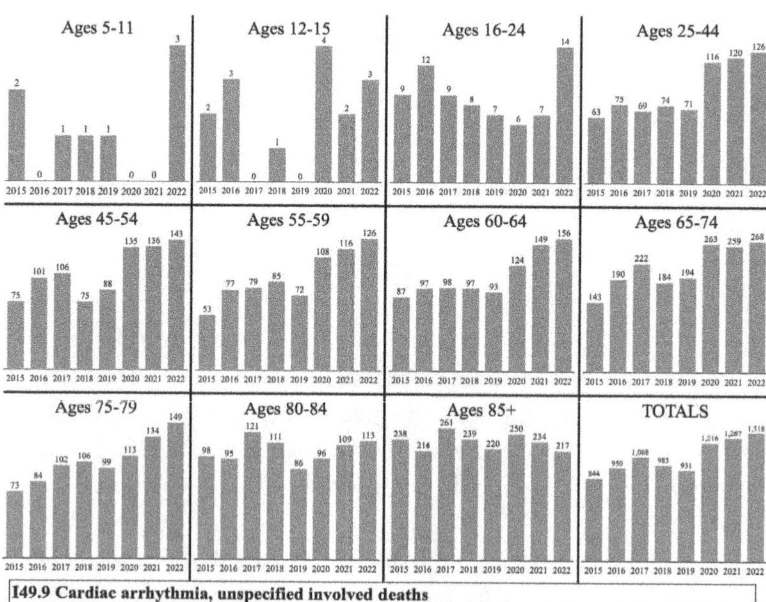

Data Source: VITAL Records of The Commonwealth of Massachusetts dated April 2023
Compiled by: John Paul Beaudoin, Sr.

Figure 14.29

Please view each age group in Figure 14.29 in context of the other graphs. Clearly something killed more people involving Cardiac arrhythmia in 2020 when there were no covid vaccines. Even though adjusting for All-Cause deaths in Figure 14.27 showed that year 2020 resembled normalcy, that does not explain the elevated number of 2020 Cardiac arrhythmia-involved deaths for ages 25 through 64. This mystery is not answered in this book. One hypothesis might be the sharp rise in fentanyl use or another drug causing bradycardia. The graphs beg for a public health investigation.

If covid declined by 45% from 2020 to 2021, why did Cardiac arrhythmia-involved deaths increase from 2020 to 2021? Why did Cardiac arrhythmia-involved deaths increase even more from 2021 to 2022? ACP decreased from 2020 to 2021, while Cardiac arrhythmia increased. There is an inverse relationship between the two categories. Clearly something other than covid is responsible for much of the increase in Cardiac arrhythmia-involved deaths.

I8 VEINS & LYMPH VESSELS DEATHS

"I8" is a group of all ICD-10 codes using "I8" as a prefix. These include phlebitis and thrombophlebitis of lower extremity veins, portal vein thrombosis, other venous embolism and thrombosis, varicose veins, esophageal varices, other vein disorders, lymphadenitis, other noninfective disorders of lymphatic vessels and lymph nodes.

I8 deaths involving clots in veins and other vessels are depicted in the following figures beginning with the annual bar graph in Figure 14.30.

Massachusetts Annual Deaths involving I8 Prefix - Diseases of veins, lymphatic vessels & lymph nodes, not elsewhere classified
All Ages

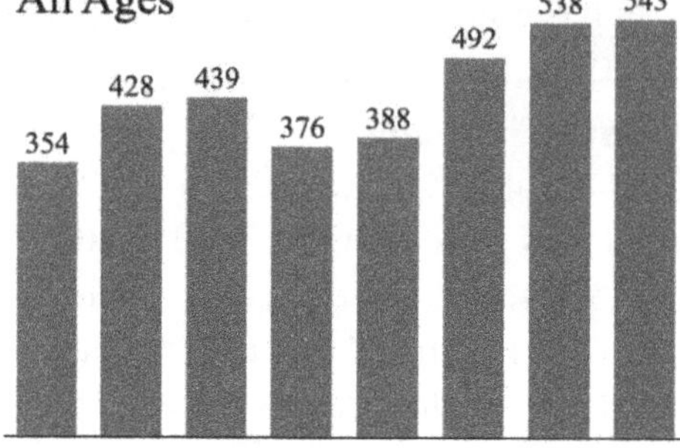

Source: Massachusetts Department of Health, Office of Vital Records
Compiled by: John Paul Beaudoin, Sr. || Data Received April 2023

Year	Excess	Excess % over Expected
2020	90	22.4%
2021	135	33.4%
2022	138	34.1%

Figure 14.30

An *excess* 273 deaths occurred in Massachusetts involving I8 veins and lymph vessels in 2021 and 2022.

Again, while there is an elevation in I8-involved deaths in 2020 compared to the baseline years 2015 through 2019, adjusting for percentage of total All-Cause deaths provides a different perspective. Figure 14.31 shows excess I8 deaths as a percentage of All-Cause deaths for the respective years.

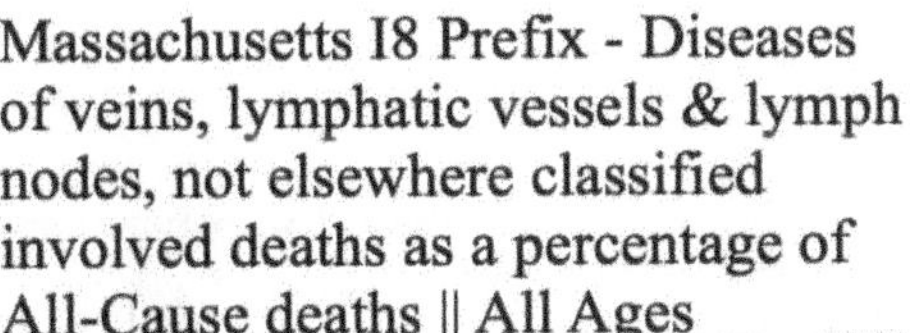

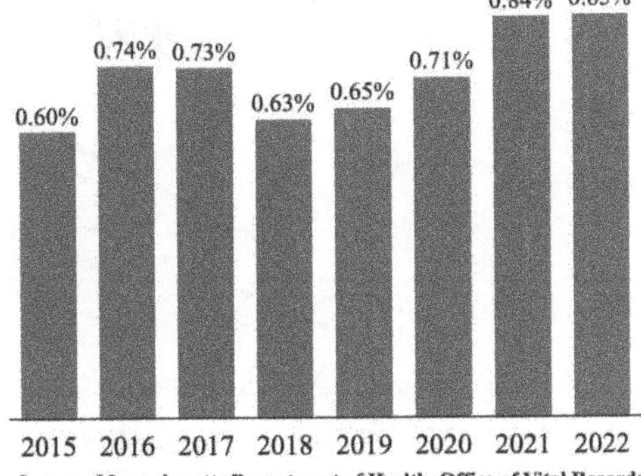

Figure 14.31

The 2020 I8 Veins and lymphatic vessels-involved deaths apparent *excess* in Figure 14.30 raw data disappears when adjusted for All-Cause deaths. In fact, I8-involved deaths in 2020 are below the levels in both 2016 and 2017. Year 2020 I8-involved deaths does not look anomalous at all.

The behavior was different in 2021 and 2022 when I8 deaths were significantly above the level in the baseline years despite the fact that covid deaths were lower in those years. The pattern is becoming increasingly familiar. Something other than covid was responsible for elevated levels of I8 deaths.

I8 deaths involving pathologies in veins and lymphatic vessels is a major issue that a prudent department of health would study is sufficient detail to enable the public to be timely informed.

Apparently, Massachusetts does not have such a prudent health department. One must wonder what they do with all the data they are responsible for collecting and archiving. Over the past three years, the Massachusetts Department of Public Health (MA DPH) seemed to prioritize programs to market covid "vaccines" and provide infrastructure to facilitate administering multiple covid shots in every arm. **Does the MA DPH work for The People or for the pharmaceutical corporations headquartered in Massachusetts?**

The semi-monthly plots in Figure 14.32 show when the I8-involved deaths occurred.

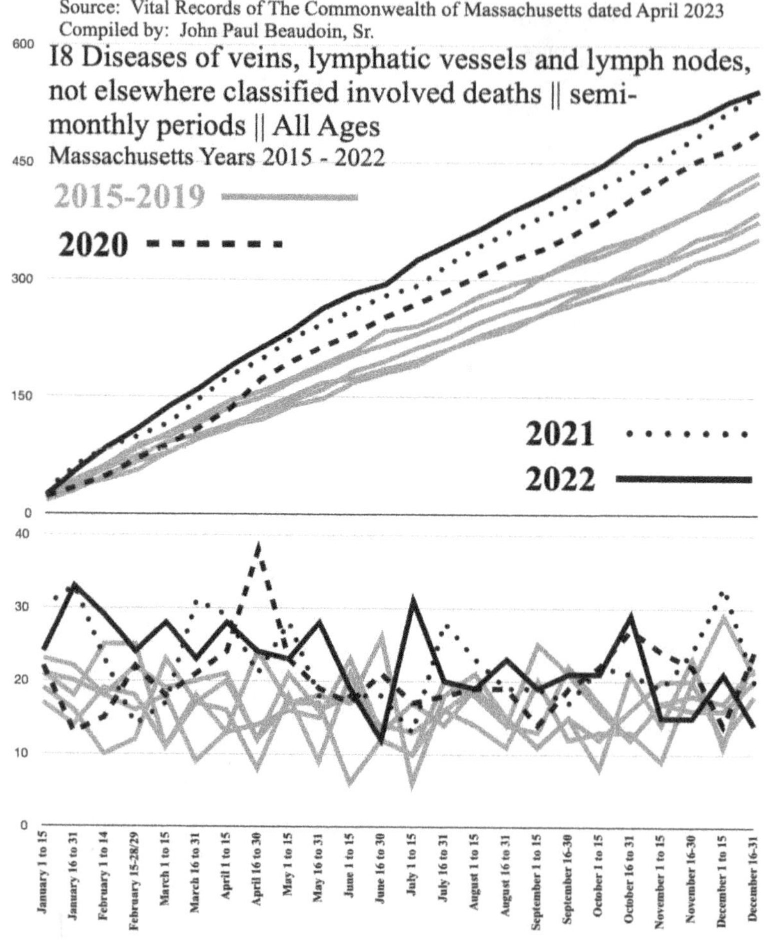

Figure 14.32

Again, there is a familiar pattern of behavior for I8 deaths. Whereas 2021 and 2022 appear to have a non-seasonal elevation of I8 deaths during the entire year with additional elevations from second and third covid waves, 2020 I8 deaths are consistent with the baseline years 2015 through 2019, except for elevated levels coincident with the first covid wave in spring 2020. Some additional elevation toward the end of 2020 is apparent as the second wave of covid begins.

Whatever is causing all these circulatory system deaths is consistent across the "I" code causes and is inversely related to ACP graphs.

The I8-involved deaths by age groups are depicted in Figure 14.33.

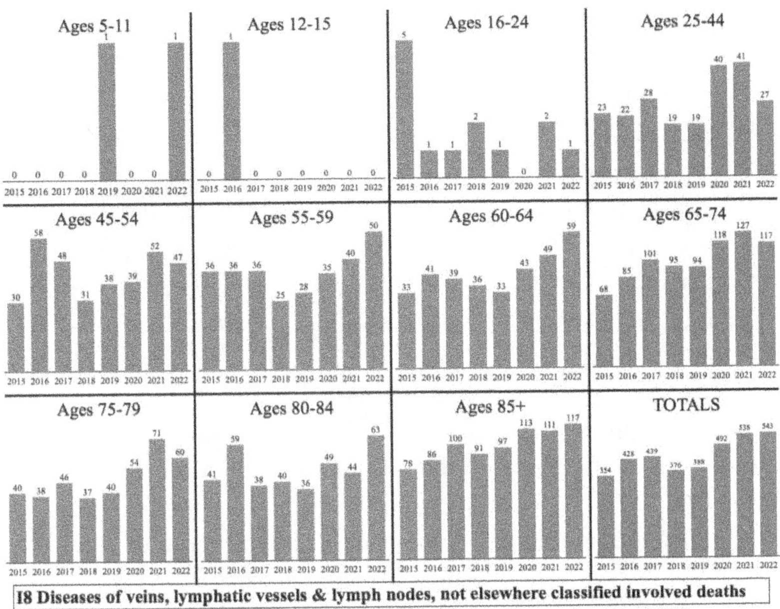

Figure 14.33

Figure 14.33 shows that the patterns of I8-involved deaths also behave inversely to the ACP patterns. Deaths involving I8, veins and lymph vessels, increased from 2020 to 2021 for ages 25 through 79. The switchover in the pattern of I8 deaths is at around age 80—twenty years older than for ACP. More younger people died from a blood transport system cause of death in 2021 after the incidence of covid-involved deaths had substantially declined from 2020, when they were at their highest levels.

SUMMARY OF ICD-10 CODES WITH PREFIX "I"

The behavior pattern of ICD-10 codes with prefix "I" shown in this section (I26.9, I46.9, I49.9, I8) is inversely related to the pattern of ACP-involved deaths.

In Substack articles under the name Coquin de Chien ("The Real CdC") from 2022, a common thesis is, "*It's all about the blood.*" Articles such as *C19 "vaccine" - the cause of causes, Circulatory attack continues,* and *Mors ex cruentum sanguinem - Death from bloody blood,* found at coquindechien.substack.com, laid the foundation for this chapter. It really is all about the blood.[5]

Pharma companies and the U.S. government claimed that covid "vaccines" stay in the deltoid muscle despite the fact that their internal documents, which the courts ordered them to disclose, clearly showed that this is not true. "Muscles keep the action localized." reported North Carolina Health News and many others.[6] They accepted and reported a lie.[7]

Big Pharma and our government claimed that covid vaccines do not enter the cell nucleus.[8,9,10] That was a lie.[11]

Big Pharma and our government said that covid vaccines are rigorously quality tested. Kevin McKernan showed that to be a lie.[12]

Three-word phrases are a great tool to program the human mind. Those who wish to nudge the public into the outcome they desire use catch phrases to effect the programming.

"Safe and effective" is such a three-word nudge.

"Trust the science" is another three-word nudge.

"Two weeks to flatten the curve" is a nudge of six words.

The hard evidence of the Massachusetts death certificates reported in this book confirm that covid vaccines are deadlier than SARS-CoV-2 viral infections. They are certainly not safe; nor do they prevent infection, nor transmission. However, they are clearly effective, if the desired effect is death, disability, and possibly sterilization or spontaneous abortion.

"D" CODES BLOOD & IMMUNE DEATHS

ICD-10 codes beginning with the prefix "D" cover a range of blood and blood-forming disorders and diseases. The immune mechanism is also heavily represented in "D" codes. Although "D" codes also include benign neoplasms, there are so few of them on the Massachusetts death certificates that they can be ignored for the purposes of these analyses.

Notwithstanding the heterogeneity of the category, "D" codes, in the aggregate, are a good indicator of deaths involving blood, circulation, and immune function.

The D codes considered in this section are:

- D62 – Acute posthemorrhagic anemia
- D69.5 – Secondary thrombocytopenia
- D8 category – Certain immunodeficiencies and other disorders involving the immune mechanism

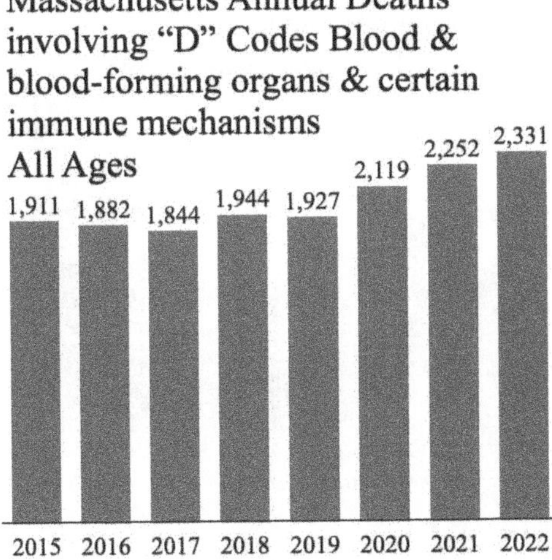

Year	Excess	Excess % over Expected
2020	189	9.8%
2021	313	16.1%
2022	382	19.6%

Figure 14.34

Figure 14.34 provides an initial overview of the entire category of D codes.

Figure 14.34 shows that in 2021 and 2022 "D" codes *excess* deaths amounted to 695 people in Massachusetts whose deaths involved disorders of blood, blood formation, or an immune mechanism. Families and friends will miss these 695 souls. May God rest their souls and make known the true causes of their deaths, whatever that truth may be.

Again we see a familiar pattern. D code-involved deaths in 2021 and 2022 are inversely related to ACP deaths in those years and continue to increase year over year.

Adjusting the D code-involved deaths in proportion to All-Cause deaths provides a perspective that normalizes the first wave of covid deaths in spring 2020. Figure 14.35 depicts D code-involved deaths as a percentage of All-Cause deaths. Note that the x-axis is positioned at y = 2.90% in order to emphasize the differences among the years.

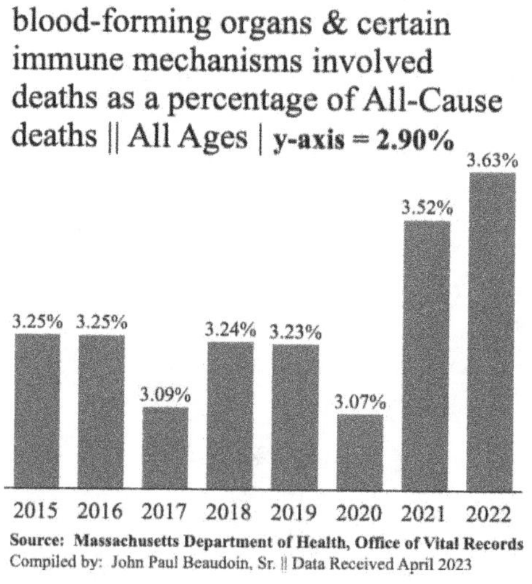

Figure 14.35

It is clear in Figure 14.35 that ICD-10 D code-involved deaths were unremarkable during 2020 despite the high number of deaths during the first wave of covid. It is also clear that there was a drastic change beginning in 2021, the year that mass administration of the covid vaccines began.

Figure 14.36 shows the semi-monthly plots of D code-involved deaths for 2015 through 2022.

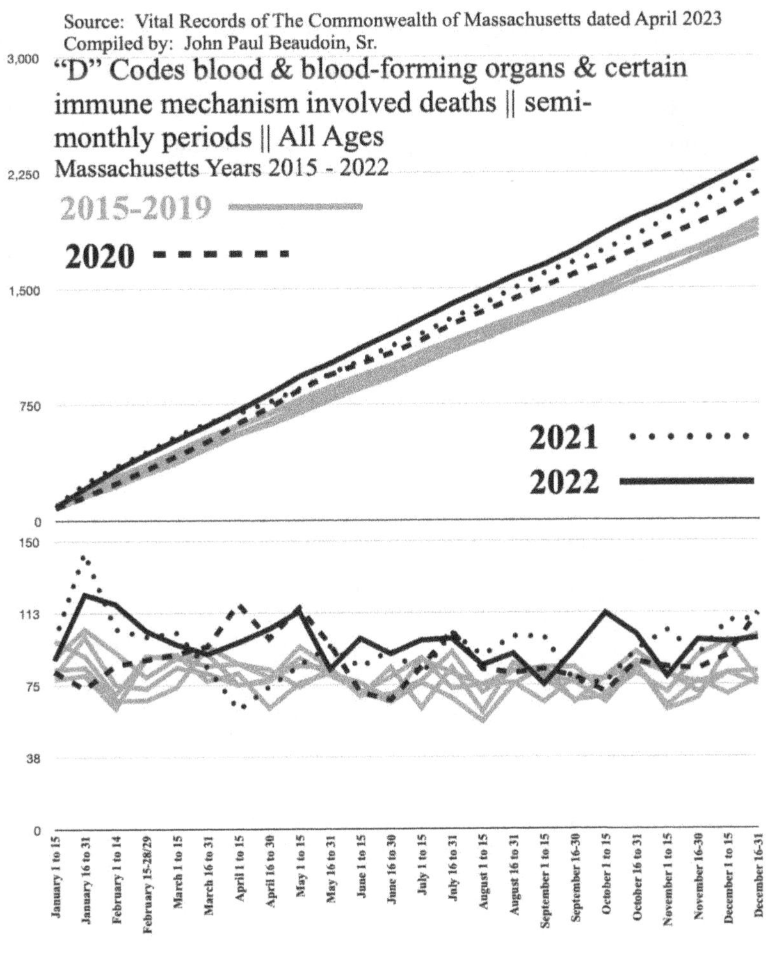

Figure 14.36

The lower plot in Figure 14.36 shows that during the first quarter of 2020, D code-involved deaths followed the behavior of the baseline years, 2015 through 2019.

An *excess* of D code-involved deaths emerged in sync with the first covid wave, from March through May 2020 and returned to the baseline level in June, concurrent with the end of the first covid wave.

D code-involved deaths were elevated again during the second covid wave in the winter 2020/2021. Note that this second wave of D code deaths is larger than the first wave in 2020 even though the second covid wave was significantly lesser than the first wave.

Note also that during 2021, D code-involved deaths fail to return fully to the baseline level. The top panel shows that in 2021, cumulative D code-involved deaths exceeded 2020 deaths in a non-seasonal manner. From June to the end of the year, the gap between the 2020 and 2021 plots widens, showing more 2021 deaths every semi-monthly period.

Finally, note that the cumulative D code deaths in 2022 surpassed the 2021 levels in a non-seasonal manner. The gap between all other years' plots widens from April through the end of each year. Clearly, something other than covid was killing more people on an ongoing basis in D Code causes after the first wave of covid was over and coincident with the introduction of mass administration of the covid gene therapy immunizations.

The plots in Figure 14.37 of D code deaths by age group provide additional insights.

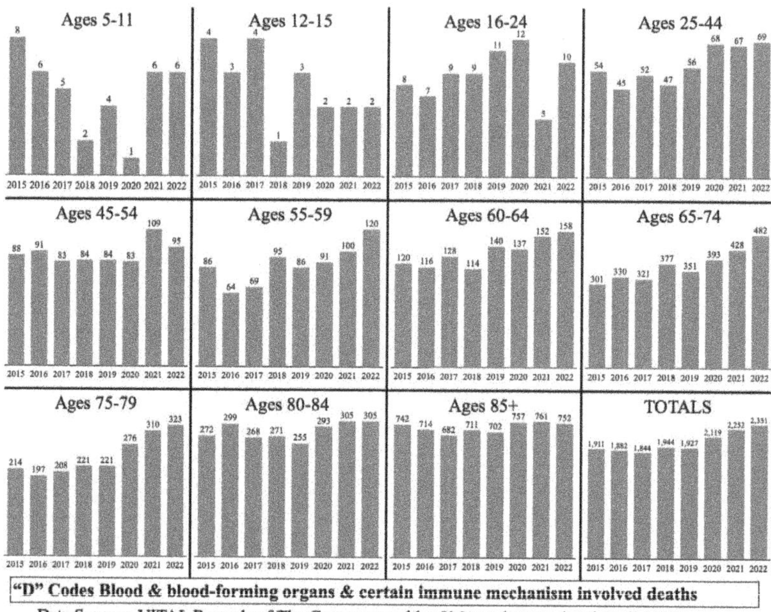

Figure 14.37

There is a clear trend of steadily increasing *excess* D code-involved deaths for all ages above 54. It is virtually impossible for trends that are this broadly consistent across time and age to be coincidental. Something other than *seasonal* and diminishing covid must be responsible for this worsening mortality.

Why are so many people dying with blood issues since the covid vaccine was introduced? And why are "D" code-involved deaths inversely related to the rates of covid-involved deaths year over year from 2020 to 2021? The fact that these plots are inversely related to the ACP pattern decisively refutes the claims by CDC and state health departments, incessantly amplified by the credulous media, that this increased mortality is somehow related to covid *per se*.

D8 IMMUNE MECHANISM INVOLVED DEATHS

The ICD-10 codes using prefix "D8" are analyzed as an aggregate group because the number of deaths within each of the individual D8x sub-codes are quite small, which makes it difficult to discern any patterns. All of these D8 codes are related to immune mechanism disorders. By considering them together in a single group, patterns are seen to emerge from the data.

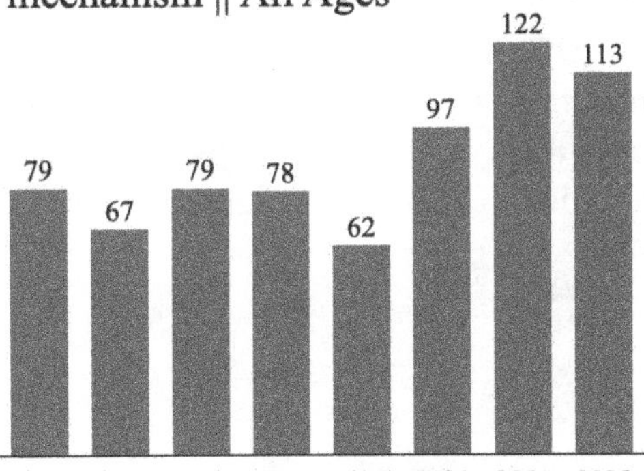

Year	Excess	Excess % over Expected
2020	24	32.9%
2021	49	67.1%
2022	40	54.8%

Figure 14.38

The D8 grouping includes: various immunodeficiencies such as familial and non-familial hypogammaglobulinemia, IgG and IgM deficiencies, antibody defects, T-cell and B-cell deficiencies, defective response to Epstein-Barr, lymphocyte function antigen defect, sarcoidosis of lung or lymph nodes or skin, or other immune mechanism disorders. Figure 14.38 depicts the annual totals of D8-involved deaths.

Figure 14.38 clearly shows that the ACP pattern is again broken. D8 immune mechanism-involved deaths are higher in 2021 and 2022, well after the major first wave of covid in 2020 had abated.

Covid is obviously not the trigger for D8 immune mechanism-involved deaths since it is 67.1% higher than expected in 2021 and 54.8% higher than expected in 2022. If covid infection is not responsible for the elevated level of D8-involved deaths, could the covid "vaccinations" be the culprit? Mass administration of the covid gene therapy shots began in 2021. Fewer shots were administered in 2022. While the correlation between "vaccine" administration and D8-involved deaths is not absolute proof that the shots are responsible, it is certainly highly persuasive evidence.

Another 89 excess deaths in 2021 and 2022 manifest in families and friends grieving for lost loved ones. I continue to write these sentiments of grieving families because this is a long chapter of data, and it is important to remember that all these *excess* deaths are very likely caused not by covid, but rather by covid "vaccines." The Massachusetts Department of Public Health, the CDC, the FDA, and all government entities owe "We The People" the results of an investigation that would take only one week in any state. More on this is explained in *QUARTA PARS.*

Adjustment for All-Cause deaths is depicted in Figure 14.39.

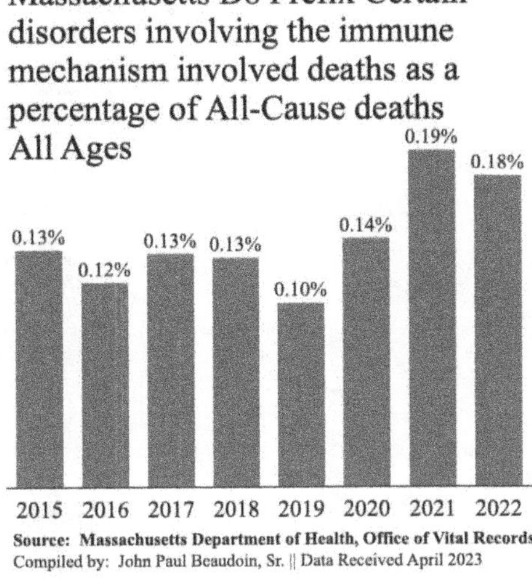

Figure 14.39

Figure 14.39 depicts the D8 immune mechanism-involved deaths during 2015 through 2022 as a percentage of annual All-Cause deaths, respectively.

Again, the pattern is familiar. It is clear in Figure 14.39 that D8 deaths were unremarkable during 2020 despite the high number of deaths during the first wave of covid. It is also clear that there was a major change beginning in 2021, the year that mass administration of the covid "vaccines" began and continued through 2022.

Figure 14.40 shows the semi-monthly plots of D8 codes deaths for 2015 through 2022.

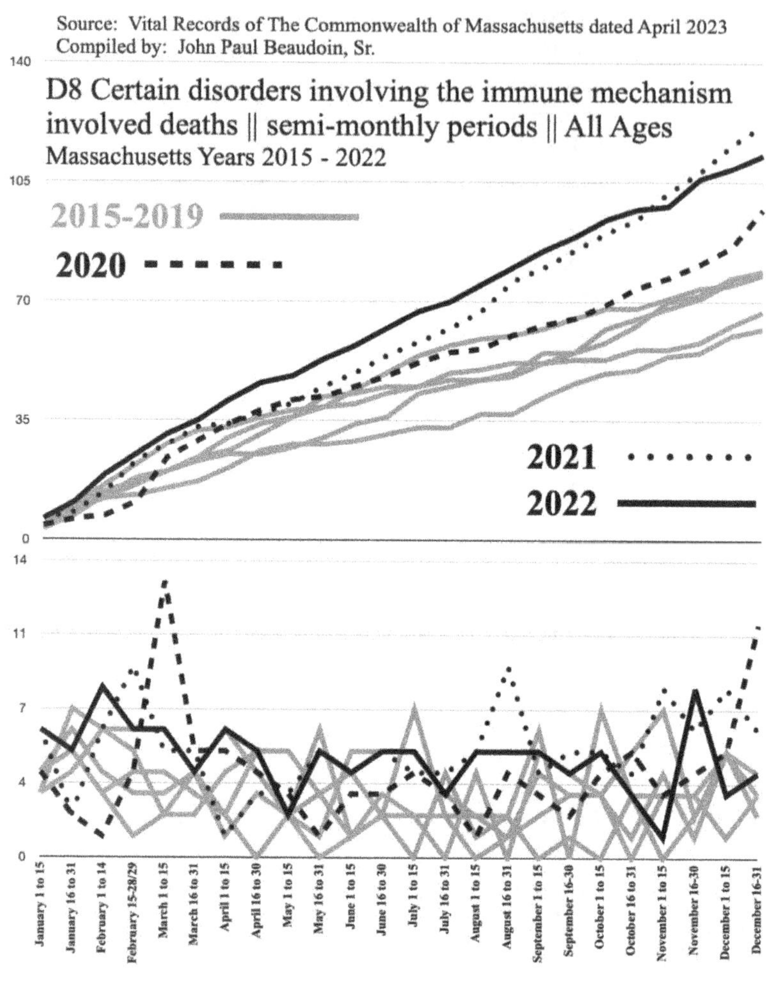

Figure 14.40

The plots in the upper panel of Figure 14.40 leave no doubt that 2021 and 2022 D8 immune mechanism-involved deaths climb steeply from April 2021 all the way through the end of 2022. **That's some twenty straight months of excess D8-involved deaths.**

With each additional cause of death examined, it becomes increasingly clear that something other than covid was killing more people on an ongoing basis after the first wave of covid had ended. For each cause of death, the elevation in *excess* deaths coincided with the introduction of the mass administration of the covid gene therapy "vaccination."

The fact that no government agency is pursuing any of this data, at least not publicly, should make everyone wonder what taxpayers are paying for. What is the Massachusetts Department of Public Health doing? What is the CDC doing? All we hear from them is sophisticated psychologically manipulative mass marketing of "vaccines" based on inducing fear in a credulous public. What little data they release is aggregated in a way that conceals the serious indications revealed here in this book.

The bar graphs by age group in Figure 14.41 provide additional insights into whose deaths involved D8 Immune mechanism.

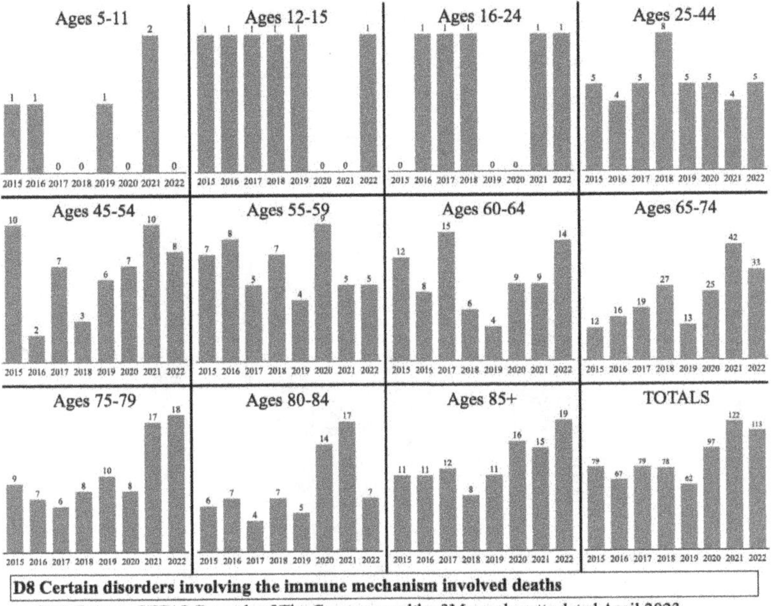

Figure 14.41

The patterns in the D8 immune mechanism age groups are less distinct. This is a natural result of working with smaller numbers comprising this category. It appears that the increased D8-involved deaths fell mainly on "Ages 45–54" and ages 65 through 84. The pattern for these age groups shows an inverse relationship to the ACP pattern, but the relationship is weaker than in the other ICD-10 "I" and "D" code groups.

D62 ACUTE POSTHEMORRHAGIC ANEMIA

D62 Acute posthemorrhagic anemia is usually an acute blood loss from trauma, after a surgical procedure that was complicated by an error, or simply bad luck.

However, manual inspection of the records associated with some two hundred deaths involving D62, sudden blood loss, in 2021 and 2022 reveal an epidemic of internal bleeding from other issues such as gastrointestinal hemorrhages or vessel ruptures. Figure 14.42 depicts annual totals and *excess* Acute posthemorrhagic anemia-involved deaths.

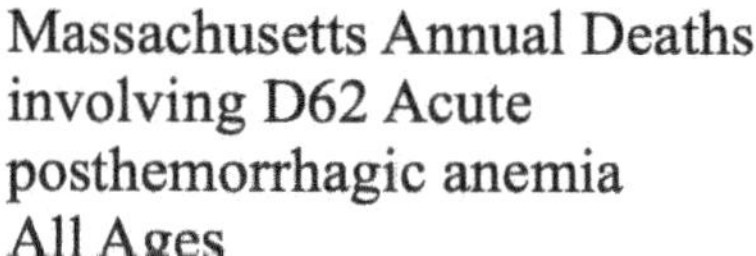

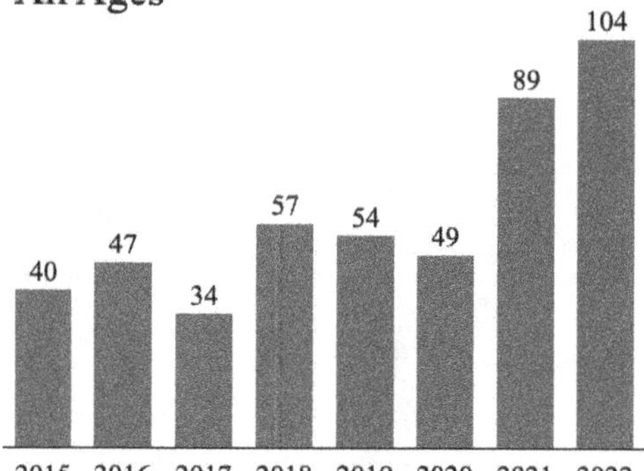

Source: Massachusetts Department of Health, Office of Vital Records
Compiled by: John Paul Beaudoin, Sr. || Data Received April 2023

Year	Excess	Excess % over Expected
2020	-9	-15.2%
2021	27	44.5%
2022	39	59.0%

Figure 14.42

Figure 14.42 shows 66 *excess* deaths in 2021 and 2022 involving acute blood loss.

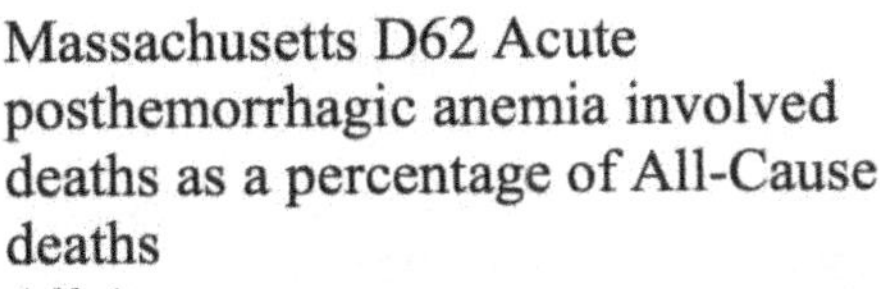

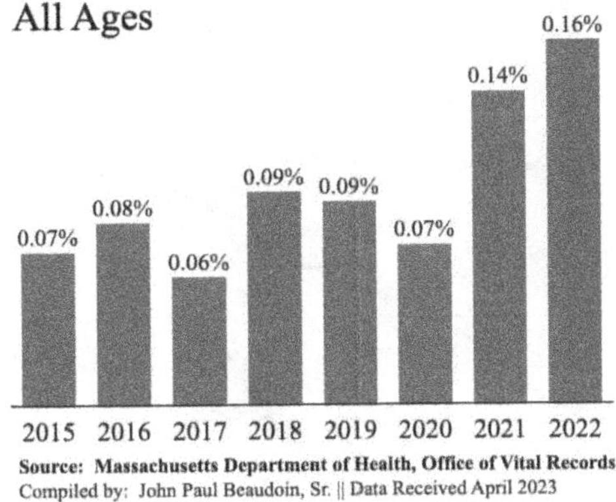

Figure 14.43

Figure 14.43 also reveals the now familiar pattern. Adjusting for All-Cause deaths by dividing D62 sudden blood loss-involved deaths by All-Cause total deaths reveals that 2020 is indistinguishable from the baseline years 2015 through 2019, while 2021 and 2022 are much higher than all others.

Years 2021 and 2022 D62 acute blood loss-involved deaths are a disaster amounting to 66 *excess* lives lost in the Commonwealth of Massachusetts.

The semi-monthly plots are shown in Figure 14.44.

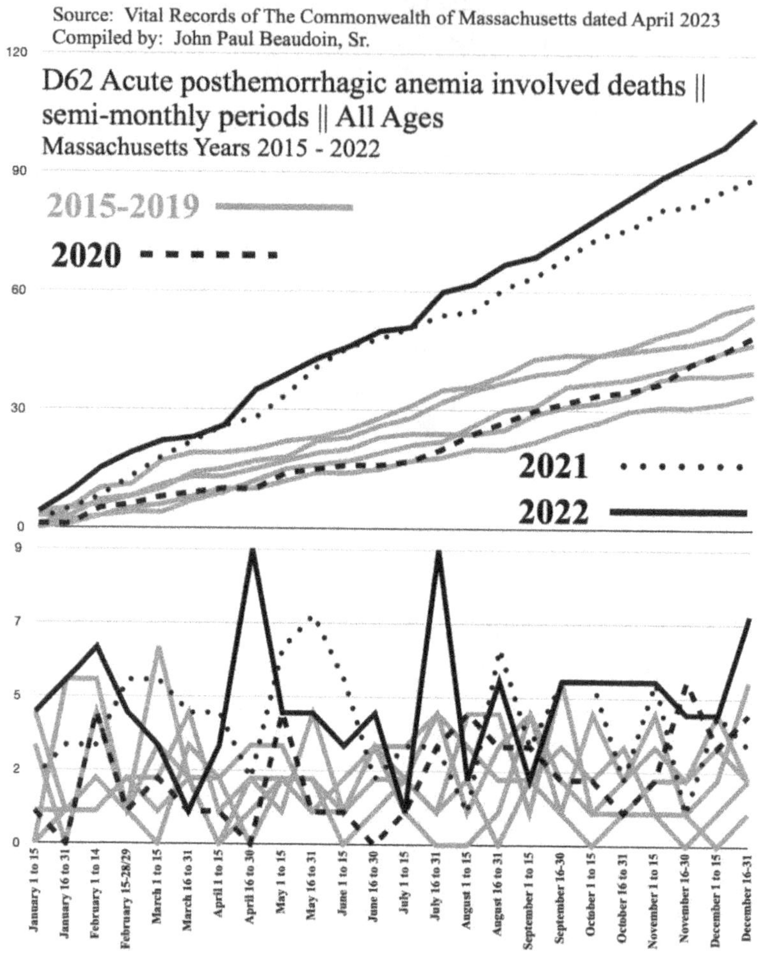

Figure 14.44

The top panel of Figure 14.44 makes quite a statement!

While D62 Acute posthemorrhagic anemia-involved deaths were at completely normal levels in 2020, when covid infections were at their peak, D62-involved deaths raged out of control in 2021 and 2022, years of mass administration of covid "vaccines." Does the Commonwealth of Massachusetts or the CDC even know about this? Do they track these causes? **The People are dying younger and dying of different things than normal and in *excess*; yet governments do not know, do not care,**

are deliberately concealing this information, or perhaps all three alternatives apply.

The world must know that something occurred beginning in 2021 in Massachusetts that is not covid and that is killing thousands of people per year. D62-involved deaths are a relatively small fraction of the *excess* deaths in 2021 and 2022.

Figure 14.45 shows deaths by age group involving D62 sudden blood loss.

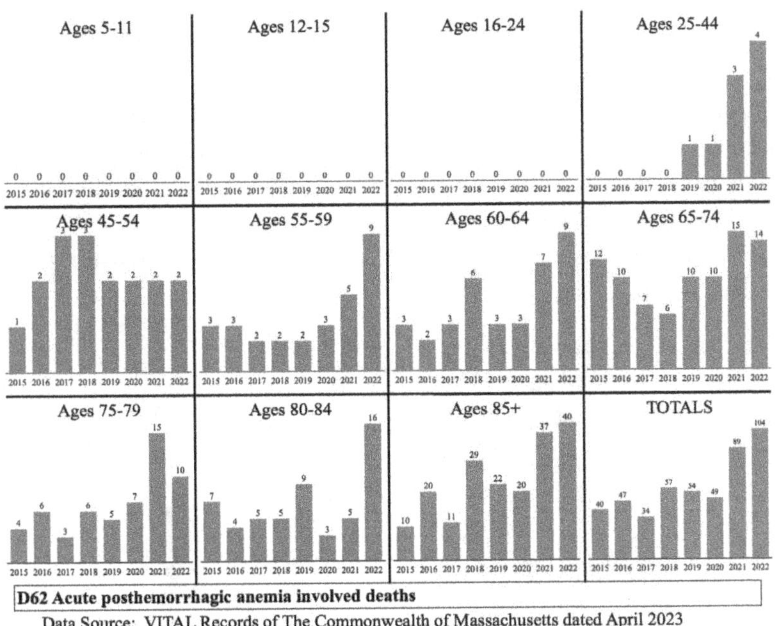

Figure 14.45

The age group graphs in Figure 14.45 make one wonder if the booster doses are related to the 2021 and 2022 spikes in the lower graph of Figure 14.44.

The Figure 14.45 age group graphs of D62 Acute posthemorrhagic anemia depicts the damage to all ages. Not much more needs to be written. D62 Acute posthemorrhagic anemia is involved with many *excess* deaths since covid "vaccination" began. **This can be described quite literally as a bloody massacre.**

D69.5 SECONDARY THROMBOCYTOPENIA

Chapter 2, *Three Strokes*, includes notes from a *Brief Report* entitled *Fatal Post COVID mRNA-Vaccine Associated Cerebral Ischemia* written by six doctors on Brianna's case from Beth Israel Deaconess Medical Center and Harvard Medical College. In that report, they stated "*thrombocytopenia is frequent*" in the setting of CVST stroke from covid vaccines. Eden, age 17, died from a Cerebral Venous Sinus Thrombosis (CVST) hemorrhagic stroke. Diane, age 62, died from an intracranial hemorrhage in the setting of thrombocytopenia.[13]

Thrombocytopenia is a condition of low platelet count. Platelets are required for clotting. If one's platelet count is too low, dangerous internal bleeding can occur. A significant *excess* of deaths from clotting and bleeding emerged in 2021 and 2022.

Figure 14.46 depicts annual totals and *excess* deaths involving D69.5, Secondary thrombocytopenia.

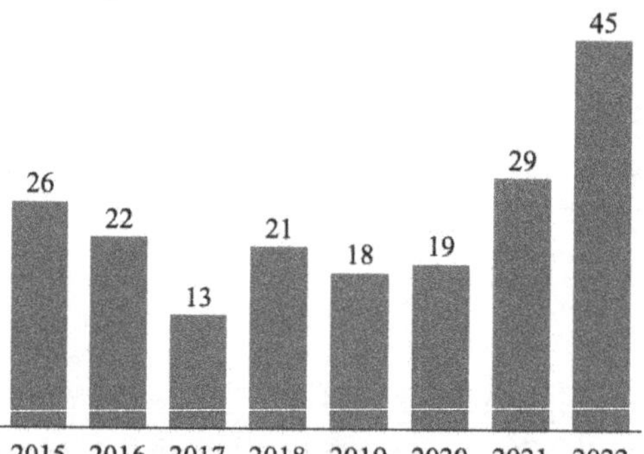

Year	Excess	Excess % over Expected
2020	-1	-5.0%
2021	9	45.0%
2022	25	125.0%

Figure 14.46

Figure 14.46 shows that there are no *excess* Secondary thrombocytopenia-involved deaths in 2020.

Year 2021 Secondary thrombocytopenia is significantly in *excess* by 45.0%. When the numbers are small, as they are in this category, elevation of *excess* in a single year might be due, in part or wholly, to statistical noise. Any statistical doubt is dispelled by 2022 in which the *excess* is an outrageous 125.0%.

One of the 2022 Secondary thrombocytopenia records includes Cause A "*ACUTE HEART FAILURE*," Cause B "*ACUTE LIVER FAILURE*," Cause C "*ACUTE KIDNEY FAILURE*," and Cause D "*ANEMIA THROMBOCYTOPENIA*," all occurring in "*DAYS*." In other words, the patient suddenly encountered these issues only days prior to death.

Many Secondary thrombocytopenia-involved death records also included "*BRAINSTEM HERNIATION*," which is a stroke, and pulmonary embolism, heart attack, other types of stroke, intracranial hemorrhages, and gastrointestinal hemorrhages.

D69.5 Secondary thrombocytopenia as a percentage of All-Cause is shown in Figure 14.47.

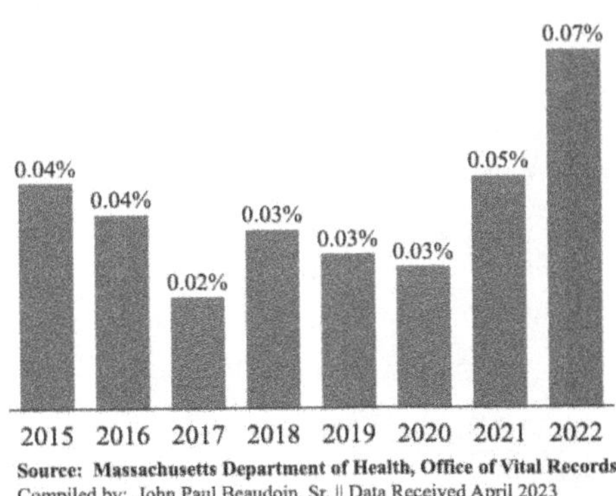

Figure 14.47

While there is no significant signal in 2021, there is a clear safety signal in 2022 when thrombocytopenia-involved deaths rose to 225% of *expected* level.

The semi-monthly plots for thrombocytopenia are shown in Figure 14.48.

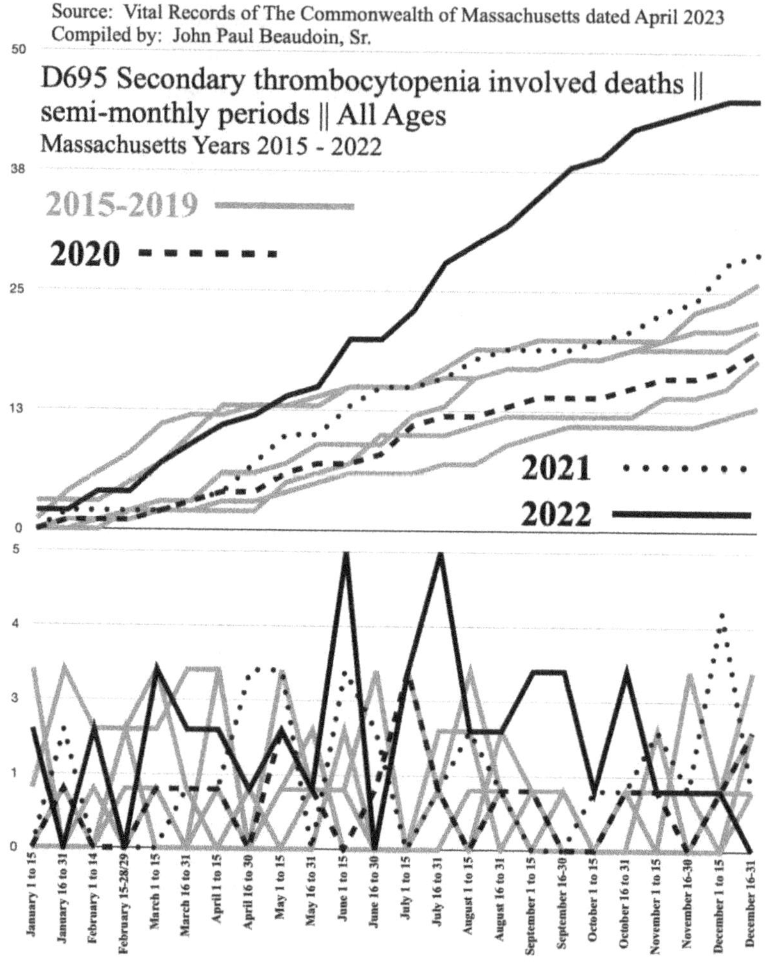

Figure 14.48

Figure 14.48 shows D69.5 Secondary thrombocytopenia-involved deaths in 2022 to be a health emergency.

The numbers may be low, but 34 *excess* deaths in 2021 and 2022 add to the stack of blood-involved deaths since covid "vaccination" began.

For the sake of completeness, Figure 14.49 shows the age groups affected by thrombocytopenia-involved deaths.

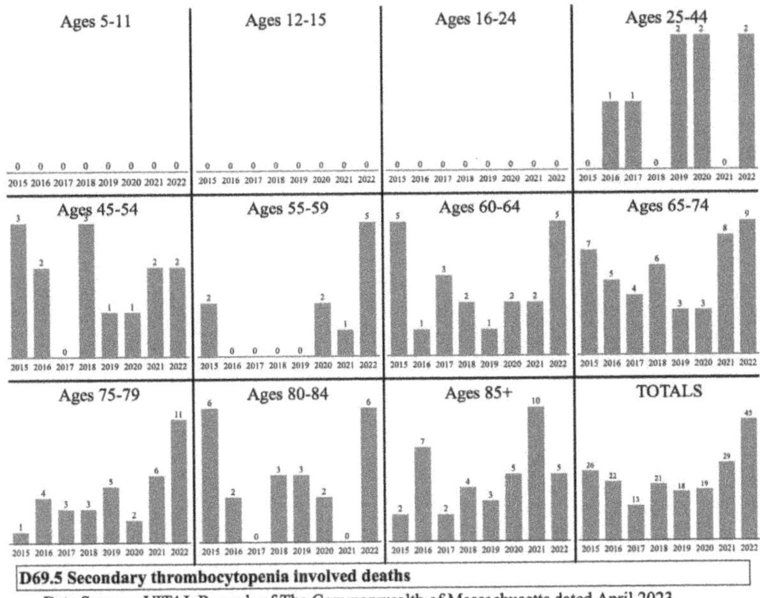

Figure 14.49

When the total numbers are this small as in Figure 14.49, distributing them by age group results in even smaller numbers. Statistical noise obscures any signals that might be embedded in these small numbers.

This Chapter 14 extensive parade of specific causes of death is surely wearisome, but the conclusions are highly alarming. The weight of the accumulated evidence, based on unbiased analyses of primary Record-Level Source Data, extracted from actual Massachusetts death certificate records, is irrefutable. Something other than covid is responsible for thousands of *excess* deaths in Massachusetts; and the covid gene therapy shots are the primary suspect, more likely the sole suspect. It is important to remember that each one of these *excess* deaths involved a human being and impacted countless friends and family of the unfortunate decedent. It is important to remember that most of these deaths were easily avoidable. And it is important to remember that our governments lied, and people died.

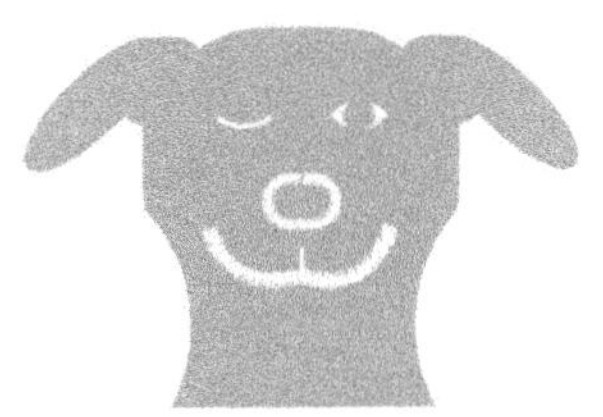

Chapter 15
Which Cancers?

Cancers take longer to manifest and contribute to death than the acute bleeding and clotting adverse events considered in Chapter 14. For that reason, the numbers for *excess* cancer deaths would be expected to be smaller than the adverse events analyzed in the previous chapters. Accordingly, cancer related safety signals would be expected to be harder to confirm. Nonetheless, cancer related safety signals are visible in the Record-Level Source Data extracted from the Massachusetts death certificates.

The term "Turbo Cancer" is used with increasing frequency among those who follow or report on covid and covid vaccines. There are many reports of cancer patients who were expected to survive an additional five years after their cancer diagnoses, but who perished in a few weeks or a few months after receiving a covid shot. There are also reports of initial diagnoses of fast growing cancers in people who did not have cancer prior to vaccination. Indeed, in some of these cases, the cancer had already progressed to stage three or fully metastatic stage four when initially diagnosed. This is extremely unusual.

The cancer-related ICD-10 codes begin with the letter C. When the C category is examined in the aggregate comprising all C code cancers, no clear signals emerge. However, some specific C codes tell of quite a calamity unfolding:

- C77.9 Secondary and unspecified malignant neoplasm: lymph node
- C79.5 Secondary malignant neoplasm of bone and bone marrow

C77.9 LYMPH NODE CANCER

Figure 15.1 shows annual totals of Secondary lymph node cancer-involved deaths. *Res ipsa loquitur* means "the thing speaks for itself."

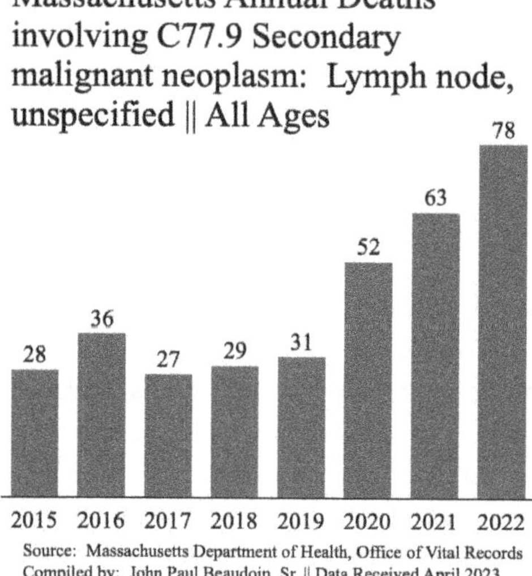

Year	Excess	Excess % over Expected
2020	22	72.2%
2021	33	108.6%
2022	48	158.3%

Figure 15.1

Some will say that the *excess* cancer related deaths in 2020 were due to delays in cancer screening and treatment. Medical evaluations and treatments were delayed due to closures, fear, and apprehension of hospitals and clinics. Without medical procedures such as chemotherapy to retard growth, cancers were allowed to mature and outpace one's immune response. Others might say that covid itself is the cause of *excess* lymph node cancers in 2020. There may be some truth to this given the known impact of the covid spike protein on immune function. However, covid declined in 2021 and 2022, yet *excess* lymph node cancers continued to climb during these years when covid vaccines were administered en masse.

Other factors support a causal relationship between secondary lymph node cancer and covid vaccines. It is a fact that the immune mechanism is immediately affected by covid vaccines as manifested by a sharp drop in leukocytes and neutrophils after injection.[1] Also, "sore armpit" (lymph node pain) is a frequently reported adverse event after covid vaccines.[2] The data presented in Chapter 14 for the combination of ICD-10 codes D8 and I8 strongly suggest severe negative impacts on the immune mechanism beginning in 2021, coincident with the commencement of mass covid vaccination.

Given strong evidence of a causal relationship between maladies of the lymph nodes and covid vaccines, people should consider what is causing a 158.3% increase in 2022.

Figure 15.2 shows secondary lymph node cancer-involved deaths by year adjusted by dividing by total All-Cause deaths in the respective years.

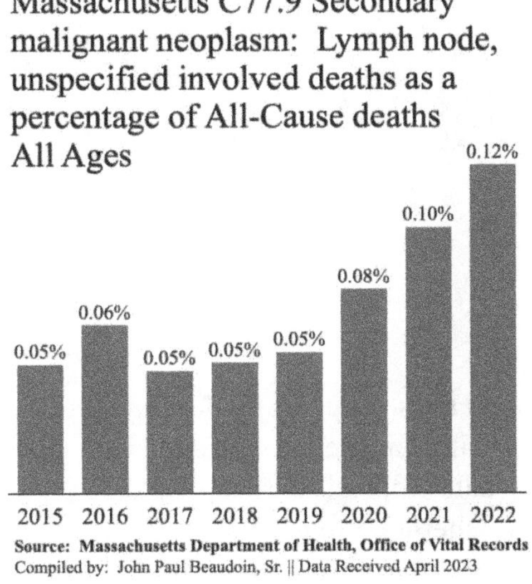

Figure 15.2

The semi-monthly plots in Figure 15.3 show an alarming trend over time. While the familiar seasonal pattern is difficult to discern in the bottom panel, the cumulative excess lymph node-involved deaths is clearly alarming.

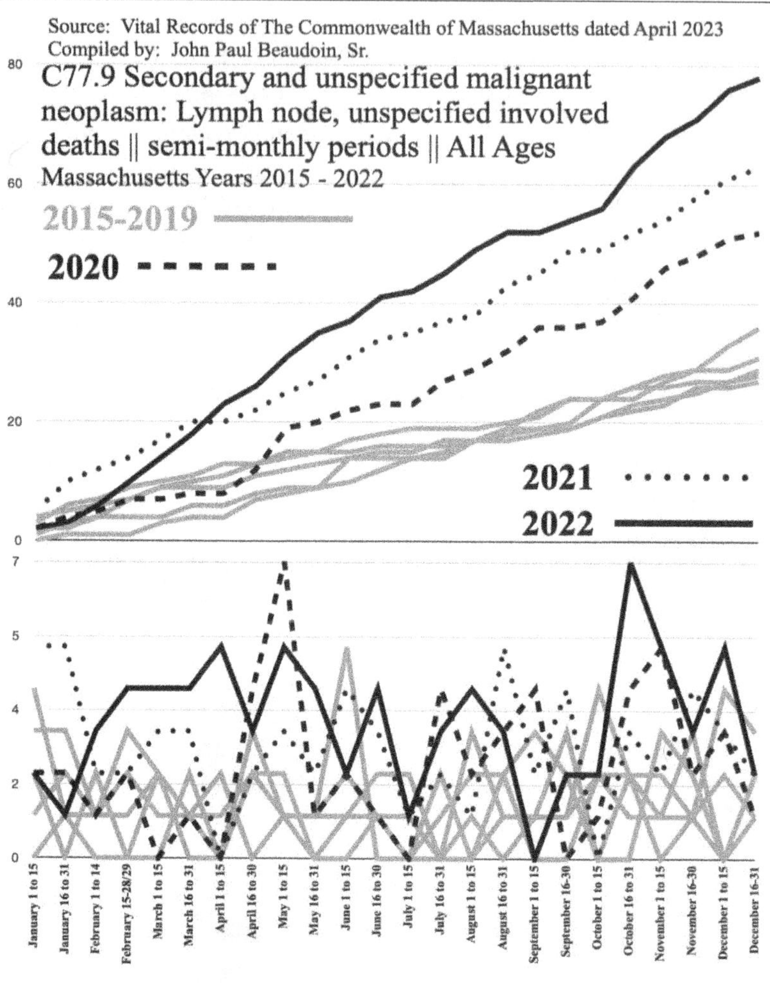

Figure 15.3

Eighty-one *excess* lives were lost in 2021 and 2022. These people were real human beings with families and friends. We must keep reminding ourselves that this "data" represents real people.

Regardless of whether covid infections or covid vaccines or a combination of the two are causing this alarming trend, the Massachusetts Department of Public Health, the CDC, and other health agencies are failing to report on these dramatic increases in causes of death. Are they failing to monitor for significant adverse events from the covid vaccines, or are they aware of the situation but purposely concealing it from the public? What is their job? Do they protect the public or do they protect pharmaceutical companies?

In the lower panel of Figure 15.3, we see the familiar peak in secondary lymph node cancers during the spring of 2020 wave of ACP. This is also evident in the upper panel given the sharp increase in slope in April 2020, which raised the plot of cumulative deaths above the baseline years, 2015–2019.

The entirety of *excess* C77.9 Lymph node cancer in 2020 cannot be blamed on that short spring event because the gap between 2020 and the baseline years 2015–2019 continued to widen thereafter.

Something during 2020 was responsible for a continuing increase in the rate of *excess* deaths involving secondary lymph node cancer. This began before the introduction of covid vaccines and continued after the rate of ACP declined. This suggests that there may be more than one reason for the increases.

Figure 15.4 shows the secondary lymph node-involved deaths by age groups.

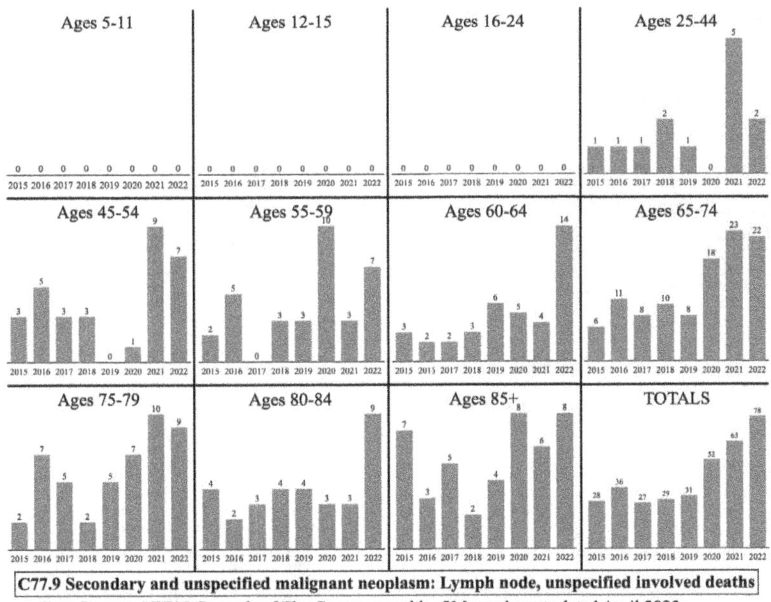

Figure 15.4

In Figure 15.4, the "Ages 25–44" group depicts seven total deaths involving secondary lymph node cancer in 2021 and 2022, which is more than double any other two years shown. Year 2020 shows zero.

The "Ages 45–54" group depicts sixteen total deaths involving secondary lymph node cancer in 2021 and 2022, which is double the next highest two-year total. Year 2020 only shows one.

Age groups 55–59, 65–74, and 85+ show spikes in 2020. In all other age groups, 2020 is among baseline years 2015–2019.

There was only one secondary lymph node cancer-involved death in 2020 under the age of 55. Compare this to 14 in 2021 and 9 in 2022.

In terms of life-years-lost due to secondary lymph node cancer-involved deaths, 2020 pales in comparison to the massive increase in *excess* in 2021 and 2022. Death in great *excess* involving lymph node cancer among those ages 25–54 represents a massive number of life-years-lost compared to deaths among the elderly from co-morbidities while battling lymph node cancer. The impact of the loss of adults during their prime years leaves deep, dark holes in the hearts and psyches of the surviving children and families.

At the time of this writing, the death certificate dataset for 2023 is not yet stabilized. It takes months for the death certificates to be completed, especially when the queue of autopsy reports can extend up to six months. The dataset contains many "PENDING" causes of death. However, once something is entered in Parts I or II, it is rarely removed from the death certificate.

The alarming trend of C77.9 secondary lymph node cancer-involved deaths prompted a preliminary compilation of the 2023 data. For an equitable comparison, deaths involving secondary lymph node cancer in the first quarter of each year from 2015 through 2023 are shown in Figure 15.5.

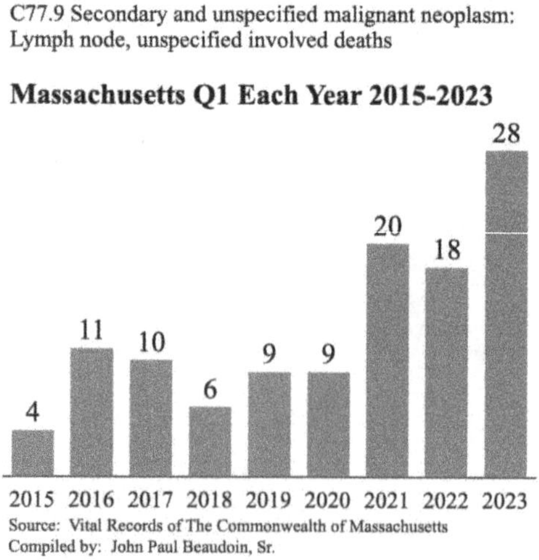

C77.9 Secondary and unspecified malignant neoplasm:
Lymph node, unspecified involved deaths

Massachusetts Q1 Each Year 2015-2023

4 11 10 6 9 9 20 18 28

2015 2016 2017 2018 2019 2020 2021 2022 2023

Source: Vital Records of The Commonwealth of Massachusetts
Compiled by: John Paul Beaudoin, Sr.

Figure 15.5

In Figure 15.5, Q1 of the year 2023 for secondary lymph node cancer-involved deaths is alarmingly higher than Q1 of the prior years.

Q1 deaths in 2021 and 2022 almost look reasonable compared to 2023; but they're not reasonable at all. By Q1 2023, C77.9 secondary lymph node cancer-involved deaths are a health emergency in their own right extending over a period of three years.

This Massachusetts disaster manifests in a single ICD-10 code. Regardless of whether the cause is covid vaccines, covid infections, or some combination, the MA DPH and CDC have a legal duty to investigate C77.9 secondary lymph node cancer increases.

One man, a humble volunteer with a computer, uncovered significant *excess* deaths involving multiple ICD-10 codes at a level indicating the biggest public health crisis in the Commonwealth of Massachusetts since the 1918 Spanish flu. Where are the Massachusetts officials who are charged with protecting the public health?

The MA DPH has reported nothing related to an investigation of these causes of death despite the August 23, 2022 lawsuit I filed against them in U.S. District Court. The lawsuit does not seek financial compensation. The lawsuit seeks relief by a court order for the Commonwealth of Massachusetts to report honestly to the The People of the Commonwealth. **I requested that the judge order the Commonwealth to announce the true causes of death of those individuals mentioned in *PRIMA PARS* and to provide confidential access to data so that researchers may study the correlation between immunizations and causes of death without violating the privacy of the persons concerned.**

C79.5 BONE AND BONE MARROW CANCER

Like the lymph nodes, bone marrow produces blood components. The marrow produces platelets, white blood cells, and red blood cells (RBC).

Since the bone marrow is instrumental in creating blood components and the circulatory system transports these blood components throughout the body, any dysregulation of the bone marrow can induce problems, including possibly lethal issues, anywhere in the body.

Figure 15.6 shows annual totals for C79.5 secondary bone and bone marrow cancer-involved deaths.

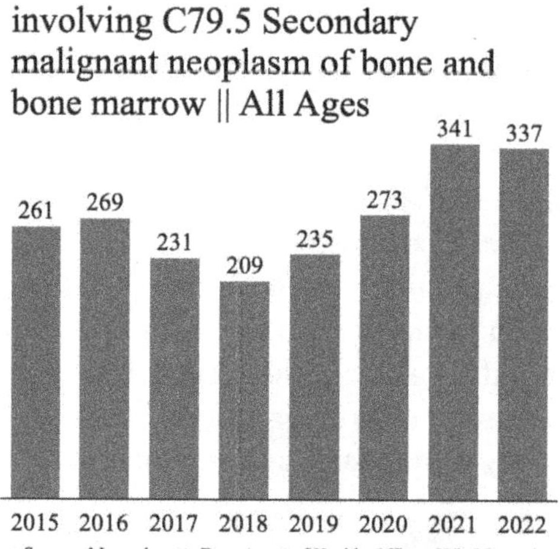

Year	Excess	Excess % over Expected
2020	32	13.3%
2021	100	41.5%
2022	96	39.8%

Figure 15.6

In early 2020, governments imposed restrictions on freedom of movement, ordered closure of small businesses, and recommended people avoid hospitals and healthcare facilities unless an acute emergency arose.

That may be the reason for more deaths involving C79.5 marrow cancer. Or it could be another externality that occurred in 2021 and 2022 such as covid vaccines.

One would think that a forty percent rise in marrow cancer that took nearly two hundred lives in 2021 and 2022 is worthy of investigation by the Massachusetts Department of Public Health or the CDC.

Figure 15.7 shows marrow cancer-involved deaths as a percentage of All-Cause, not that the adjustment for All-Cause is even needed to see this obvious signal.

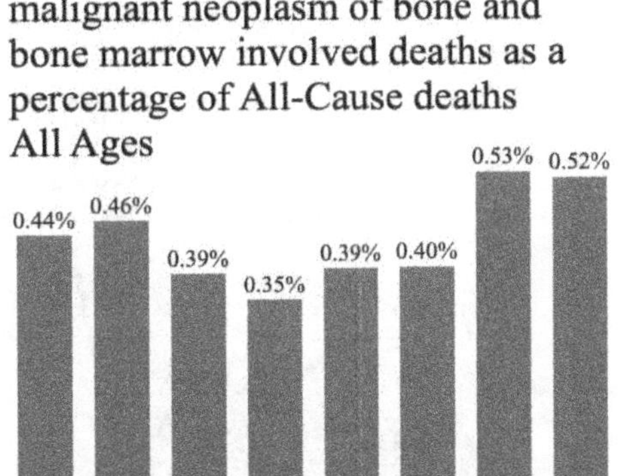

Figure 15.7

In Figure 15.7, again, the 2020 *excess* disappears when adjusted for the total number of people who died that year. Bone and marrow cancer-involved deaths are flagrantly high in years 2021 and 2022.

How is it possible that we have heard nothing whatsoever from the Massachusetts Department of Public Health or the CDC about these alarming increases in death?

The semi-monthly plots for bone and marrow cancers is shown in Figure 15.8.

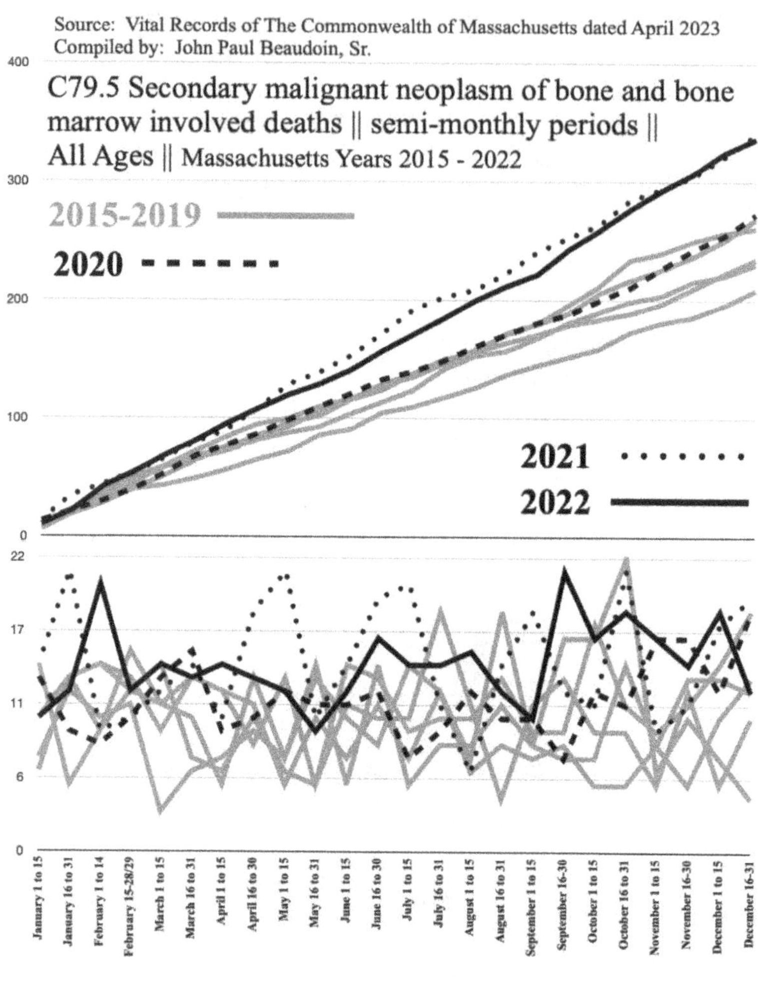

Figure 15.8

It is clear in the upper panel of Figure 15.8 that bone and marrow cancer-involved deaths rose alarmingly in 2021 and 2022. Two consecutive years of non-seasonal excess deaths are a strong signal which should trigger an urgent investigation by departments charged with protecting public health.

Figure 15.9 shows bone and marrow cancer-involved deaths by age group. These excess cancers are not confined to the elderly.

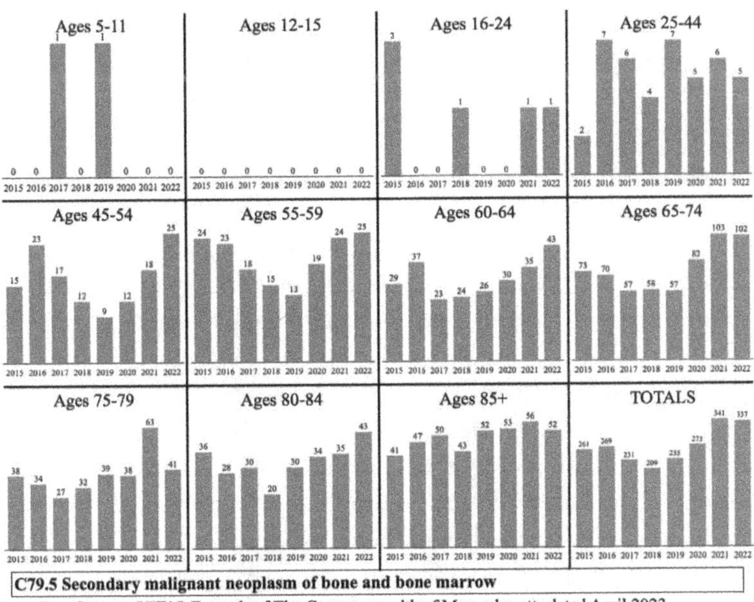

Figure 15.9

There is no question there is an issue with bone and marrow cancers. It is not seasonal and impacts a wide range of ages.

OPINION

It isn't practical to analyze all ICD-10 cancer codes in this book. There are simply too many. When all of these cancer codes are considered in the aggregate, the overlap of the individual signals mask one another. The two codes discussed individually in this chapter are among those which show clear signals of significant *excess* since covid vaccines were introduced in 2021.

My website, https://viaveravita.com, presents the data for other ICD-10 malignant neoplasm codes such as peritoneum and retroperitoneum cancer and B-cell lymphocytic leukemia. These were significantly in *excess* in 2021 and 2022.

Regardless of my biases while authoring this book, the raw data and case studies scream for investigation. The reason public health agencies exist is to monitor, study, and raise alerts regarding causes of death and injury.

None of our public health institutions at the federal or state levels seem to be interested in public health data analyses. This is not likely a matter of incompetence. The truth uncovered in this book is very damaging to public trust in government. It seems that government agencies, whose specific mission is to protect the public health, do not want the public to know the truth. Their apparent ignorance of this tragic data seems to be willful.

People are still talking about the Pfizer trials more than two years into the covid vaccination campaign. Meanwhile, billions of vaccinated people comprise readily available data. The databases of every state health department contain immensely more data than the Pfizer and Moderna trials combined. It seems clear that the state health departments and the CDC must be deliberately ignoring these data troves.

The purported covid pandemic was used by governments to instill public fear. Our military psyop manuals explain the methodology. Fear makes the mass of people compliant. People were programmed to accept what they were told. Fear was employed to induce the people to accept loss of freedom for a purport of safety. Useless, absurd measures such as arrows on supermarket aisle floors, plexiglass on lecterns, and masking the entire population were imposed to train people using the same methods that are successful with any other animal. We were told to accept shut downs to "flatten the curve." Then the shutdowns were extended indefinitely. We were told that we could go back to normal if we took the experimental gene therapy injections. Yet the gene therapy injections were fraudulently marketed as "safe and effective vaccines" to trick the public into ready acceptance of these dangerous, experimental interventions. "Vaccine" was accompanied by the useful propaganda label, "antivaxer," conveniently applied to anyone curious or skeptical about an experimental gene therapy product that bypasses the mucosal lung defenses and is injected directly into the body.

These are my opinions, but the graphs stand on their own as factual depictions of government's own data. There is no way that governments can get around the carnage they've wrought upon the credulous innocent.

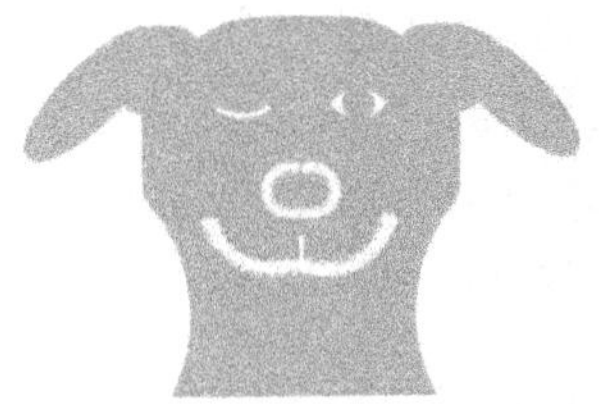

Chapter 16
Strokes and Neurological Maladies

Several people sent me stories of their loved one's stroke deaths as I became known for understanding ICD-10 codes and death certificates. For several months, I searched the circulatory system ICD-10 code categories expecting them to be listed under "I" codes because they involve hemorrhage (bleeding) or ischemia (from clotting).

Hemorrhagic stroke occurs from ruptured blood vessels that service the brain. Ischemic stroke occurs from clots in blood vessels that service the brain, thereby depriving the brain of oxygenated blood or thereby allowing pressure to build up behind the clot, causing brain swelling. This paragraph does not represent medical terms or medical descriptions. The situations are much more complicated than a few sentences.

The "I6" prefix of ICD-10 codes represents "Cerebrovascular diseases." These include subarachnoid hemorrhages, intracerebral hemorrhages, intracranial hemorrhages, cerebral infarctions, stroke not specified as hemorrhage or infarction, and others.

Two terms are important to know for this chapter. *Ischemia* is a decrease in blood supply from a blockage, obstruction, or restriction in a vessel. *Infarction* is the resultant tissue death from inadequate blood supply to a region.

If your cells cannot get oxygen passed to them from oxygenated blood flowing through nearby capillaries, then they die. Too much cellular death will manifest in tissue death in that area. These terms commonly apply to heart and brain deaths but may also be applied for any part of the body.

Upon reflection on the death certificate of 17-year-old Eden MacDonald, who was mentioned in Chapter 2, I learned that these stroke deaths are often not certified as I6 prefix code deaths. Eden was certified using only one code, G08 "Intracranial and intraspinal phlebitis and thrombophlebitis." "G" codes represent "Diseases of the nervous system."

While investigating all the "G" codes, I found a trove of evidence that depicts 2021 and 2022 *excess* stroke and neurological-involved deaths. This is consistent with anecdotal reports of neurological issues in the living as well as the dead.

Given that the reader is now familiar with the graph formats, commentary is light.

G08 INTRACRANIAL THROMBOPHLEBITIS

Figure 16.1 shows annual deaths involving G08 Intracranial and intraspinal phlebitis and thrombophlebitis-involved deaths.

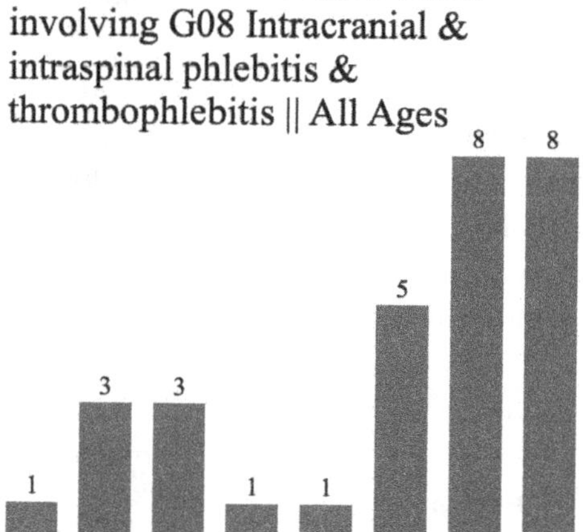

Source: Massachusetts Department of Health, Office of Vital Records
Compiled by: John Paul Beaudoin, Sr. || Data Received April 2023

Year	Excess	Excess % over Expected
2020	3	177.8%
2021	6	344.4%
2022	6	344.4%

Figure 16.1

Twelve *excess* deaths involving G08 "Intracranial and intraspinal phlebitis and thrombophlebitis" occurred in Massachusetts in 2021 and

2022. These few deaths are worthy of individual record investigation. Agents at the MA DPH and CDC can easily read the medical reports of these decedents to find commonalities. Even though the quantities in G08 are low, the signal is obvious and strong.

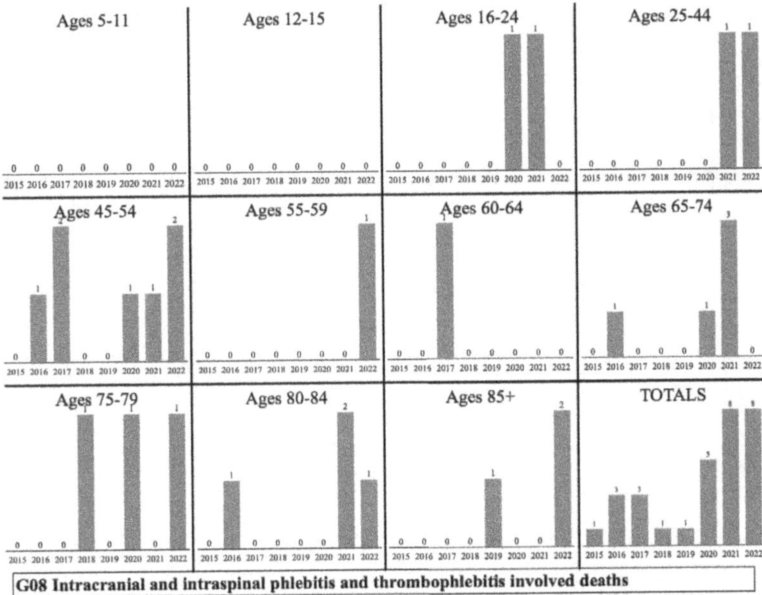

Data Source: VITAL Records of The Commonwealth of Massachusetts dated April 2023
Compiled by: John Paul Beaudoin, Sr.

Figure 16.2

The Figure 16.2 age group graphs are shown to satisfy curiosity. There is not much that can be gleaned from such low numbers except that they happen to the young and the old.

G90 AUTONOMIC NERVOUS SYSTEM

The term “
” spikes in internet searches every October as shown in Figure 16.3.[1] Other than October, there is a linear and steadily growing baseline trend from 2013 through 2021.

At the beginning of 2022, both the troughs and the October peak of internet searches for “dysautonomia” effectively doubled.

The October spikes may coincide with an annual research paper or conference related to dysautonomia.

Even if one research paper caused the October 2022 spike, that does not explain the year-long baseline increase in Figure 16.3. There was definitely a large increase in interest in dysautonomia in 2022.

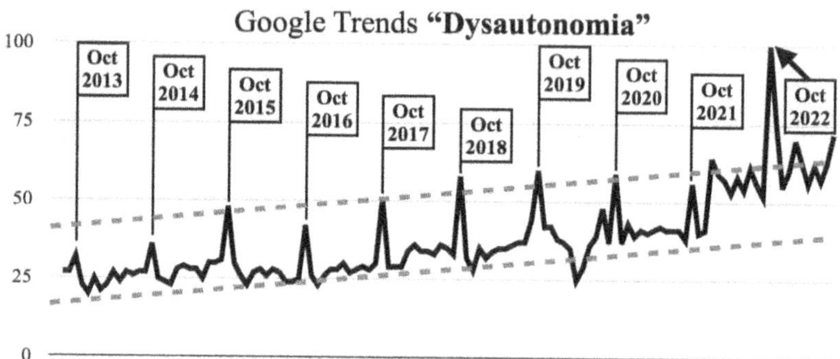

Figure 16.3

Dysautonomia is a disorder of the autonomic nervous system (ANS). Your ANS includes functions you don't have think about in order for them to continue operations. The beating rhythm of your heart, your breathing rate and volume, and digestion are autonomic functions.

The G90 ICD-10 code prefix includes:[2]

- G90.0 Idiopathic peripheral autonomic neuropathy
- G90.1 Familial dysautonomia [Riley-Day]
- G90.2 Horner syndrome
- G90.4 Autonomic dysreflexia
- G90.5 Complex regional pain syndrome type I
- G90.6 Complex regional pain syndrome type II
- G90.7 Complex regional pain syndrome, other and unspecified type
- G90.8 Other disorders of autonomic nervous system
- G90.9 Disorder of autonomic nervous system, unspecified

Figure 16.4 shows the annual totals for deaths involving G90 "Disorders of the autonomic nervous system."

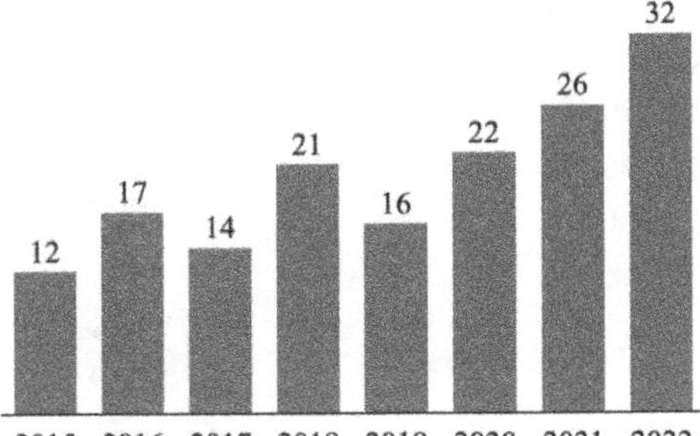

Year	Excess	Excess % over Expected
2020	2	12.2%
2021	5	25.0%
2022	10	45.5%

Figure 16.4

Excess deaths involving the autonomic nervous system total 15 in Massachusetts in 2021 and 2022, a substantial 45.5% increase over *expected* in 2022.

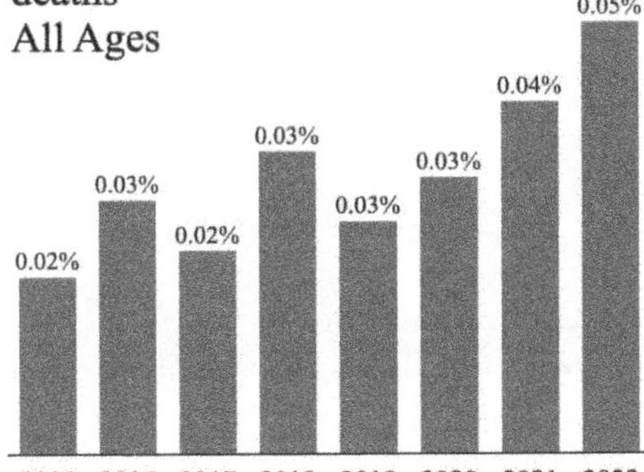

Figure 16.5

Adjusting for All-Cause deaths, Figure 16.5 depicts that G90 was indeed normal in 2020. Only 2021 and 2022 are substantially higher than baseline years and 2020.

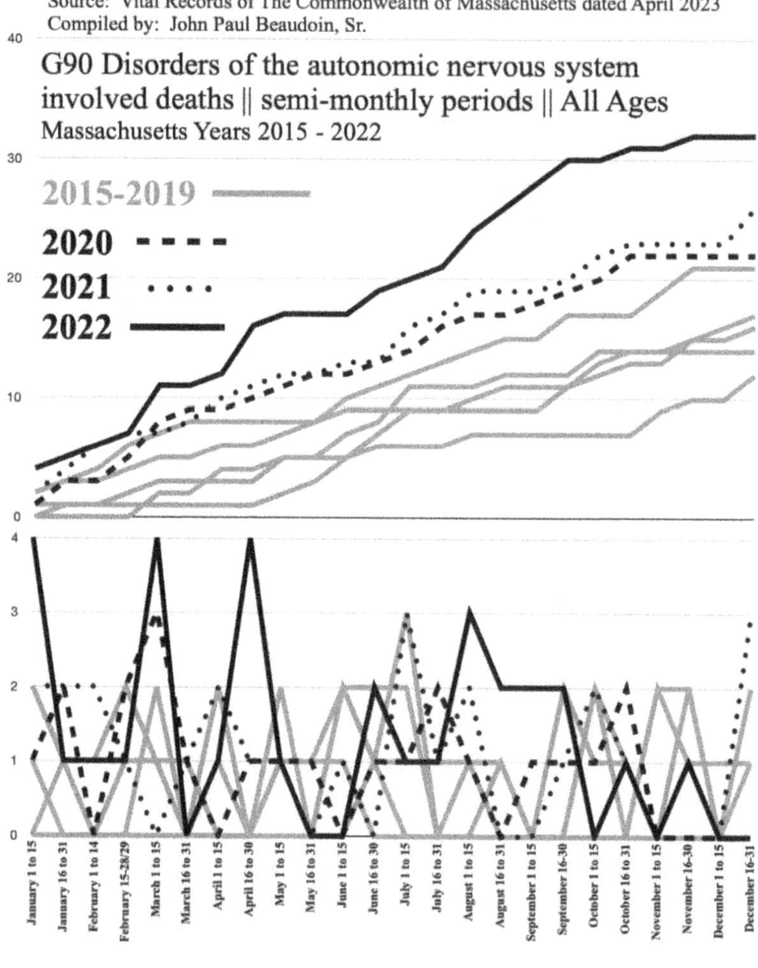

Figure 16.6

The timeline of G90 autonomic nervous system-involved deaths in Figure 16.6 depicts the year 2022 to be an unrestrained, unstable system causing more deaths as time continues.

Please note that while these "G" codes have few deaths in total compared to some of the "I" and "D" codes, there are more than a dozen of these "G" codes that are in substantial *excess*. Many tens of Massachusetts citizens lost their lives to causes involving stroke and neurological maladies.

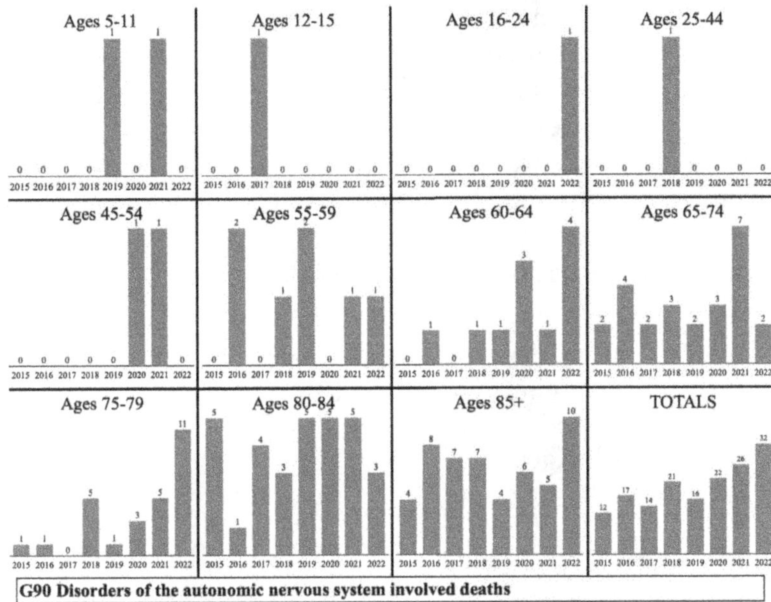

Figure 16.7

Figure 16.7 shows that *excess* G90-involved deaths seem to be over the age of 60 years old.

G96 OTHER CENTRAL NERVOUS SYSTEM

The difficulty with small quantities of deaths involving each prefix "G" code is that if they do represent stroke or neurological issues, the massive aggregate signal is lost among all these different small totals in individual codes. Each one, however, tells a story of death involving the nervous system in a pattern of extreme *excess* in 2021 or 2022, or both years.

Figure 16.8 shows the total of deaths involving G96 prefix "Other disorders of central nervous system." Following the totals, Figure 16.9 shows the G96 percentages of All-Cause deaths by year.

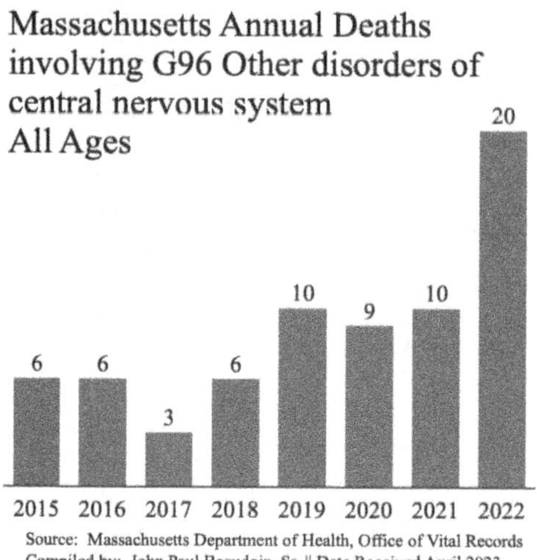

Year	Excess	Excess % over Expected
2020	0	4.7%
2021	1	6.4%
2022	10	96.1%

Figure 16.8

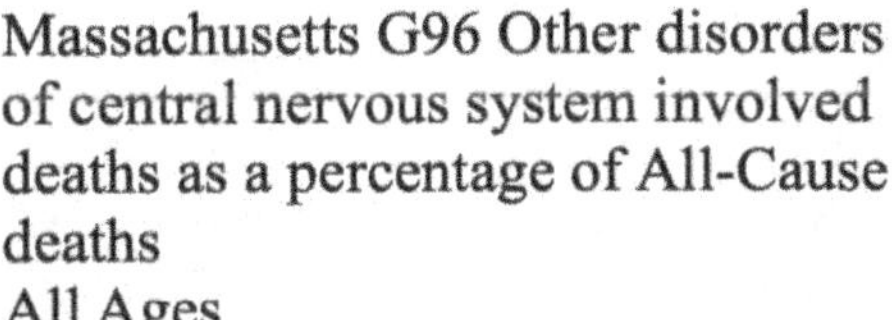

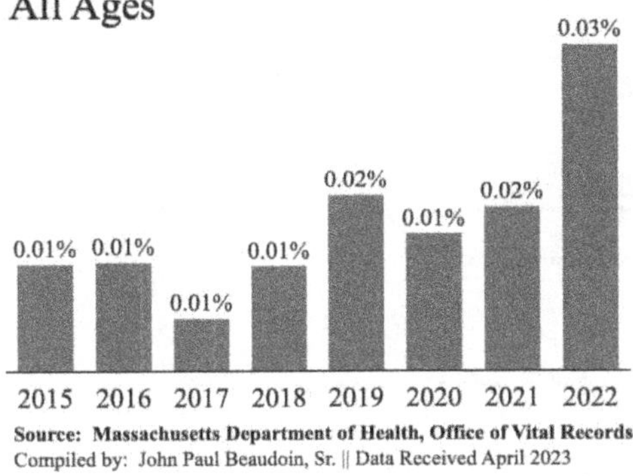

Figure 16.9

Figures 16.8 and 16.9 depict a massive 2022 increase in deaths involving "Other disorders of central nervous system." The *excess* 11 deaths should not be dismissed as a low number. These graphs represent deaths in one state from one small "G" prefix category. Extrapolated across the USA, this one small number ICD-10 code would be involved in ~ 540 deaths and would have caused any other vaccine to be pulled from the market.

Covid immunizations get a free pass from all government scrutiny as these tens of deaths per code category add up to thousands of *excess* deaths in one state.

How do the MA DPH and the CDC dismiss ~ 100% increase in G96-involved deaths in Massachusetts 2022? What do they do with all this incredibly important and rich data that provides a look into the health of society on a weekly basis? Death certificate analysis such as is in this book leads research papers by at least a year. Later in this book will be explained how death certificates can be an early warning system to society.

As a percent of All-Cause deaths in Figure 16.9, note that 2020 fades again into baseline normal. Only the covid immunization booster year, 2022, stands out.

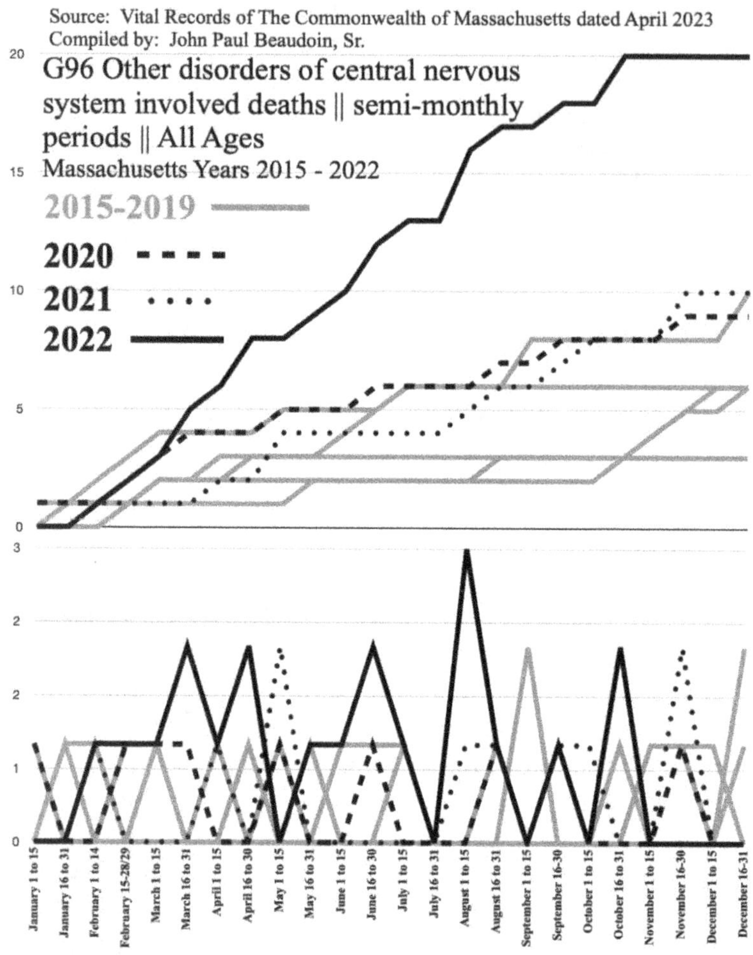

Figure 16.10

There is no seasonality expression in Figure 16.10. G96-involved deaths occur at any time of year in the years shown.

Year 2022 is an unstable system causing a massive increase in *excess* deaths continuing into 2023.

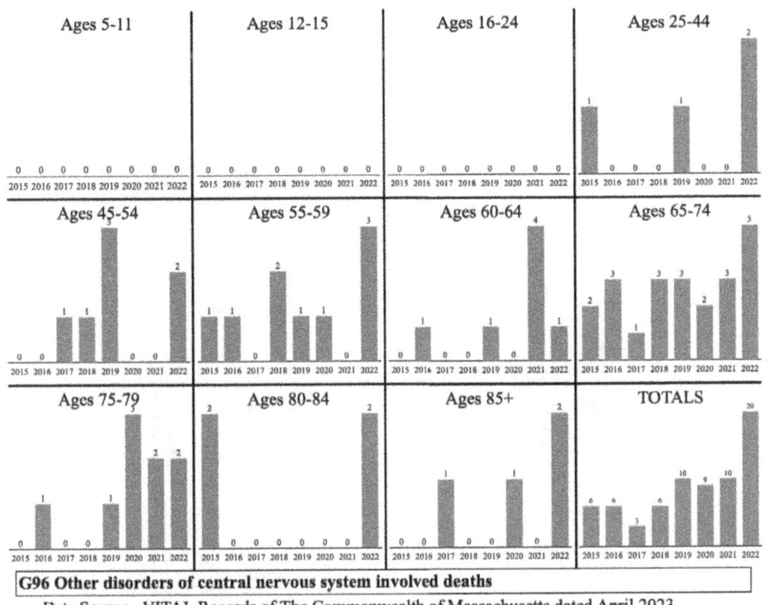

Figure 16.11

The age groups in Figure 16.11 show *excess* G96-involved deaths in various ages down to 25 years old.

Young and middle-aged people who survived two years of covid *per se* died in 2022 from stroke and neurological issues after 2 to 5 covid immunizations. The evidence is overwhelming.

G93.4 ENCEPHALOPATHY

If someone dies with a clot in their lungs, it is a pulmonary embolism for which there are only two ICD-10 codes. If someone dies with a clot in their head, more than twenty different ICD-10 codes can be applied, depending on the vessel, the brain area, hemorrhage or ischemia, swelling or no swelling, and other variables.

G93.4 Encephalopathy merely means disease of the brain, or any various condition affecting the brain.[3]

Encephalopathy-involved deaths annual totals are shown in Figure 16.12 and the percentage of All-Cause adjustment graph is shown in Figure 16.13.

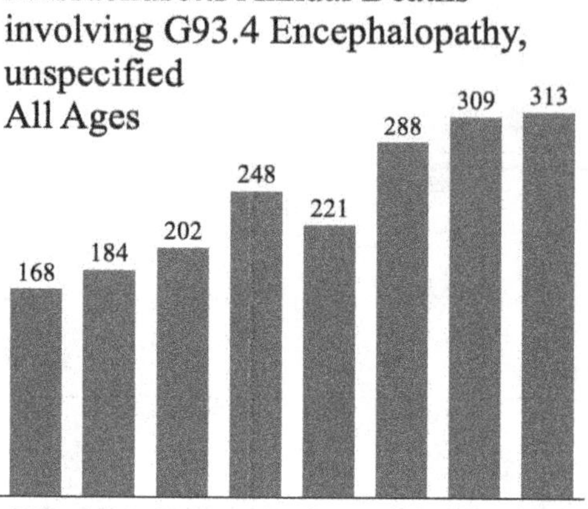

Source: Massachusetts Department of Health, Office of Vital Records
Compiled by: John Paul Beaudoin, Sr. || Data Received April 2023

Year	Excess	Excess % over Expected
2020	32	12.7%
2021	36	13.4%
2022	23	8.1%

Figure 16.12

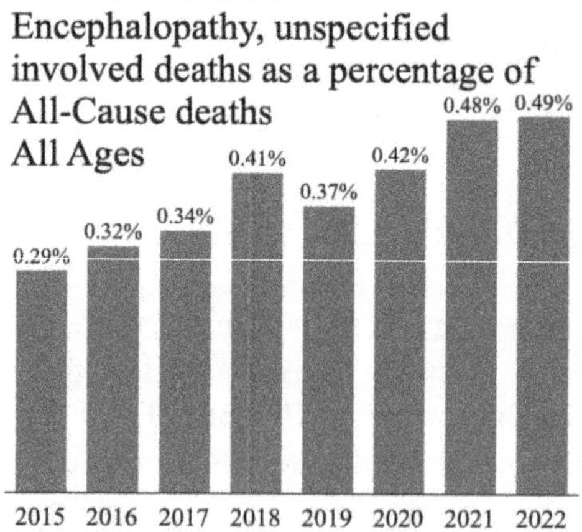

Source: Massachusetts Department of Health, Office of Vital Records
Compiled by: John Paul Beaudoin, Sr. || Data Received April 2023

Figure 16.13

Figure 16.12 shows a shocking 59 *excess* Encephalopathy-involved deaths occurred in 2021 and 2022 in Massachusetts.

The 2020 deaths, though totaling 32, are an artifact of the ~9,000 *excess* deaths that occurred in the spring first wave in very old people.

The graph in Figure 16.13, adjusted for total All-Cause deaths, depicts the true trend and the *excesses* of 2021 and 2022. Year 2020 again fades into 2015–2019 baseline years when adjusted for All-Cause deaths.

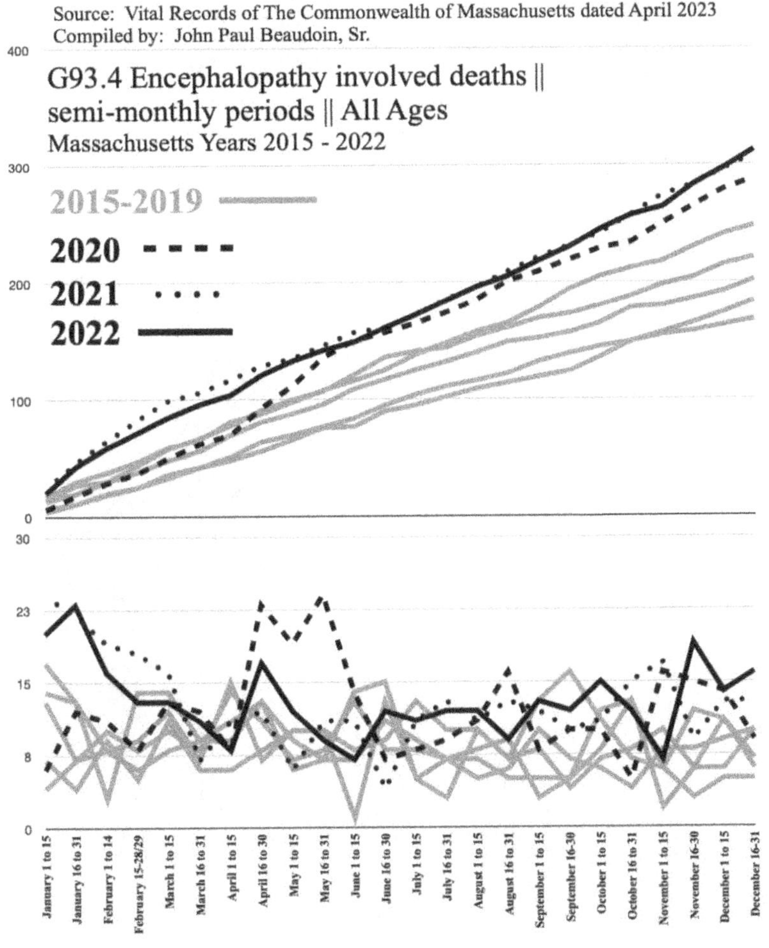

Figure 16.14

Figure 16.14 shows the timing of Encephalopathy-involved deaths. They are indeed excessive in 2020 only during that spring wave April through June.

The Simpson's paradox that the first wave in spring 2020 created across age groups and causes of death is why so many researchers worldwide have failed to find the smoking gun evidence as is depicted in this book. RLSD is necessary to untangle the paradoxes.

Note the steady slopes of 2021 and 2022 plots in the upper graph. The gap widens between the 2020 plot and the 2021 plot and also widens between the 2020 plot and the 2022 plot after the 2020 spring wave of deaths. It is subtle, but visible. This means that more deaths involving encephalopathy were occurring throughout 2021 and 2022 than throughout 2020, except for that first spring wave of purported covid deaths from around March to June 2020.

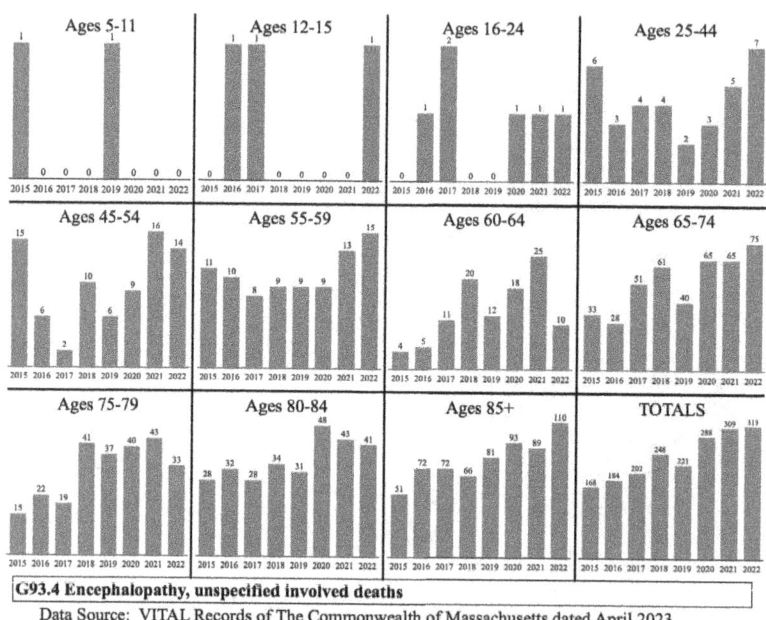

Figure 16.15

Most age groups in Figure 16.15 show strong increases in 2021 and 2022. Only the "Ages 80–84" group shows the greatest overall number in 2020.

What happened in 2015 in the two age groups "Ages 25–44" and "Ages 45–54"? What caused such an anomalous increase in Encephalopathy in middle-aged people?

This is why I continue to raise the point that the MA DPH and CDC hoard and hide data from the public. They gain little utility from such a valuable resource as the RLSD of the death certificate database. I have found anomalies that could have been caused by a new medicine or some other externality. The cause could possibly have been a contaminated recreational drug lot sold into a community. Again, death certificates lead research papers by more than a year. Death certificates are a robust and valuable early warning system.

It is surely sad to see how many younger people in *excess* lost their lives involving Encephalopathy in 2021 and 2022. People in their 20s through 60s should not be losing their lives to stroke and neurological issues caused by clots and bleeds in their heads.

OPINION

Again, it is important to remind the reader that all these *excess* deaths are people who have families who love them. They will be missed by many.

Many of the dead did what they thought was right in taking covid immunizations. They took a new gene therapy drug platform the government called a "vaccine." Why would adults take an experimental drug made on an experimental platform never before injected en masse into human beings? Some did so because they were made fearful by media and politicians and thought the injection would protect them from covid. Some took it because it was required to maintain employment or matriculation in university. Some took it because government schools required it for enrollment. Some were solicited into a moral barter as they were told they were good citizens and cared about others if they submitted to the experimental gene drug.

In Figure 16.15, the "Ages 12–15" group of G93.4 "Encephalopathy" depicts one 2022 death. RLSD allows me to quickly examine the record.

Syeisha was a 12-year-old girl who died in September 2022. Part I of her death certificate only states Cause A as "*PROBABLE SEIZURE*" and Part II states, "*EPILEPTIC ENCEPHALOPATHY (GABRB2 MUTATION), ASTHMA.*"

Syeisha had a genetic condition of epilepsy, severity unknown from her death certificate.

We The People need to know if and when 12-year-old Syeisha was vaccinated for covid. Maybe she was not vaccinated. Maybe she was. The People deserve to know what harm may be done to their children.

Amaya was age 12 upon her death and she was vaccinated in the same month of her ultimate stroke death from "*cerebellar tonsillar and bilateral uncal herniation*." (See Chapter 3)

When I looked for the record representing the one bar in the 12–15 age group, I expected to find the record of Amaya. I suppose I'm not surprised to see a different name there. There are many deaths of children who have disorders from birth or from accidents years earlier. These people at the margins of health do not fare well during diseases. And it seems they fare even worse when they are injected with the experimental drug cocktail called a "covid vaccine." The state should verify the dates of immunization of the decedents.

Why do the MA DPH and CDC seemingly never investigate young deaths for immunizations as the cause of death? Why do they willfully ignore the death data in deliberate indifference to child and adult losses of life? Why do they ignore a mass scale *excess* death signal across specific causes related to covid vaccines? Why do they ignore the literature and case studies of vaccine deaths and injuries such as Brianna's?

One obvious and manipulative propaganda tactic in the research papers and manufacturers' literature is to write "rare" or "extremely rare" without defining those subjective terms.

What is *rare*? What is *extremely rare*? Would you accept an injection death risk of *rare* that is 1 in 100? Or rare that is 1 in 1,000? Or 1 in 1,000,000? Given that no healthy children died from covid in three years in Massachusetts that we know for sure, and knowing that Cassidy's death certificate is likely fraudulent, then would you risk your child's life on a covid vaccine? Knowing what you now know from the facts brought forth in this book, would you take a covid gene drug immunization?

To close Chapter 16, please take time to review a few selected individual "G" codes in Figures 16.16 and 16.17.

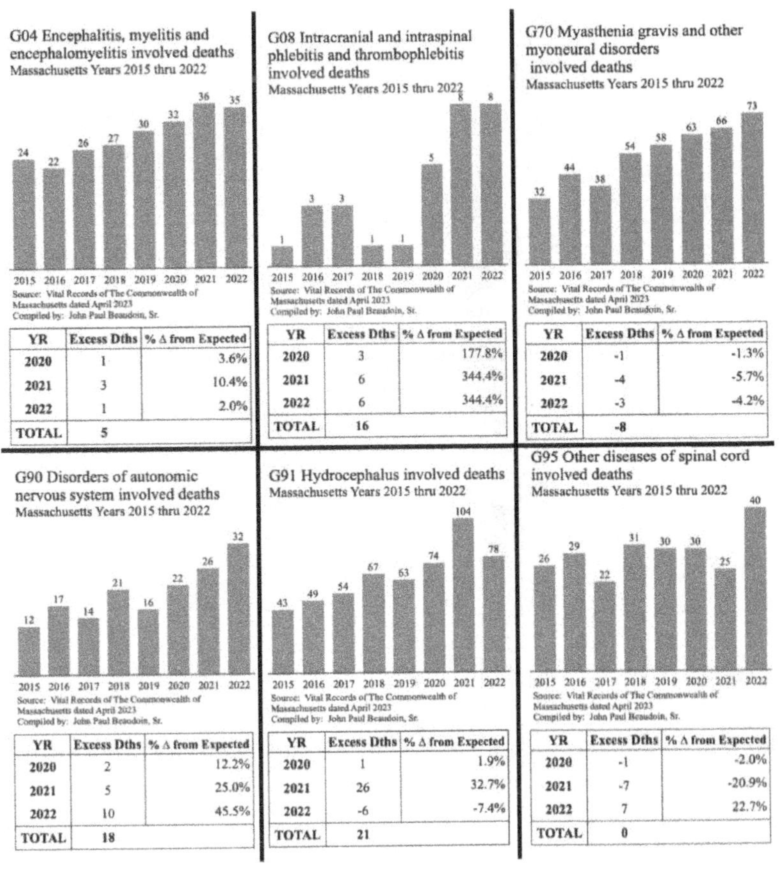

G04

YR	Excess Dths	% Δ from Expected
2020	1	3.6%
2021	3	10.4%
2022	1	2.0%
TOTAL	5	

G08

YR	Excess Dths	% Δ from Expected
2020	3	177.8%
2021	6	344.4%
2022	6	344.4%
TOTAL	16	

G70

YR	Excess Dths	% Δ from Expected
2020	-1	-1.3%
2021	-4	-5.7%
2022	-3	-4.2%
TOTAL	-8	

G90

YR	Excess Dths	% Δ from Expected
2020	2	12.2%
2021	5	25.0%
2022	10	45.5%
TOTAL	18	

G91

YR	Excess Dths	% Δ from Expected
2020	1	1.9%
2021	26	32.7%
2022	-6	-7.4%
TOTAL	21	

G95

YR	Excess Dths	% Δ from Expected
2020	-1	-2.0%
2021	-7	-20.9%
2022	7	22.7%
TOTAL	0	

Figure 16.16

Figure 16.16 depicts the following"G" codes.

- G04 Encephalitis, myelitis and encephalomyelitis
- G08 Intracranial and intraspinal phlebitis and thrombophlebitis
- G70 Myasthenia gravis and other myoneural disorders
- G90 Disorders of the autonomic nervous system
- G91 Hydrocephalus
- G95 Other diseases of the spinal cord

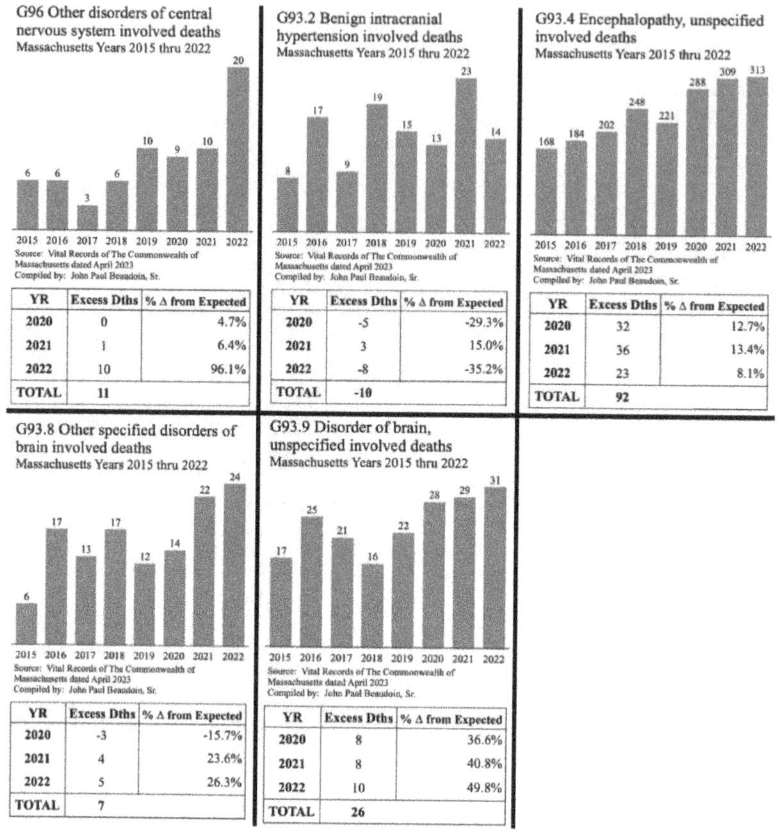

G96:

YR	Excess Dths	% Δ from Expected
2020	0	4.7%
2021	1	6.4%
2022	10	96.1%
TOTAL	11	

G93.2:

YR	Excess Dths	% Δ from Expected
2020	-5	-29.3%
2021	3	15.0%
2022	-8	-35.2%
TOTAL	-10	

G93.4:

YR	Excess Dths	% Δ from Expected
2020	32	12.7%
2021	36	13.4%
2022	23	8.1%
TOTAL	92	

G93.8:

YR	Excess Dths	% Δ from Expected
2020	-3	-15.7%
2021	4	23.6%
2022	5	26.3%
TOTAL	7	

G93.9:

YR	Excess Dths	% Δ from Expected
2020	8	36.6%
2021	8	40.8%
2022	10	49.8%
TOTAL	26	

Figure 16.17

Figure 16.17 depicts the following "G" codes.

- G96 Other disorders of the central nervous system
- G93.2 Benign intracranial hypertension
- G93.4 Encephalopathy
- G93.8 Other specified disorders of the brain
- G93.9 Disorder of the brain, unspecified

A reasonable person cannot look at these graphs and deny that there is a significant public health crisis and emergency in deaths involving neurological issues.

The MA DPH and the CDC are willfully ignoring this public health crisis. It is an undeniable fact.

What is causing these neurological *excess* deaths? We will not know unless government steps aside and lets The People access the data that the government is hoarding and hiding.

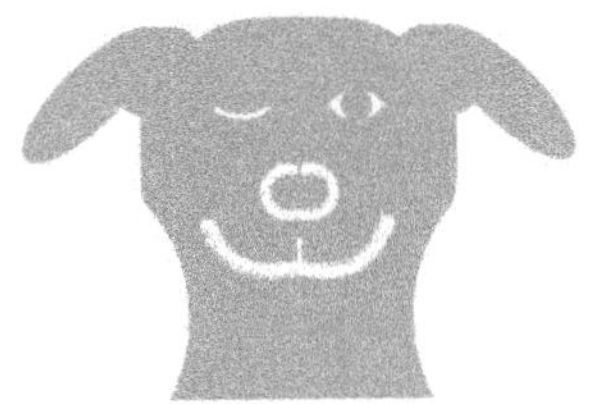

Chapter 17
Acute Renal Failure

Of all ICD-10 codes, N17.9 "Acute renal failure, unspecified" (ARF) -involved deaths shows one of the greatest increases in causes of death in 2021 and 2022. In Massachusetts alone, *excess* ARF-involved deaths in 2021 and 2022 total nearly 2,000 souls. ARF is a pandemic in its own right. Has the Massachusetts Department of Public Health or the CDC even noticed this calamity?

The CDC should be aware of this epidemic because it is not confined only to Massachusetts. Chapter 10, *The Minnesota Memorandum*, proves that this epidemic of kidney death is also similarly manifest in Minnesota.

"Acute" means sudden. Most ARF-involved decedents did not have a kidney issue, then they suddenly developed a kidney issue and died. Only around 11% of ARF-involved deaths in Massachusetts also involved "Chronic kidney disease" (CKD). *Id est*, almost 90% of ARF-involved decedents, an overwhelming majority, did not have CKD before ARF killed them.

The N17.9 ARF story evinces a brutal truth about our health systems. Please pay close attention to this chapter. The information herein may save your life or the life of a beloved. Do not let doctors and hospital staff coerce you into taking a drug called remdesivir, brand named, "Veklury." Demand to know what they are hooking up to you or anyone whom you want to survive their hospital stay. The hundreds of thousands of *excess* deaths in the United States involving ARF should immediately be investigated. A careful review of ARF-involved deaths is required for all combinations and timing of medicaments administered, including remdesivir, baricitinib, vancomycin, covid immunization, and covid *per se*.

Our society is rife with some who lack empathy. Doctors and other health professionals are not immune to this character trait. Some will follow orders, which they rationalize to be recommendations, guidelines, or "the standard of care," knowing that the results that flow from their actions may end someone's life. They prescribe procedures and medications that they would not themselves take nor would allow to be administered to their loved ones.

They do this for a few reasons. They are solicited through monetary incentives in the CARES Act and other legislation. They are coerced by medical certification boards, state medical licensing boards, and hospital administrators by threats of medical license investigation, suspension, or revocation. They are protected from scrutiny, lawsuit, and prosecution by the liability shield in the PREP Act and other policies that protect them, their employers, and the government agent enforcers.

Some physicians, hospital administrators, and staff know there will be no punishment for an immoral fatal act. They also know that failure to cooperate with the imposed "standard of care" could be a career-ending act. They then prescribe the administration of a fatal medicament seemingly without suffering internal conflict. We, who know the evidence, are left with a struggle to accept this ugly, sad truth about our broken health systems and the immoral professionals who act in deliberate indifference to human life.

Figure 17.1 shows ARF-involved deaths in Massachusetts for 2015 through 2022. There were 1,940 *excess* N17.9 ARF-involved deaths in 2021 and 2022.

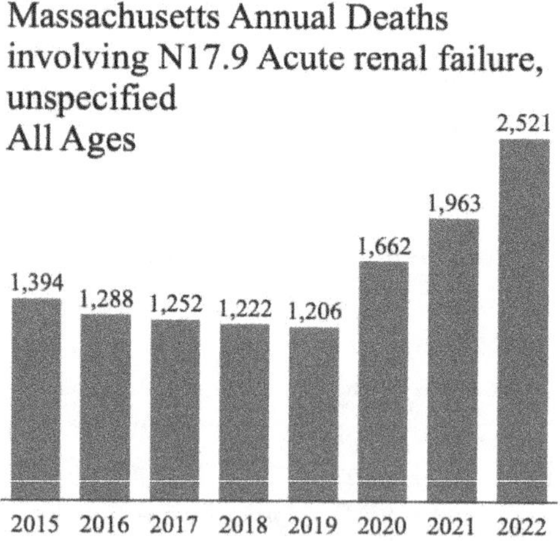

Year	Excess	Excess % over Expected
2020	390	30.6%
2021	691	54.3%
2022	1,249	98.1%

Figure 17.1

Some have suggested that the *excess* ARF-involved deaths may have resulted, in part, from covid immunizations. However, many believe the large majority of *excess* ARF-involved deaths are due to remdesivir, a drug issued, like covid vaccines, under Emergency Use Authorization (EUA). Thus, the 2020 *excess* ARF-involved deaths tallying 390 should also be investigated because remdesivir was approved in 2020 and the financial incentives for hospitals to administer it began November 2, 2020.[1]

> *CMS issued an Interim Final Rule with Comment Period that established the New COVID-19 Treatments Add-on Payment (NCTAP) under the Medicare Inpatient Prospective Payment System (IPPS). The NCTAP, designed to mitigate potential financial disincentives for hospitals to provide new COVID-19 treatments, is effective from November 2, 2020, until September 30, 2023.*[1]

This text from the Center of Medicare and Medicaid Services (CMS) government website aligns with a longstanding business concept. "The pay plan defines the behavior." If remdesivir is the culprit in kidney failure, responsible for killing more than 100,000 people in USA in two years, then the CMS remdesivir incentive is a behavior modification tactic that proved very effective on hospital administrators and the doctors they employed. They will probably never admit that they never looked at side effects and just prescribed it because the government said to prescribe it.

Prior to covid, remdesivir was tested in comparison to a few other drugs as an antiviral treatment during Ebola outbreaks in Africa. Of all drugs tested, remdesivir had the highest day 28 mortality rate at 53.1%.[2] The testing of remdesivir was halted when interim analysis showed this large number of people who had died. In another study, liver and kidney cells were shown to have unique sensitivity to remdesivir, and it was indicated that updosing would likely result in hepato- (liver) and nephro- (kidney) toxicity.[3] Yet, remdesivir was pulled out of mothballs as a response to covid.

CMS has never explained why the financial incentive was issued. And CMS never explained how the incentive advanced the wellbeing of covid patients and the taxpayers. Does the CMS financial incentive have any relationship to the fact that Dr. Anthony Fauci receives a royalty every time remdesivir is administered?

Figure 17.2 shows ARF-involved deaths in Massachusetts for 2015 through 2022 adjusted for All-Cause deaths.

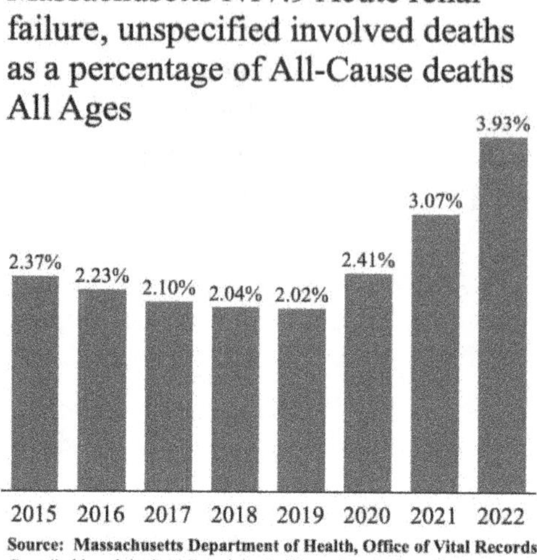

Figure 17.2

Figure 17.2 shows that, when adjusted for the increased number of All-Cause deaths during the first covid wave, 2020 ARF-involved deaths fall in line with the baseline years 2015 through 2019. During the first covid wave in spring of 2020, many may have died "with" ARF rather than "from" ARF.

Figure 17.3 shows semi-monthly plots of the Massachusetts N17.9 ARF deaths.

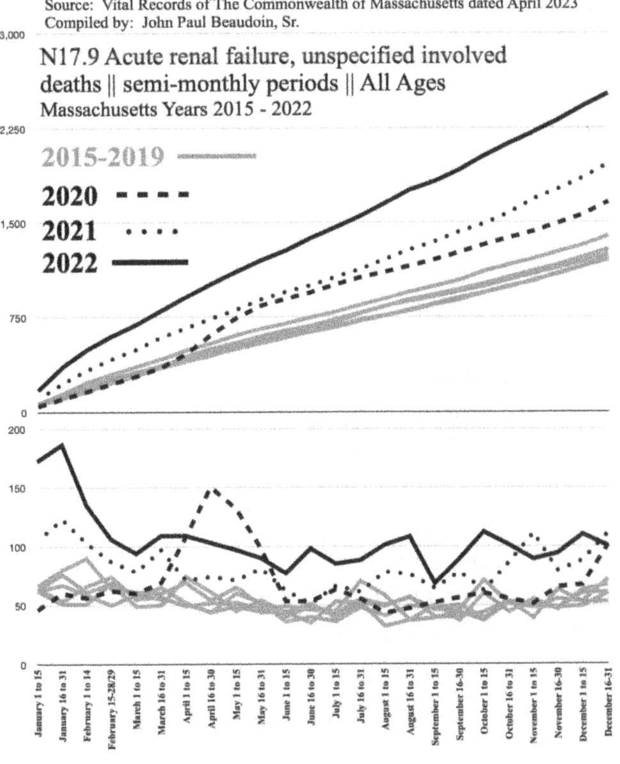

Figure 17.3

The bottom panel of Figure 17.3 shows that ARF-involved deaths start out normally at the beginning of 2020 running at the same rate as the baseline years, 2015–2019 (gray plots). They then rise to a peak in April concurrent with the first covid wave. This supports the idea that some people may have died from covid with ARF rather than from ARF. After the first wave concluded, ARF deaths returned to the level of the baseline years.

Notice also in the bottom panel of Figure 17.3 that the 2020 dashed line shoots up in December, only a few weeks after the CMS financial incentive.

The story is different in 2021 and 2022. To be sure, there are peaks in ARF deaths concurrent with the second covid wave during winter 2020/2021 and the third way during winter 2021/2022. However, it is significant that when the seasonal peaks wound down, ARF deaths did **not** return to the level of the baseline years. Also significant is the fact that the peak of ARF deaths during winter 2021/2022 greatly exceeded the peak in spring 2021 and the level of ARF deaths continued significantly above the baseline levels through the end of 2022. Covid deaths were much lower that winter than they were during the first wave. Clearly, this drastic increase in ARF-involved deaths cannot be related to covid. Something else was responsible for killing so many people. Remdesivir is the most likely culprit. Covid immunization side effects may share responsibility.

There is a sustained, epidemic level of ARF deaths in 2021 and 2022. Excluding cardiac arrest, these *excess* ARF deaths comprise the biggest single cause of death in decades. Two thousand *excess* deaths occurred from one cause in one state; yet the CDC and Massachusetts Department of Public Health are asleep at the wheel. If they noticed this serious safety signal, they have not alerted the public to it. **Are they willfully ignoring it, or even actively trying to cover it up?**

How does one explain such depraved indifference exhibited by healthcare professionals? Such callous inaction concurrent with legal and moral duties to act is nothing short of manslaughter and is more likely murder en masse.

The death toll at the Jonestown cult massacre in French Guyana in 1978 was greater than nine hundred.[4] More than double that number died needlessly in Massachusetts in 2021 and 2022 likely from government-incentivized administration of a so-called "medicine" known to cause kidney failure. These facts are not going away. The adverse effects of remdesivir are known. Yet remdesivir was one of the few approved treatments for covid. Why?

The CARES Act and FEMA in combination with a complex network of other regulations pays hospitals and care providers enormous sums of money to prescribe and administer remdesivir.

Figure 17.4 shows Massachusetts ARF-involved deaths in 2015 through 2022 by age group.

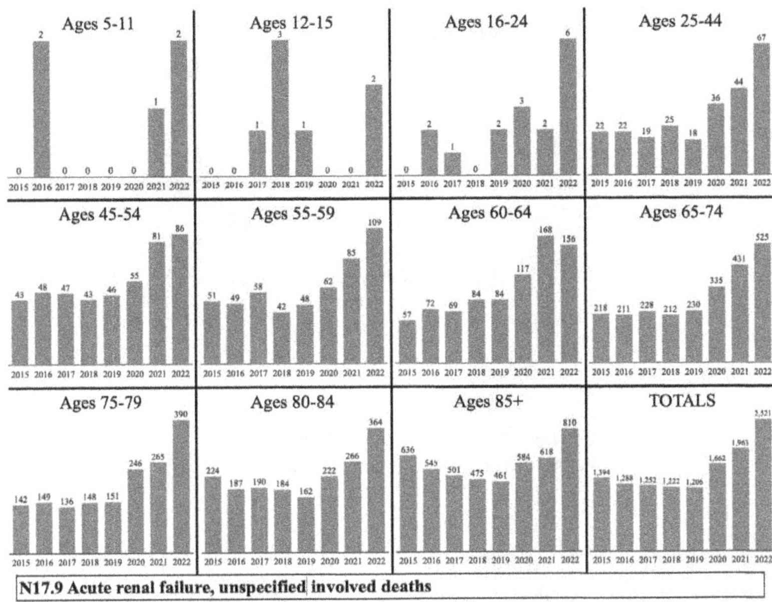

N17.9 Acute renal failure, unspecified involved deaths

Data Source: VITAL Records of The Commonwealth of Massachusetts dated April 2023
Compiled by: John Paul Beaudoin, Sr.

Figure 17.4

Figure 17.4 shows absolute carnage. Death in young people should not ever happen like this. It did not happen like this from covid in 2020 in Massachusetts, and yet some of these ARF-involved deaths are labeled covid deaths.

Three deaths in 5 to 11 year olds in 2021 and 2022 is difficult to fathom. Almost every age group shown is alarmingly high in ARF-involved deaths in years 2021 and 2022. Remember that ACP (All-Cause, covid, and pneumonia) *excess* deaths were cut in half from 2020 to 2021. ARF-involved deaths increased 100%.

This massive number of *excess* ARF deaths is not caused by covid or long covid, notwithstanding official government propaganda.

Figure 17.5 shows how ACP-involved deaths decreased from 2020 to 2021. Figure 17.6 shows how ARF-involved deaths increased from 2020 to 2021. The relationship between ACP and ARF is quite clearly inverted.

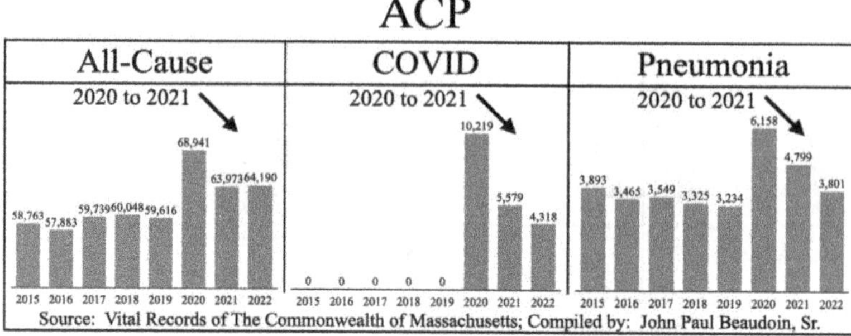

Figure 17.5

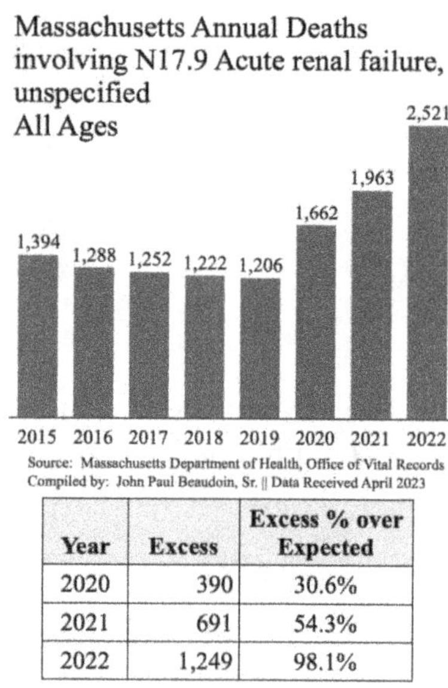

Year	Excess	Excess % over Expected
2020	390	30.6%
2021	691	54.3%
2022	1,249	98.1%

Figure 17.6

COMBINATIONS

In 2020–2022, there were {10219, 5579, 4318} U07.1 covid-involved deaths, {1662, 1963, 2521} N17.9 ARF-involved deaths, and {399, 388, 362} deaths involving both.

The respective percentages of covid-involved deaths of people who also had ARF involvement in 2020–2022 are {3.9%, 7.0%, 8.4%}. Clearly the incidence of ARF effectively doubled following the introduction of financial incentives to hospitals for the administration of remdesivir.

The respective percentages of ARF involved deaths of people who also had covid in 2020–2022 are {24.0%, 19.8%, 14.4%}. Contraction occurred over time.

Covid-involved deaths as a percentage of All-Cause deaths each year are {14.82%, 8.72%, 6.73%}. Contraction occurred over time.

ARF deaths as a percentage of All-Cause deaths each year are {2.41%, 3.07%, 3.93%}. Expansion occurred over time.

Deaths involving both covid and ARF as a percentage of total All-Cause deaths each year are {0.58%, 0.61%, 0.56%}.

No one can know for sure what caused and is causing massive *excess* ARF death numbers in 2021 and 2022 unless investigations are conducted. Start with the youngest decedents and look through their medical history for what changed in their lives just before ARF and death. Were they given a covid immunization? Did they test positive for covid? Did they have covid symptoms? Were they given remdesivir or baricitinib or vancomycin? How much? What dosage and schedule?

Will the Massachusetts Department of Public Health or the CDC conduct these simple and easy investigations to learn why some 100,000 *excess* people were killed by ARF in USA in 2021 and 2022? Demand they do so. Please do not allow your family or friends or yourself to fall victim to government incentivized lethal injection of "medication."

WHY CDC NUMBERS ARE DIFFERENT

CDC Wonder is a publicly accessible system for disseminating public health data and information.[5] Some may wonder why count totals in this book may differ from those found on CDC Wonder. If you look up "Acute renal failure" on CDC Wonder for Massachusetts, it will give you numbers for UCD, meaning "underlying cause of death" and MCD, meaning "multiple cause of death." The UCOD is the last entered cause in Part I of death certificates and is considered the root cause that began the causal chain of events leading to death. The MCOD's are all other causes mentioned in Parts I or II of the death certificate. Most of my data analyses include all ICD-10 codes used on death certificates because of the disparate behaviors among death certifiers in how they author death certificates. Here is an example regarding N17.9 ARF.

A 76-year-old man died in February 2023.

Cause A (Immediate Cause)
"*CANCER UNKNOWN PRIMARY SOURCE*" in "*MOS.*"

Cause B (Underlying Cause)
"*METASTATIC TO LIVER, SPLEEN, LYMPH NODES, BONES*" in "*MOS.*"

Part II (Other Significant Conditions Contributing to Death)
"*SYMPTOMATIC ANEMIA, ACUTE KIDNEY INJURY, 1 PACK PER DAY SMOKER*"

Causes C and D are empty fields, making Cause B the purported UCOD root cause of the man's death.

This death certificate does not make sense. It is backward and discombobulated. The Immediate Cause should be immediate. The other causes in Part I should be listed in backward time order with the UCOD root cause being last. And the Conditions Contributing should be relevant and contributing.

First of all, Cancer of "unknown primary source" in months seems strange. This is not just turbo cancer. This is mystery turbo cancer. The primary source cancer should likely be the UCOD root cause.

In my opinion, using only the causes given, and following the CDC instructions of how to fill out a death certificate, below is what this death certificate should look like.

Cause A "*ACUTE RENAL FAILURE*" in "*DAYS*"
Cause B "*SYMPTOMATIC ANEMIA*" in "*WKS.*"
Cause C "*METASTATIC LIVER, SPLEEN, LYMPH NODES, BONES CANCER*" in "*MOS.*"
Cause D "*NEOPLASM PRIMARY SOURCE UNKNOWN*" in "*MOS.*"
Conditions Contributing "*1 PACK PER DAY SMOKER*"

The above example is why I analyze all ICD-10 codes on a death certificate, and I do not differentiate between Parts I and II unless I have a specific reason to do so.

"Acute" renal failure should not be on Part II. "Acute" means sharp, severe, and sudden. If a kidney injury contributes to death, then clearly it is a cause and not just a contributing factor like alcoholism, family genetic history of renal failure, diabetes, obesity, or smoker, which are common Part II listings.

My version is a logical ordering per the CDC instructions. An unknown primary cancer occurred months ago, then it metastasized to the liver, spleen, and lymph nodes, which caused symptomatic anemia, and also caused the final and immediate cause of death, sudden kidney failure. Smoking contributes to general unhealthiness and probably should have been omitted unless they believed that it may have contributed to causing the cancer.

OPINION

This chapter should be a series of books all its own. As I tried to decide what information to include, the outline got very big, very fast. Instead of referencing the many scientific papers detailing the effects of remdesivir on organs, especially kidneys, and the Gilead stock holdings of that Fauci guy and his wife, I opted to keep the chapter targeted to data and analyses that depict a health emergency in Massachusetts, and, by extension, the entire USA.

People should demand that government agencies adhere to their stated missions, *exempli gratia*, "public health."

Fauci's wife works for the National Institutes of Health Clinical Center as a "bioethicist." She has a master's degree in nursing and PhD in Philosophy.[6] It is ethically improper and possibly illegal that she became the head of the Department of Bioethics in the same organization where her husband works as Director. Fauci promotes remdesivir as one of the few treatments for covid; and simultaneously was working behind the scenes to suppress all cheaper medications. These unethical acts were evaluated by his own wife. How does that happen in government?

How many died because other treatments were withheld so Fauci could sell remdesivir? How many died from remdesivir? Whatever is killing people by ARF is likely caused by man, not by nature. My answer, based on some 500,000 Massachusetts death certificates and some 420,000 Minnesota death certificates, extrapolated to the whole of USA, is that far more than 100,000 people died in U.S.A. in 2021 and 2022 involving ARF as a result of remdesivir, covid immunizations, baricitinib, vancomycin, or any combination of them.

From hard evidence and an understanding of the elements of the crime, I conclude that NIH, CDC, and FDA are clearly a RICO crime syndicate that caused the deaths of hundreds of thousands of Americans and millions of people worldwide.

I was invited to present to a group mostly comprising widows and widowers. Their stories were all similar with regard to hospital protocols killing their spouses. After I presented about 80 slides, Q &A ensued. Each person told their story. It was difficult to listen to their painful recollections. As they spoke, I often glanced at the picture of my eldest son on my desk. Grief and anger cycled through me seconds apart as I listened to them.

Their stories merge into the following montaged anecdote. Many walked into a hospital with oxygen saturation levels (%) in the mid-90s. They tested positive for covid, then were put on a covid protocol even if they only had a cough. They were sedated, put on remdesivir, often contrary to their explicit instructions, restricted from visitors, even spouses, and eventually they were ventilated. The hospital receives CARES Act money for declaring a patient to have covid, for putting a patient on a ventilator, and for prescribing remdesivir. People who walked into the hospital upright without assistance and had normal oxygen levels, then died from needless protocols and drug administration incentivized by the CARES Act. The shock of hearing these stories from genuine people who can provide medical files and evidence was enough to drive depression to the fore of thought.

Again, the saying from my career comes to mind, "The pay plan defines the behavior." Walter E. Williams often stated an old economic principle, "If you subsidize something, you will get more of it." [7] The idea is fairly obvious to anyone who takes the time to think about it. Thomas Sowell and Milton Friedman also likely made the same types of statements.

If you want more people diagnosed with covid, then subsidize covid diagnoses. The CARES Act does that.

If you want more people on ventilators, then subsidize the use of ventilators. The CARES Act does that using exorbitant bonuses for covid patients on ventilators.

If you want patients to receive remdesivir, whether they need it or not, then subsidize it. The CARES Act does that.

Remdesivir, a purported antiviral drug, is rumored to be several hundred dollars per dose, while ivermectin, a proven antiviral drug, is pennies per dose. Far greater than that, hospitals receive an additional twenty percent (20%) of the entire hospital bill, which often amounts to hundreds of thousands of dollars per patient, if remdesivir is used. Twenty percent (20%) of a $500,000 bill for a long ICU stay is a $100,000 bonus on a patient's bill if it includes remdesivir.[1]

Again, ARF-involved deaths, extrapolated from Massachusetts and Minnesota data, amount to an *excess* of around one hundred thousand *excess* people killed across the United States.

If the intent was to sell a medication, known to cause ARF and death, in place of safer medications such as ivermectin or Hydroxychloroquine, then each of these deaths is a murder for profit.

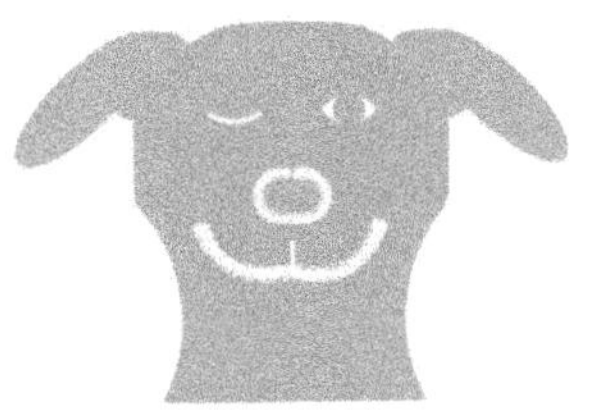

Chapter 18
Age Spectrum Profiles

The ***symptom spectrum profile*** of anomalous differences, expressed as *excess* deaths over the past eight years, is the focus of the prior five chapters of *TERTIA PARS*.

The conclusions thus far are:

- 2020 is a year of *excess* deaths predominantly respiratory system "J" code involved
- 2021 & 2022 are years of *excess* deaths predominantly circulatory system "I" code, blood-related "D" code, nervous system "G" code, and select blood-related cancers C77.9 & C79.5 involved (all related to blood *per se*, blood formation, and blood transport). These codes share underlying causal mechanisms related to clotting and autoimmunity. (Other cancers are also increasing in incidence rate.)

Viral and bacterial pandemics do not suddenly change how they kill you (mechanism of action) on a year boundary. The data is overwhelmingly clear and convincing that something else besides covid caused significant deaths beginning in 2021.

Chapter 18 focuses on changes in the ***age spectrum profile*** and the ***seasonality profile***. Beginning in 2021, the ***age*** and ***seasonality profiles*** also exhibit sharp changes from the ***profiles*** of 2020.

The average ages of death for All-Cause, covid, and *excess* deaths are compared. If they differ significantly, it suggests that the cause of *excess* deaths is likely something else besides covid.

The table in Figure 18.1 contains the numbers and average ages of All-Cause Massachusetts deaths for the years 2015 through 2022.

Year	Total Deaths	Average Age
2015	58,764	75.7
2016	57,883	75.3
2017	59,739	75.6
2018	60,048	75.7
2019	59,616	75.8
2020	68,941	76.2
2021	63,974	75.0
2022	64,191	75.4

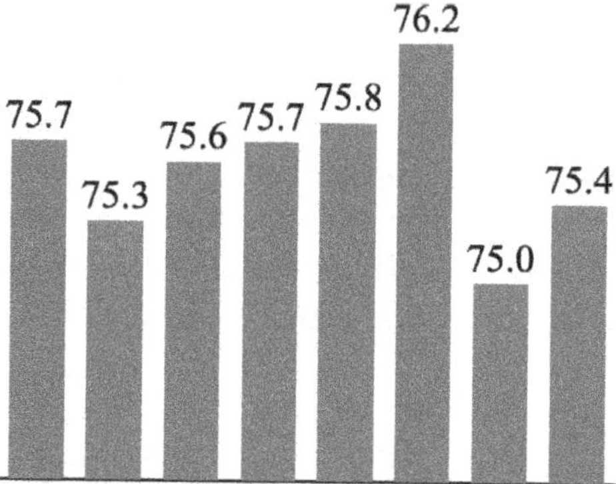

Source: Vital Records of The Commonwealth of Massachusetts; obtained April 2023
Compiled by: John Paul Beaudoin, Sr.

Figure 18.1

The table and bar graph in Figure 18.1 show that the average ages of All-Cause deaths for baseline years 2015 through 2019 range from 75.3 to 75.8. Hereinafter, this is called the "baseline range."

The average age of All-Cause deaths in the first year of covid, 2020, is 76.2, well above the baseline range.

The average age of All-Cause deaths in the first year of covid "vaccines," which is the second year of covid, 2021, is 75.0, well below baseline range.

The average age of All-Cause deaths in the second year of covid vaccines and third year of covid, 2022, is 75.4, which is within baseline range.

The table in Figure 18.2 contains the total annual numbers and corresponding average ages of deaths involving covid for years 2020, 2021, and 2022.

COVID-19 DEATHS & AVG AGES

Year	Total Deaths	Average Age
2020	10,219	81.3
2021	5,579	75.8
2022	4,318	78.0

Source: Vital Records of The Commonwealth of Massachusetts
Compiled by: John Paul Beaudoin, Sr.

Figure 18.2

In Figure 18.2, the average age of covid-involved (U07.1) deaths in 2020 is 81.3, which is much older than the baseline range. It mathematically follows that deaths labeled as involving covid likely caused the 2020 average age of All-Cause deaths to rise to 76.2, which is well above the baseline range.

The 2021 average age of covid-involved (U07.1) deaths is 75.8, exactly on the upper end of the baseline range. However, the 2021 All-Cause average age of deaths is 75.0, well below the baseline range.

Since the 2021 covid average age is within the baseline range, but the 2021 All-Cause average age is much lower than the baseline range, covid cannot mathematically have caused the 2021 All-Cause average age of deaths to be lower than baseline range. There must be something else killing younger people in 2021. The same reasoning applies to 2022.

Next, the All-Cause deaths for the baseline years is used to estimate the *expected* numbers of All-Cause deaths for 2020 through 2022. Recall that the more conservative estimate for *expected* All-Cause deaths uses the TREND method if the baseline years show a trend of a positive slope, or AVERAGE method, if the estimated slope of baseline year values is negative.

By using the conservative (higher) of the numbers derived from each method for *expected* deaths, the resulting calculations for *excess* deaths are conservatively lower than if either TREND or AVERAGE were solely used over the baseline years.

The table in Figure 18.3 shows TREND method applied to the data for baseline years, 2015 through 2019, in order to determine the *expected* and *excess* deaths totals in years 2020 through 2022.

	TOTALS
2015-2019 SLOPE	387
2015-2019 INTERCEPT	58,436
2020 TREND Expected	60,371
2021 TREND Expected	60,758
2022 TREND Expected	61,145
2020 EXCESS	8,570
2021 EXCESS	3,216
2022 EXCESS	3,047

Source: Vital Records of The Commonwealth of Massachusetts
Compiled by: John Paul Beaudoin, Sr.

Figure 18.3

To remind the reader of the TREND method, the 2020 *expected* value is the INTERCEPT plus five times the SLOPE. For 2021, the *expected* value is the INTERCEPT plus six times SLOPE; and for 2022, the *expected* value is the INTERCEPT plus seven times the SLOPE.

The following explanations for Method I and Method II are provided for those who may wish to follow and/or confirm the calculations. Readers may safely skip these explanations if they wish.

The basis for Methods I and II is the simple understanding that:

Excess = *Actual* minus *Expected*, or
Actual = *Excess* plus *Expected*

Add the weighting factor, average ages of deaths, for each variable in the latter equation. The equation then expands to:

Actual deaths * Average Age of *Actual* deaths = (*Expected* deaths * Average Age of *Expected* deaths) + (*Excess* deaths * Average Age of *Excess* deaths)

Then, solve the equation for "Average Age of *Excess* deaths."

Average Age of *Excess* deaths = ((Actual deaths * Average Age of Actual deaths) - (*Expected* Deaths * Average Age of *Expected* deaths)) ÷ *Excess* deaths

Method I

The first method answers the following question. Within what range would the "Average Age of *Excess* deaths" in each of the years 2020 through 2022 have to lie in order to bring the All-Cause *Actual* deaths for each of the years 2020 through 2022 within the range of "Average Age of *Expected* deaths," which is the baseline range (average age of deaths in years 2015 through 2019) in Method I?

Inputs

- Age range of the baseline years (Average Age of *Expected* deaths) is 75.3 to 75.8 (see Figure 18.1)
- In year 2020, *Actual* All-Cause deaths total 68,941 at an *Actual* Average age of 76.2 (see Figure 18.1)
- *Expected* 2020 deaths total 60,371 (see Figure 18.3)
- *Excess* deaths total 8,570 (see Figure 18.3)

Calculations

Year 2020 calculations are shown in detail.

The calculations follow these summary equations.

In order to calculate the age range of *excess* deaths for each of years 2020 through 2022, first the lower bound of baseline range (75.3) is used in the calculation, then the upper bound of baseline range (75.8) is used.

First, calculate the total *actual* person-years for 2020 by multiplying 68,941 (total *actual* deaths) by 76.2 (*actual* average age).

76.2 * 68,941 = 5,253,304.2 *actual* person-years

Next, calculate the *expected* person-years for 2020 by multiplying 60,371 (*expected* 2020 total deaths) by 75.3 (lower bound baseline range, or the *expected* lower bound age).

75.3 * 60,371 = 4,545,936.3 *expected* person-years

Lastly, subtract the two products to get the *excess* person-years and divide that difference by 8,570 (total *excess* deaths).

(5,253,304.2 - 4,545,936.3) ÷ 8,570 = 82.5 years of age

The process is repeated using the upper value of the age range for the baseline years (75.8).

((76.2 * 68,941) - (75.8 * 60,371)) ÷ 8,570 = 79.0 years of age

Results

- The "Average Age of *Excess* deaths" in 2020 must range between 79.0 to 82.5.
- The "Average Age of *Excess* deaths" in 2021 must range between 59.9 to 69.3.
- The "Average Age of *Excess* deaths" in 2022 age must range between 67.4 to 77.4.

The left two columns of Figure 18.4 and Figure 18.5 depict the results thus far.

	Excess Range			C19 Avg
Year	**High**	**Low**	**5yr Avg 2015-2019**	**minus 5yr Avg**
2020	82.5	79.0	80.3	1.0
2021	69.3	59.9	63.3	12.5
2022	77.4	67.4	70.9	7.1

Source: Vital Records of The Commonwealth of Massachusetts
Compiled by: John Paul Beaudoin, Sr.

Figure 18.4

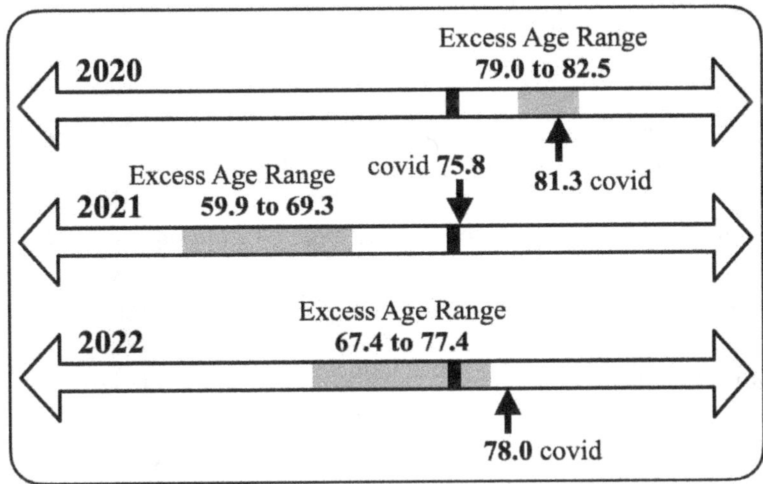

Figure 18.5

In Figure 18.5, the gray bar for each year is the age range of *excess* deaths calculated using Method I. The thin, black bar for each year is the baseline range (75.3–75.8) of All-Cause deaths. The average age of covid deaths for each year as calculated from recorded Massachusetts death certificates is represented as a black arrow.

Method I Conclusions

2020 - The average age of covid death (81.3) is consistent with the range calculated by Method I. *Id est*, the average age of covid deaths is well within the gray bar range of *excess* deaths. This is a strong indication that the method is reliable. Thus, for 2020, it is reasonable to conclude that covid, or the protocols in response to covid, or a combination of these two factors, was responsible for most of the *excess* deaths in 2020. ***Age Spectrum Profile*** equivalency is evinced.

2021 - The average age of covid deaths, as calculated from recorded death certificates (75.8) is considerably higher than the range of average ages of *excess* deaths calculated by Method I (59.9 to 69.3). *Id est*, the average age of covid deaths is far afield from the range of average age of *excess* deaths (gray bar). Since the reliability of Method I was confirmed by the 2020 data, this is a strong indication that covid was not responsible for the *excess* deaths in 2021. In 2021, people died at much younger ages from something other than covid. ***Age Spectrum Profile*** equivalency fails terribly.

2022 - The average age of covid death (78.0) as calculated from recorded death certificates is somewhat higher than the calculated range of average age of *excess* deaths (67.4 to 77.4). Since the reliability of Method I was confirmed by the 2020 data, this indicates that it is unlikely that covid was responsible for the *excess* deaths in 2022. It is more likely that something other than covid was responsible for the *excess* deaths in 2022.

Some critics may claim that the average age of death in 2021 would be expected to drop below baseline range because so many elderly were killed in the 2020 pandemic wave. The dry tinder, connoting a large group of vulnerable elderly persons, was gone.

However, the number of *excess* deaths in 2021 was quite large. The base equation holds because the *excess* would actually be a negative number, or a deficit. If the reduction in average age of death in 2021 were the result of a "dry tinder phenomenon," then the SARS-CoV-2 virus that killed the elderly dry tinder in 2020 would have had to completely change behavior to attack and kill much younger persons in 2021. We know this was not the case from the data on infections by age group.[1,2]

By extracting the "Average Age of *Excess* deaths" in 2020 through 2022 from the RLSD, Method I provides strong evidence that covid could not have caused the significant *excess* deaths in 2021 and 2022. The ***age spectrum profile*** is consistent with the ***symptom spectrum profile*** in revealing that significant *excess* deaths in 2021 and 2022 are not from covid.

Method II

A method using averages is much simpler for readers who may be confused by Method I, which is understandable. Please focus on the last two columns in the Figure 18.6 table repeated here again.

	Excess Range			C19 Avg
Year	**High**	**Low**	**5yr Avg 2015-2019**	**minus 5yr Avg**
2020	82.5	79.0	80.3	1.0
2021	69.3	59.9	63.3	12.5
2022	77.4	67.4	70.9	7.1

Source: Vital Records of The Commonwealth of Massachusetts
Compiled by: John Paul Beaudoin, Sr.

Figure 18.6

Instead of using a range for baseline years 2015–2019, the average age of deaths for all five baseline years was calculated as a single number, which is 75.6.

Using the same base equation and solving for the "Average Age of *Excess* deaths" in year 2020, the difference between the "Average Age of Covid deaths" and "Average Age of *Excess* deaths" is only 1.0 year. *Excess* and covid are very close in age, consistent with Method I results.

In year 2021, the difference between the "Average Age of Covid deaths" and "Average Age of *Excess* deaths" is 12.5 years. *Excess* deaths are much younger than covid deaths. Again, this is consistent with Method I and it sadly shows that much younger people died in 2021 from something that was very unlikely covid.

In year 2022, the difference between the "Average Age of Covid deaths" and "Average Age of *Excess* deaths" is 7.1 years. *Excess* deaths are significantly younger than covid deaths to the extent that one must challenge the government story that covid is killing people.

Conclusions from both Methods I & II

Two different methods were used to test whether the ***age spectrum profile*** of covid-involved deaths is aligned with the ***age spectrum profile*** of All-Cause *excess* deaths. In both methods, the following statements explain the results.

In year 2020, covid or the government protocol responses to covid likely caused the *excess* deaths because the "Average Age of *Excess* deaths" aligns with the "Average Age of Covid deaths."

In years 2021 and 2022, covid likely did not cause the *excess* deaths because the "Average Age of *Excess* deaths" is disparate from the "Average Age of Covid deaths."

Ergo, something is killing much younger people in 2021 and 2022 and it is not covid *per se*.

CALCULATION OF LIFE-YEARS-LOST

Here we calculate the life-years-lost in 2020 through 2022 because of covid and other causes of death.

The average age of death from all causes during baseline years 2015 through 2019 is 75.6. For the purposes of this exercise, if a person died from a new disease at an age greater than 75.6, then the default value assigned to life-years-lost for that person is "one" because that person is already past the average age of death.

In 2020–2022, the average ages of persons who died involving covid were 81.3, 75.8, 78.0, respectively.

Since there were 20,116 deaths involving covid in Massachusetts in years 2020–2022, then there were 20,116 life-years-lost purportedly from covid because the average ages of these covid-involved deaths are older than the average age of death and "one" was used as the multiplier.

In 2021, the average age of All-Cause *excess* deaths was 63.3. The difference between this average age and that of the baseline years is 12.3. That means that 12.3 additional life-years were lost per 2021 *excess* death. All-Cause *excess* 2021 deaths totaled 3,216. *Excess* 3,216 deaths multiplied by 12.3 years per *excess* death equals 39,557 *excess* life-years-lost in 2021. The data have already shown that whatever was responsible for the *excess* deaths in 2021 was very unlikely to have been covid. Thus, in 2021 alone, 39,557 *excess* life-years were lost because of some externality or externalities, which were not covid. To be clear, I believe that the covid vaccines together with remdesivir or some other medicament or combination of medicaments caused most of these 39,557 *excess* life-years-lost in 2021. This is nearly double the 20,116 life-years-lost due to covid in 2020.

In 2022, the average age of *excess* deaths was 70.9. The *excess* deaths totaled 3,047.

75.6 - 70.9 = 4.7 life-years-lost per *excess* death in 2022

3,047 *excess* deaths multiplied by 4.7 years per *excess* death equals 14,321 life-years-lost in 2022 from causes that the data have already shown were very unlikely covid and were very likely circulatory, blood, acute renal failure, and others.

The total life-years-lost in years 2021 and 2022 is 53,878. The data show that these losses were not from covid, but rather from something else that many believe to be covid vaccines and medicaments such as

remdesivir, baricitinib, or vancomycin. 53,878 life-years-lost is more than two and a half times the losses in 2020 due to covid *per se*.

Ignoring the fact that many, if not the majority, of the deaths reported as covid-involved are proven to be fraudulent in *PRIMA PARS* and *SECUNDA PARS*, 53,878 life-years-lost from only two years and to a cause-of-death that is not covid, is far greater than the 20,116 purported life-years-lost from three years of covid-involved deaths.

Additional variables show the difference to be far worse. The additional variables pertain to life-years-**affected** of those who depend on or care for the decedent. When parents of young children or children themselves die, many lives are affected by depression, psychoses, self-abuse, self-destructive behavior, and other pathologies for years, sometimes decades. Families split apart. Suicides, drug overdoses, or other maladies of the mind occur. Several souls are left behind on Earth for each death that occurs. Some say the total is four or five people affected for twenty to fifty years per lost child or parent. That equates to a multiplier between 80 and 250.

In other words, the life-years-affected for younger people dying could be in the millions for covid vaccines, while still only being ~20,000 for covid because we expect those in their 80s to die soon. We are prepared for that rite of passage to another existence. The loss of a woman aged 98 is not the same as the loss of a woman aged 35 with four children under the age of 8.

The imbalance of harms cannot be tipped much further than it already is. The real issue is that society is ignorant of these types of calculations. Their moral calculus in deciding about vaccines or other government mandates is devoid of facts, logic, and thinking past the fear and compliance programmed into them by media and politicians.

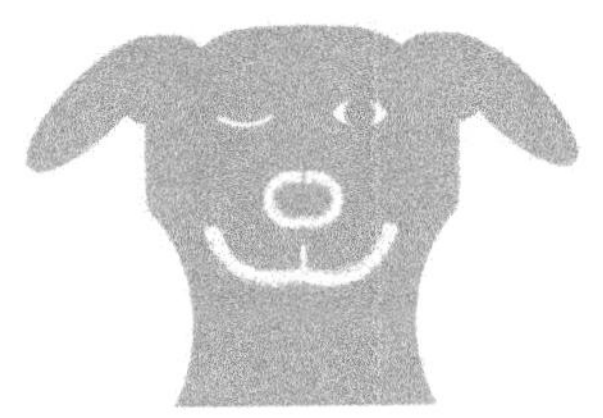

Chapter 19
Seasonality Profiles

Waveforms depict variations in a phenomenon over time. Consider the phenomenon to be the vertical position of a ball floating on a lake. A waveform depicting such a phenomenon would yield a flat line plot representing a calm lake, a diminishing sinusoidal or undulating plot representing the *externality* of waves from the wake of a passing motorboat, or a chaotic jagged plot representing the *externality* of a blustery storm. An *externality*, in this context, is something introduced into a somewhat stable or deterministic system, such as a calm lake.

Waveforms convey a tremendous amount of information. In this chapter, waveforms represent the number of deaths recorded on Massachusetts death certificates over years 2015 through 2022. Each semi-monthly total of deaths comprises a single data point. The vertical *y*-axis represents the total number of deaths that occurred during each semi-monthly time period. The horizontal *x*-axis denotes the specific semi-monthly time period within the years 2015–2019. The data points are connected with lines resulting in waveforms. Please note that curve smoothing was applied to the data streams in this chapter (for the data hounds, three and a half month smoothing was applied).

For the purpose of framing the illustrations in this section, these first waveforms in Figures 19.1 through 19.3 are ideal and theoretical waveforms meant to lay a foundation of understanding before moving to the waveforms of *actual* deaths.

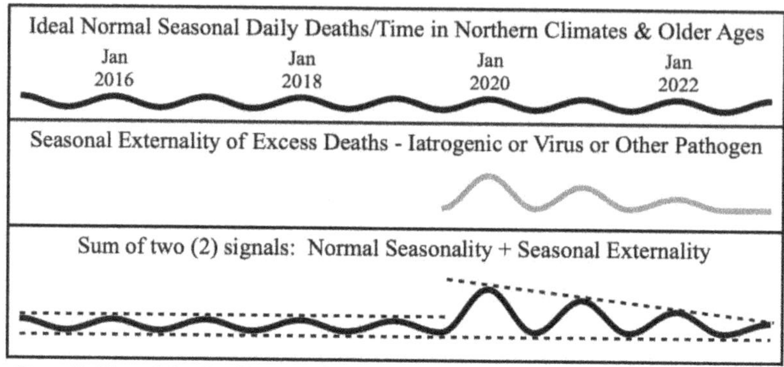

Compiled by: John Paul Beaudoin, Sr. - May 2023

Figure 19.1

In Figure 19.1, the top waveform illustrates an idealized plot of total deaths over eight years from 2015 through 2022.

The second waveform illustrates an idealized plot of a *seasonal* externality in the form of additional deaths caused by a virus, bacterium, or other pathogen. Or the additional deaths could be a consequence of changes in policies involving public spaces, economic restrictions, or some other externality that has a *seasonal* impact on deaths. Notice the diminishing peaks of the *seasonal* externality which engineers would call damped harmonic behavior. This idealized waveform models how pathogens become endemic. Society builds an immune response or tolerance to the pathogen. The peaks diminish in amplitude, but the troughs return to baseline each year or season if the externality is *seasonal.*

The bottom waveform is simply the sum of the top two waveforms. After the externality is introduced, the peaks of the wave are substantially higher than normal, but the troughs of the wave return to normal baseline because the externality is *seasonal. Id est*, every point on the waveform after introduction of the externality is greater except the trough points, which return to the baseline.

This is what one would expect from a *seasonal* respiratory virus or other *seasonal* virus introduced to a society. To illustrate the introduction of something that behaves like covid, this ideal example depicts a *seasonal* externality beginning in July 2019.

The next set of waveforms in Figure 19.2 depict the introduction of a *steady-state* externality. This externality begins to ramp in January 2021, not January 2020, and reaches steady-state in 3 months.

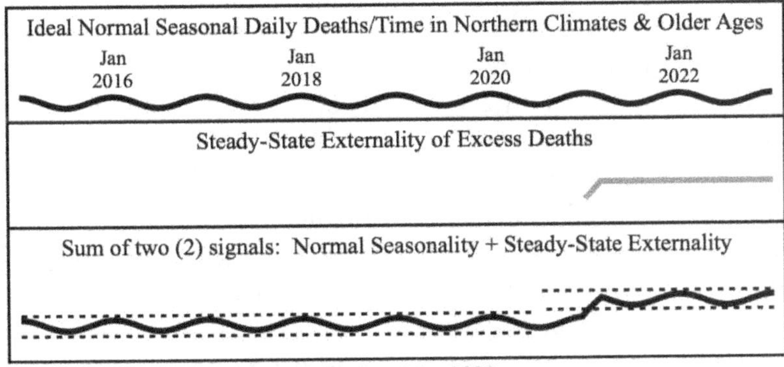

Figure 19.2

The same process is applied in Figure 19.2 as in the first *seasonal* externality waveform depiction in Figure 19.1. The top two graphs are added to produce the bottom graph.

In Figure 19.2, both the peaks and troughs of the resultant bottom graph rise equally. Remember that these are idealized graphs.

Notice the ramping period at the beginning of the externality. In the real world, the ramping period can take any shape based on delivery time of the externality. In the case of vaccines causing the externality of deaths, it likely would be similar to a distribution delivery curve. As the vaccines are delivered and administered, the externality of vaccine fatalities would likely proportionately parallel the distribution curve.

Let's take a look at a linear ramping, or *linearly increasing* externality in Figure 19.3 (a positive slope line externality).

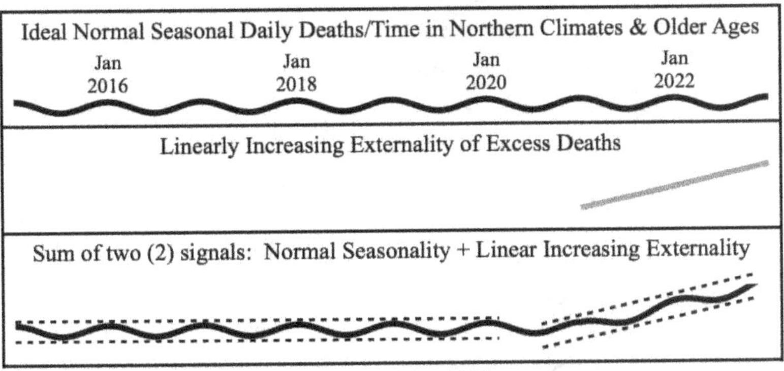

Figure 19.3

Figure 19.3 depicts the addition of a *linearly increasing* externality beginning in January 2021, not January 2020.

Before moving to real-life *actual* waveform analyses, please be aware that, in general, there may be more than one externality in play at any given time, emerging either simultaneously, or beginning at different times. Imagine that an annual and damped harmonic *seasonal* externality enters a society. Then, a year later, a *linearly increasing* externality, separate and distinct in causality from the *seasonal* externality, enters that society. Then, in the third year, the *linearly increasing* externality reaches its *steady-state* horizontal asymptote. The resulting waveform will change over time, possibly in complex ways that make it difficult to directly visualize the changes in the underlying patterns, which are responsible for the net changes in the waveform.

Actual waveforms span the baseline years 2015–2019 through the emergence of covid in 2020, and the introduction of mass administration of covid immunizations and boosters in 2021 and 2022. There are short-term causes of death such as cardiac arrest, arrhythmia, pulmonary embolism, thrombocytopenia, stroke, heart attack, etc. There are also longer term causes such as lymph node cancer, marrow cancer, Guillain Barré Syndrome, other neurological issues, and the new phenomenon called "turbo cancer." The short-term and longer-term causes of death will have different waveforms than the three ideal types used in the illustrative figures.

Finally, consider that there are iatrogenic (unintentional, physician induced) contributors besides immunization, including refusal to treat with antibiotics, refusal of early treatment with antivirals while telling people to wait at home until they are struggling to breathe, inappropriate use of ventilators on patients with O_2 saturation well over 90% purportedly to protect the medical staff from the patients' aerosolized breath, and the use of remdesivir or another medicament on patients who could not benefit from it. Each of these externalities contributed their own waveforms, some of them synchronized to dates of government financial incentive policies.

ALL-CAUSE WAVEFORMS

Figure 19.4 shows semi-monthly plots of Massachusetts All-Cause deaths spanning the eight years from 2015 through 2022 for the four older age groups.

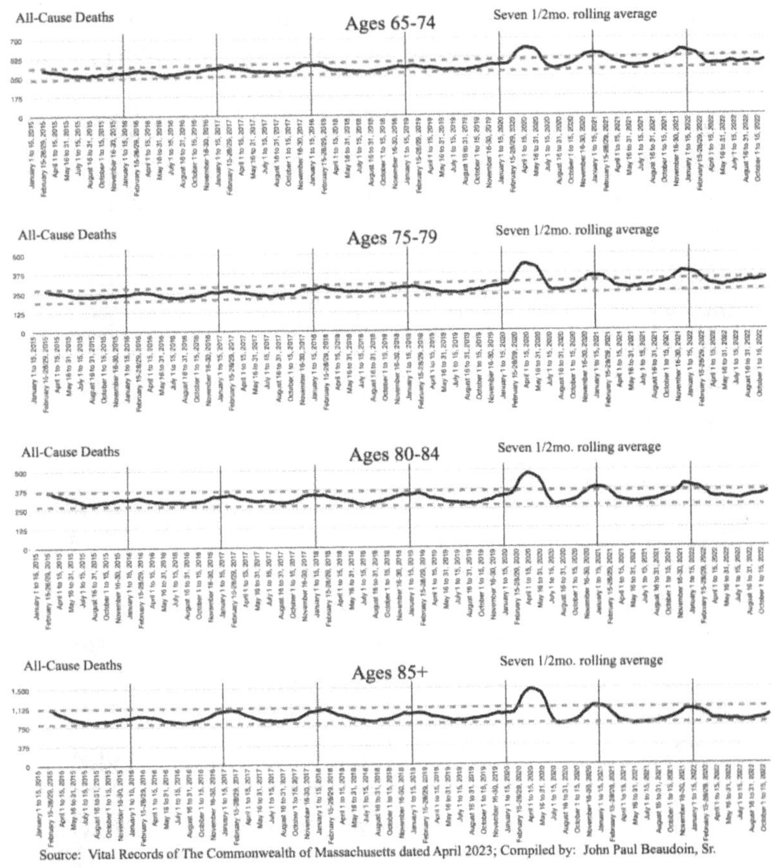

Figure 19.4

In these and all subsequent waveform plots, year boundaries are demarcated by vertical lines, and pairs of dashed gray lines as "guardrails" were added subjectively. These guardrails are approximately anchored by the top two or more peaks and bottom two or more trough points among the baseline years 2015 through 2019. The guardrails form a slope depicting the trend exhibited by the baseline years. These guardrails are extended past 2019 and into 2020 through 2022 in order for the reader to visualize any deviations from the expected behavior as exemplified during the baseline years. These guardrails were "eyeballed" manually by the author. If you, the reader, feel that the guardrails should be higher, lower, or differently sloped, then you are invited to use a straight edge to redraw them on the pages as you may prefer.

Sinusoidal waveforms depicting *seasonality* of All-Cause deaths are pronounced in northern climates, such as Massachusetts, and are generally more distinct in the very elderly age groups. The sine wave of *seasonality* is barely discernible in age groups under age 65.

Notice the bottom waveform of "Ages 85+" in Figure 19.4. What a beautiful, nearly ideal sine wave of All-Cause deaths in the baseline years 2015–2019. Then, in 2020, the amplitude jumped up dramatically in the spring, from the winter peak, indicating the influence of an externality. Notice also the return to baseline in the summers of years 2020, 2021, and 2022 after each of the three waves following the emergence of covid. The number of deaths returned toward the *expected* baseline levels after each of the *seasonal* waves. In other words, the externality responsible for the elevated winter peaks is itself *seasonal*.

The amplitudes in each of the three "Ages 85+" waves diminish over time. In fact, the third wave is relatively normal. Compare the third covid era wave to baseline years 2015–2019. This indicates that a *seasonal externality* came into society in Massachusetts and affected the 85+ age group and became endemic, or normal to society, after only two seasons. Notice also that a *non-seasonal* externality appears in the summer of 2021 in "Ages 75–84" and increases in the summer of 2022. This is visible by offsets above the bottom guardrail.

The idea that the introduction of covid vaccines was responsible for the reduction of covid deaths of those age 85 and older is clearly contradicted by the fact that the second wave during winter 2020/2021 was already sharply declining before the covid vaccines were introduced and well before the second doses, which were required to purportedly fully establish covid immunity. There is no evidence to credit covid vaccines for the classic *seasonal* behavior of an externality already on a downward trajectory. The simple truth is that covid had already run its natural course at least half a year before the vaccines were available for mass administration.

Please observe now the plots for each successive younger age group shown in Figure 19.4. In comparing age group wave- forms, notice the relative changes:

- For baseline years 2015–2019, the amplitudes of the *seasonal* waves diminish as the ages diminish. *Seasonality* ebbs in direct relation to age.
- For year 2020 springtime, the amplitudes of the first wave peaks diminish slightly as the ages diminish. *Seasonality* varies in direct relation to age.
- The amplitudes of the second wave peaks 2020/2021 winter are roughly equal irrespective of age. There are no relative changes.
- The amplitudes of the third wave peaks 2021/2022 winter actually increase in amplitude with diminishing age. This phenomenon, inversely related to age, is very concerning.
- First wave troughs of the covid era (summer 2020) return to baseline for all ages
- Second and third wave troughs (summers 2021 and 2022, respectively) of the covid era begin to rise off baseline. This *non-seasonal* externality is extremely concerning.

These anomalous, disturbing phenomena are even more pronounced in the waveforms for the younger age groups shown in Figure 19.5.

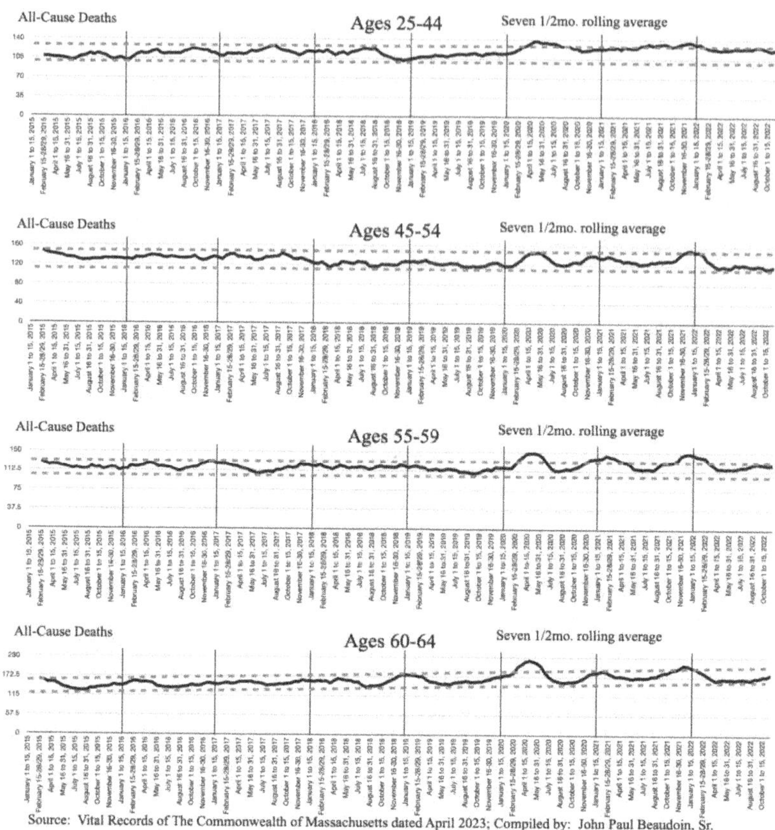

Figure 19.5

As time marches on, age group populations change. In order to adjust for age group population trending, slope is added to the guardrails (dashed gray lines) as needed. Again, the reader may have their own preferred method.

Observations of Figure 19.5, the younger waveforms:

- *Seasonal* undulations in base years 2015–2019 are much less evident in younger age groups. In some years, the *seasonality* is inverted from the norm. Younger, healthier people are not likely to die from *seasonal* illnesses.
- The amplitudes of the covid era third wave peaks are approximately equal to the respective first wave peaks and greater than the second wave peaks. What killed an equal or greater number of younger people during the third wave of purported covid disease than during

the first wave of purported covid? Did something make younger people more susceptible to death by damaging their immune mechanism? Chapter 14 presented significant evidence of increases in D8 and I8 Immune mechanism-involved deaths. Were any other causes directly responsible for some of these additional deaths?

- Year 2021 summer troughs lift off more above baseline in each younger group. This is further evidence of a *non-seasonal* externality that increases in relative severity as age decreases.
- "Ages 25–44" group stays at the high rate of death nearly all three years. It never comes down. This is alarming evidence that something other than covid is killing young people.

It appears that the "Ages 25–44" group was set to return toward baseline after the first 2020 wave, but then it turned up again, and before any major rollout of covid vaccines. The numbers are very low, which would make a state investigation very easy to conduct.

In summary, a *non-seasonal* externality appeared early in 2021. It appears to have impacted younger people more notably likely because younger people are generally healthier and stronger. That is, older people were also likely affected by the same *non-seasonal* externality, but it may not have shown because of the large numbers of deaths in older people. These plots depict All-Cause deaths. All-Cause deaths are susceptible to Simpson's Paradox. Examining some individual causes of death provides more insight.

COVID WAVEFORMS

The age group waveform plots in Figure 19.6 show the data extracted directly from Massachusetts death certificates for covid-involved deaths, ICD-10 code U07.1.

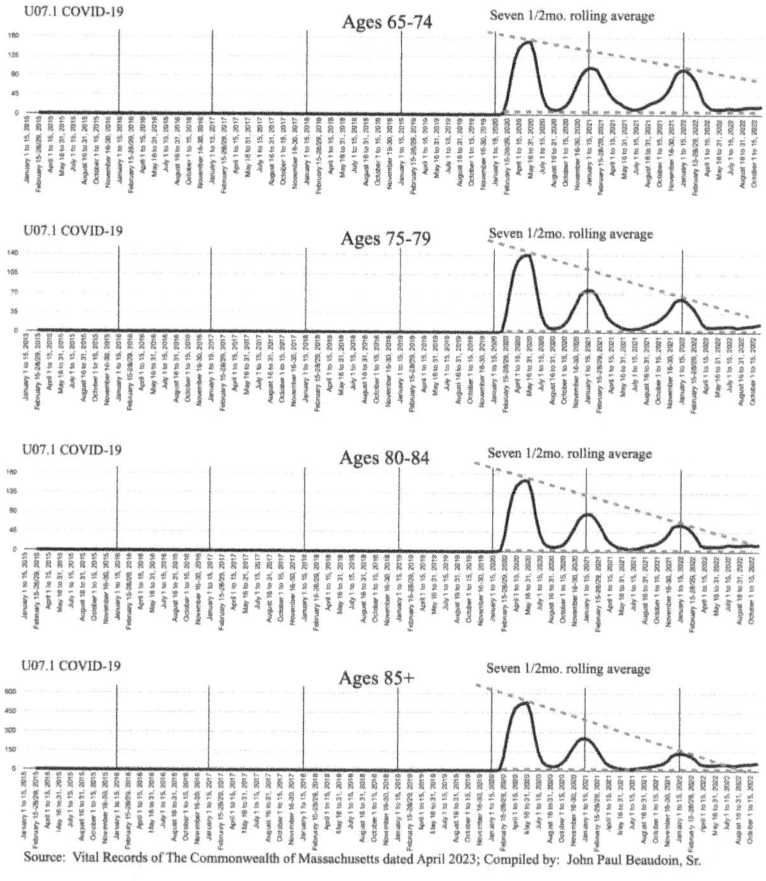

Figure 19.6

All four of these older covid-involved deaths age groups down to age 65 comprise waveforms with troughs that return to baseline during the summer off-season. *Id est*, all older covid-involved death waveforms are highly *seasonal*.

The 85+ age group closely follows the classical *seasonal* waveform for a respiratory disease. The amplitude of each successive *seasonal* wave is less than the preceding wave until this externality of *excess* death almost completely disappears.

For "Ages 85+", the ratio of amplitudes from the first wave to the third wave of covid deaths is almost four to one (4:1).

Next, look at the plot for "Ages 65–74" group. The ratio of amplitudes from the first wave to the third wave of covid deaths is only about two to one (2:1).

Figure 19.6 depicts a pattern of first to third wave diminishing ratio in each successively younger age group.

Do not confuse the amplitudes of the first wave in each age group as being the same. The graphs are automatically tuned to the largest wave. The y-axis scales are different for each age group. Far more older people die than younger people.

The waveforms in Figure 19.7 depicting the younger age groups of covid-involved deaths continue the trend of diminishing ratio of first to third waves.

The dashed line guardrails help to visualize the way the ratios change with diminishing age. The younger the age group, the more the behavior deviates from the classic behavior of an infectious respiratory disease. Instead of declining year over year, for those under age 55, deaths are increasing each successive year. It is clear from these plots that there must be one or more other externalities besides covid *per se* that are responsible for these additional deaths. A large number of these people must have been killed by something other than a *seasonal* respiratory disease.

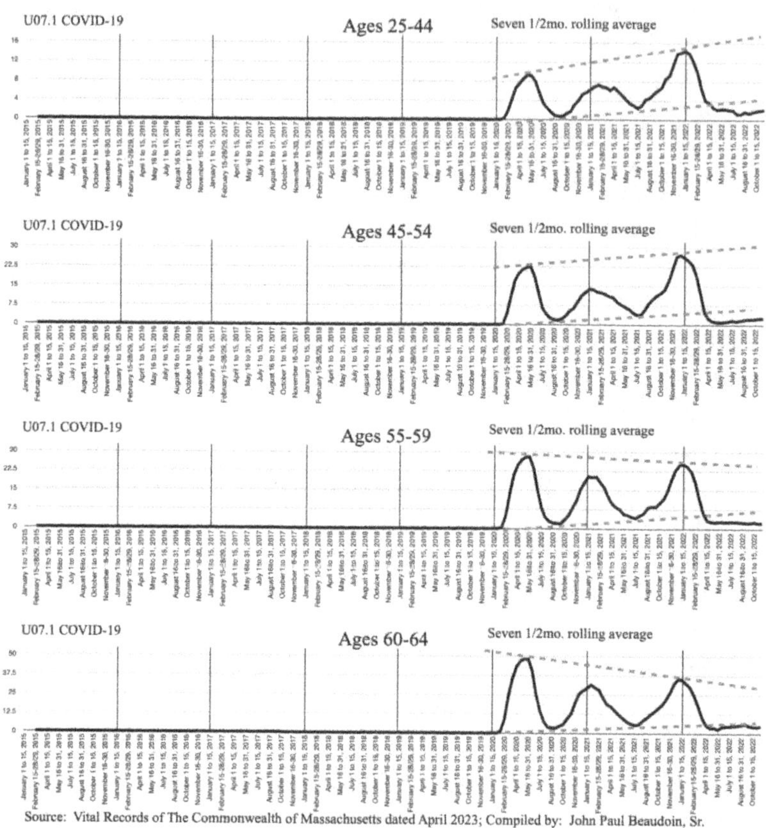

Figure 19.7

Notice that the summer 2021 troughs are farther from baseline in each successively younger age group. The troughs substantially lift off the baseline. This *trough lift-off* is evidence of a component of a *linearly increasing* externality in addition to the normal, classical *seasonal* externality.

Why did people die in the summer of 2021 purportedly from covid when they did not die in the summer of 2020 when covid was most virulent? Are their immune systems less able to handle covid after two seasons of covid or after a two-course covid mRNA immunization?

The increases in certain causes of death showcased in *TERTIA PARS*, including the immune mechanism, demand investigation. These young people previously beat one or even two years of covid? Their immune systems were intact before the covid vaccine rollouts. The immune mechanism seems to be broken in a great many people since 2021.

PNEUMONIA, UNSPECIFIED WAVEFORMS

Figure 19.8 shows the waveform plots for death from ICD-10 code J18.9 "Pneumonia, unspecified" for all eight age groups. Pneumonia, unspecified is expected to follow All-Cause and covid trends as was depicted in annual bar graphs earlier in Chapter 14.

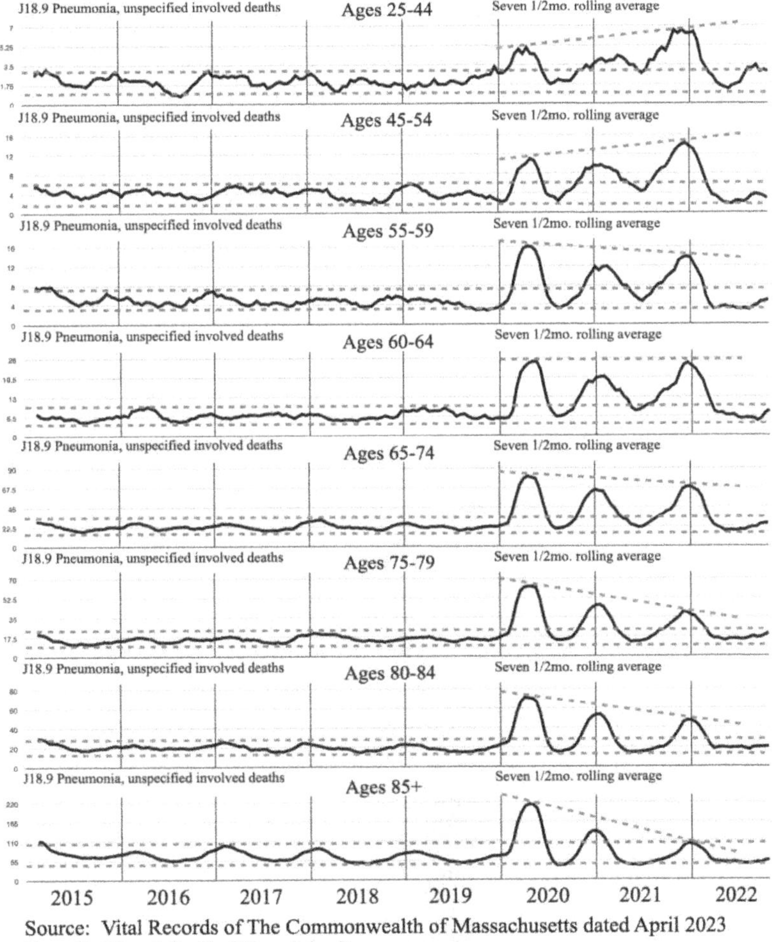

Figure 19.8

The same patterns in the All-Cause and covid waveforms are evident in the J18.9 waveforms.

Observations

- It is visually evident that the plots for summer 2021, below age 80, fail to return to the *expected* baseline levels. This alarming deviation is progressively worse in each successively younger age group. After two full seasonal waves, more people under age 75 died from pneumonia in the summer of 2021 than in the summer of 2020.
- During winter 2021/2022, more people under age 75 died from pneumonia during the third wave than during the second wave. Even more alarming, more people under age 55 died from pneumonia during the third wave than during the first wave! Why did this happen? Massachusetts has one of the highest covid vaccination rates in the United States.[2] Pneumonia was regarded as a cause of death precipitated by covid infection. If the covid vaccine works as claimed, then fewer people should have died from pneumonia during the third wave. This appears to be evidence of **negative efficacy**—the risk of dying from pneumonia secondary to a covid infection increased in proportion to the number of covid vaccinations received.
- Below age 50, *seasonal* variation of deaths in the baseline years, 2015–2019, is not discernible.
- The externality that suddenly appeared in early 2020 is highly *seasonal*. Whether it was covid, government interventions, or some combination of the two, a disastrous embedded externality killed a large and growing number of middle-aged people.

How can a virus turn off to near zero all summer long in 2020, but then not turn off after two full waves of covid and after six months of a covid vaccination campaign?

All three ACP waveforms depict similar patterns of *excess* deaths.

There is a *seasonal* externality in all of the baseline years 2015–2019 in the elderly that disappears in the younger.

There is a *seasonal* externality of deaths that switches from the elderly in the first wave to the younger in the third wave.

There is also an embedded *linearly increasing* externality.

CARDIAC ARREST WAVEFORMS

ICD-10 code prefix I46, "Cardiac arrest" is an interesting catch-all ICD-10 code. When someone dies from heart and breathing cessation, medical examiners often write, "*CARDIOPULMONARY ARREST.*" Since all deaths involve arrest of heart and breathing, the use of this code can confuse people, doctors included.

Cardiac arrest occurs at the end of a fentanyl overdose, upon impact from falling off a building, and upon succumbing to sepsis. Which of these three examples is appropriate to be labeled with I46 as Cause A, the "immediate cause," on a death certificate? The fall from a building obviously should not carry an I46 code. The arrest was not part of a heart or breathing problem. It was merely the foregone conclusion of hitting the ground. Thus, I46 is not relevant in the causality of the death. The fentanyl overdose is in the gray area. The fentanyl caused suppression of autonomic function, such as breathing. Breathing slowed until it ceased, and then the heart stopped. Some physicians use I46 on death certificates with fentanyl overdoses, but medical examiners do not seem to use I46 for fentanyl overdoses. That is what I observed while reading thousands of death certificates. The sepsis likely caused a heart infection where the heart muscle itself failed as a result of the causal chain of blood infection. The use of I46 in sepsis deaths is not uncommon, but it is not used in the majority of cases.

Notwithstanding the misuse or overuse of I46, it is still possible to use the code prefix to detect patterns in deaths involving the heart. Assuming the set of medical examiners and physicians was relatively unchanged over the past eight years, the I46 code prefix should contain a signal associated with the heart. Deaths involving I46 are numerous enough to provide robust waveforms depicted in Figure 19.9.

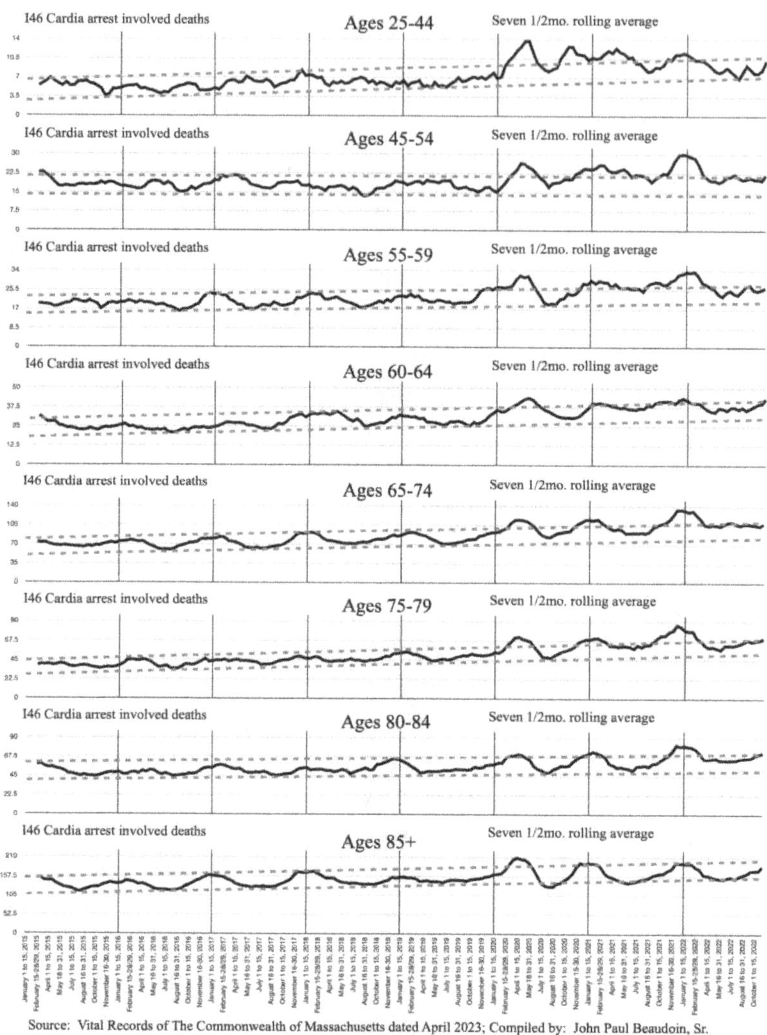

Figure 19.9

Notice that *seasonality* is discernible in some of the baseline years. "Ages 85+" and "Ages 65–74" show *seasonality* almost every year in the baseline range 2015–2019. The other age groups display *seasonality* in some, but not all of the years. "Ages 55–59" shows a significant *seasonal* peak during the winter 2016/2017 followed by a couple smaller peaks the following two winters.

As was the case for J18.9 Pneumonia, the failure of the plots to return to the *expected* baseline levels in the summers of 2021 and 2022 is visually evident. This alarming deviation is progressively worse for each successively younger age group. After two full *seasonal* waves of purported covid, more people under age 75 died from cardiac arrest in the summer of 2021 than in the summer of 2020.

Even more alarming, **more people between the ages of 44 and 80 died from cardiac arrest during the third wave than during the first wave**.

A clear *seasonal* externality appeared early in 2020 and another *linearly increasing* externality was added in 2021. Beginning in 2020, I46 Cardiac arrest contributed to *excess* deaths across all age groups, and relatively more, or comparatively more, in the younger age groups in 2021 and 2022.

I46 Cardiac arrest-involved deaths are in significant *excess* and comprise the largest health emergency in Massachusetts since 1919. Most significantly, *excess* Cardiac arrest-involved deaths disproportionately impacted much younger people than covid-involved deaths. Thus, life-years-lost is many times more than covid in the I46 Cardiac arrest cause of death.

The tremendous *excess* loss of life involving I46 Cardiac arrest demands immediate and scrutinous investigation by the Massachusetts Department of Public Health and the CDC. A cursory evaluation is not acceptable. Thousands of young and middle aged people lost their lives due to something that is not covid *per se*.

"D" CODES WAVEFORMS

ICD-10 "D" codes span a range of conditions which include blood, blood-forming organs, and some aspects of the immune mechanism. Figure 19.10 shows age group waveform plots of deaths involving an aggregated collection of individual "D" codes.

Many of the individual "D" codes assigned to the Massachusetts death certificates are insufficient in number to enable visual identification of patterns. Data, collected in a complex, sometimes chaotic world of humans, has a lot of natural variation. Variability within a small data set can overwhelm even a strong underlying signal. That is the case for inspecting waveforms of individual D codes. By assembling the data for multiple D codes into an aggregate data set, the underlying pattern can effectively become visible above the noise of variability.

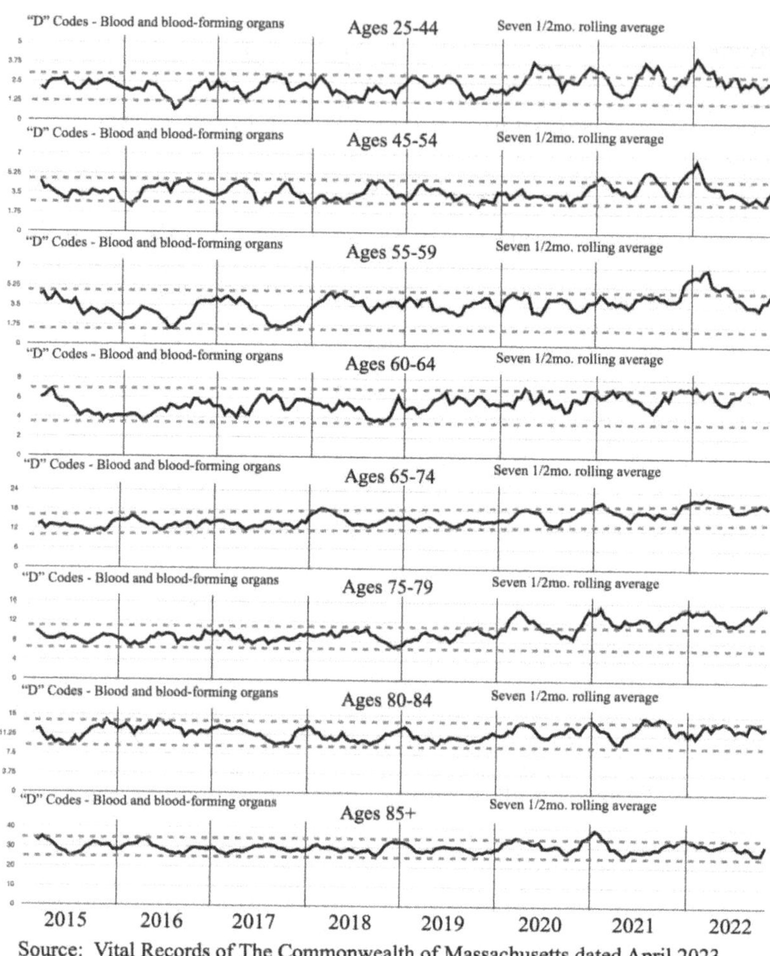

Source: Vital Records of The Commonwealth of Massachusetts dated April 2023
Compiled by: John Paul Beaudoin, Sr.

Figure 19.10

There are some very concerning peaks of *excess* deaths involving blood issues in the winters of 2020/2021 and 2021/2022 that are evident in all age groups, except "Ages 80–84".

In years 2021 and 2022, it is clear that there was introduced a non-seasonal *steady-state* or *linearly increasing* signal, or combination of multiple signals. Something other than covid killed younger people in 2021 and 2022.

No matter how the guardrails are placed, visual inspection of these plots reveals a significant and tragic issue involving the "D" codes prefix group of deaths. **All age groups under age 80 exhibit a high number of *excess* deaths in the winter of 2021/2022.**

ACUTE RENAL FAILURE WAVEFORMS

Figure 19.11 shows the age group waveform plots for deaths involving ICD-10 code N17.9, Acute renal failure (ARF).

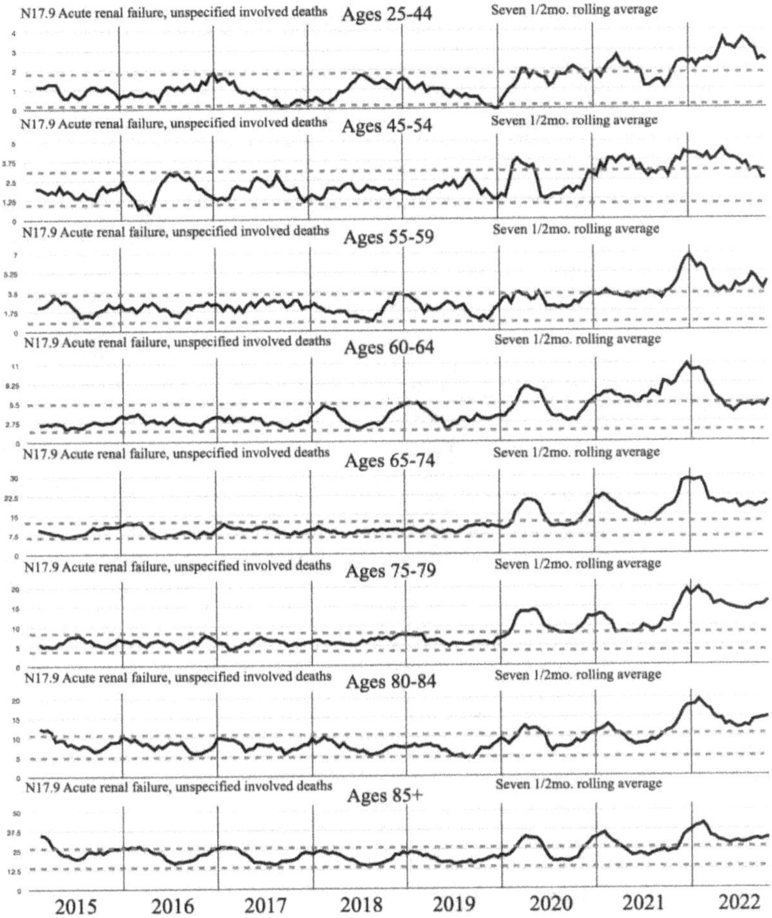

N17.9 Acute renal failure, unspecified involved deaths Ages 25-44 Seven 1/2mo. rolling average

N17.9 Acute renal failure, unspecified involved deaths Ages 45-54 Seven 1/2mo. rolling average

N17.9 Acute renal failure, unspecified involved deaths Ages 55-59 Seven 1/2mo. rolling average

N17.9 Acute renal failure, unspecified involved deaths Ages 60-64 Seven 1/2mo. rolling average

N17.9 Acute renal failure, unspecified involved deaths Ages 65-74 Seven 1/2mo. rolling average

N17.9 Acute renal failure, unspecified involved deaths Ages 75-79 Seven 1/2mo. rolling average

N17.9 Acute renal failure, unspecified involved deaths Ages 80-84 Seven 1/2mo. rolling average

N17.9 Acute renal failure, unspecified involved deaths Ages 85+ Seven 1/2mo. rolling average

2015 2016 2017 2018 2019 2020 2021 2022

Source: Vital Records of The Commonwealth of Massachusetts dated April 2023
Compiled by: John Paul Beaudoin, Sr.

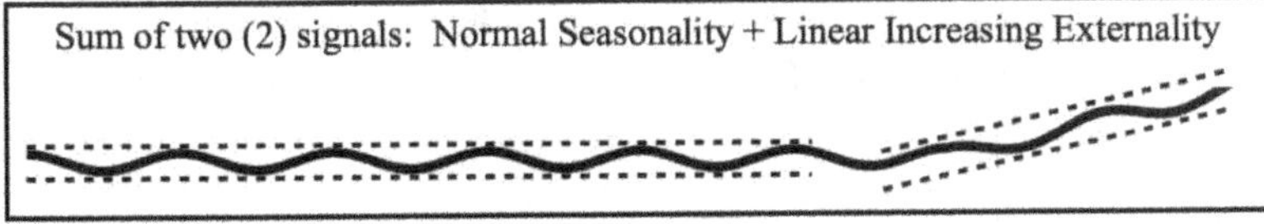

Compiled by: John Paul Beaudoin, Sr. - May 2023

Figure 19.11

The ARF waveform for "Ages 85+" closely follows that classical pattern for *seasonal* normal deaths summed with a *linearly increasing* externality. For comparison, the illustrative plot from Figure 19.3 is reproduced immediately below the plot of the 85+ age group.

In 2020 through 2022, each successive *seasonal* winter peak is higher than the prior peak and each successive summer trough bottoms out at a higher level above the baseline than the prior trough.

These graphs depict a runaway out-of-control system with no indication that deaths involving ARF are stabilizing, let alone returning to normal baseline levels.

Each of these decedents was a human being with family and friends. Many of them were mothers or fathers of young children who are left to grieve their irreplaceable losses indefinitely. Two thousand *excess* people were killed by ARF in 2021 through 2022 in Massachusetts. Some of them have parents in their 60s and 70s who may lose the will to live like many of us who have suffered the loss of an adult child in the prime of life.

The life-years-lost and lives-affected calculations are stark and depressing. Taking a reasonable estimate of 20 average years lost per *excess* ARF-involved death; this translates to 40,000 life-years-lost during 2021 and 2022 in Massachusetts alone. Estimating that an average of five extra people are affected by the loss of the decedent equates to ~200,000 life-years-affected in Massachusetts alone from this one cause of death in 2021 and 2022.

Has the Massachusetts Department of Public Health or the CDC even noticed this ongoing mass casualty ARF phenomenon?

These ***seasonality profiles*** comprise another tool to reveal externalities that contributed to *excess* deaths from 2020 through 2023. Examination of these waveform plots for various ICD-10 "D" codes, "I" codes, "G" codes, and N17.9 clearly showed that covid cannot be responsible for some thousands of *excess* deaths in Massachusetts. Something else is responsible for killing these children, siblings, mothers, fathers, grandparents, and dear friends.

If remdesivir and covid vaccines are responsible for these *excess* deaths, then many would consider it murder by officials, physicians, and researchers who exhibited deliberate indifference to life resulting in the deaths of those to whom they owed a duty of care and protection. Above all, they owed them a duty to do no harm.

The evidence presented in these pages is a serious indictment of agents of the CDC and the Massachusetts Department of Public Health for nothing less than depraved heart murder. These agents knew or should have known of the cases and data in this book. Here, I am not referencing the workers and clerical staff in these bloated government agencies. I refer to the leaders who knew what they did to The People. They compound their crimes by continuing to hoard these data and hide it from The People.

BACTERIAL PNEUMONIA & FLU DEATHS

Some have claimed there was no covid pandemic and that purported covid deaths were stolen from the pneumonia and influenza (PNI) categories. This claim is directly contradicted by the Massachusetts death certificate data. Such a statement promotes exaggerated relevance of the factual evidence.

Figure 19.12 is a montage of bar graphs, each of which presents the total deaths in each of the years 2015 through 2022 for the following individual or aggregated ICD-10 codes.

- J codes - Diseases of the respiratory system (bundle)
- J18.9 - Pneumonia, unspecified (specific code)
- J12 - Viral pneumonia, not elsewhere classified (prefix code)
- U07.1 - COVID-19 (specific code)
- J15 - Bacterial pneumonia, not elsewhere classified (prefix code)
- J10 - Influenza due to identified seasonal influenza virus (prefix code)
- J11 - Influenza, virus not identified (prefix code)

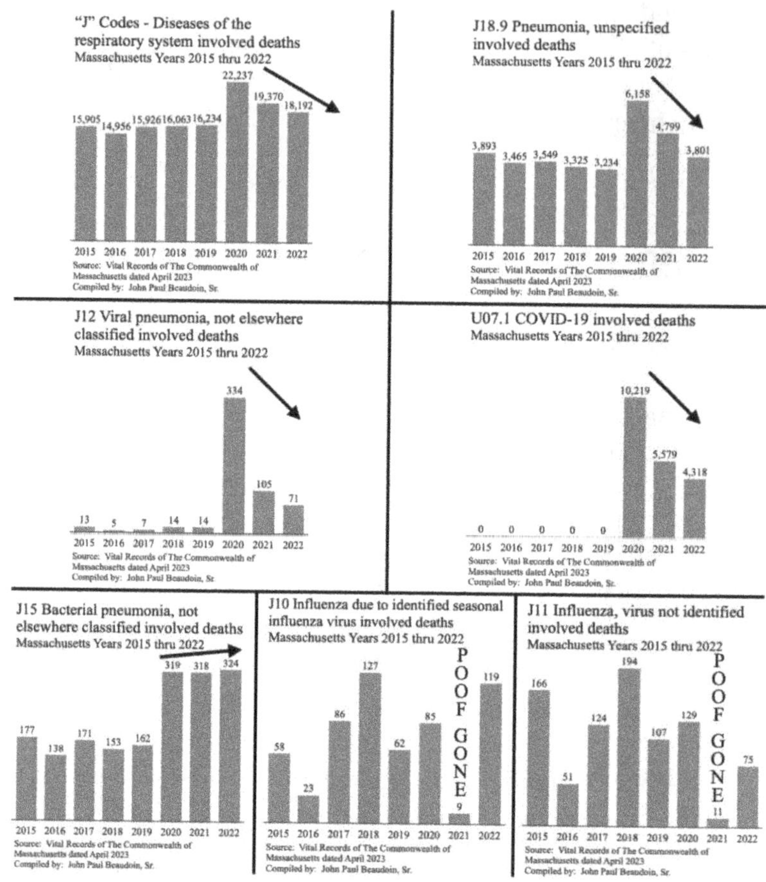

Figure 19.12

These graphs expose a number of interesting and important points.

The two influenza causes of death in the bottom right of Figure 19.12 depict a 2021 year in which influenza all but disappeared. There were only twenty total influenza-involved deaths across the two ICD-10 prefixes, I10 and I11, certified in Massachusetts in 2021. It seems virtually impossible that there could be a natural mechanism capable of causing flu to almost completely disappear precisely in sync with the appearance of covid. Proponents of the PNI theft premise claim that this is proof that covid was fabricated out of the missing PNI deaths.

Even if the PNI theft premise is true, there persist two major problems with the stolen PNI theory.

First, in 2018, the baseline year that logged the most flu deaths, there were a total of 321 flu-involved deaths (sum of ICD-10 codes J10 and J11). Even if flu deaths in 2021 were actually double the highest baseline level, that would only amount to 642 total flu deaths. Even if all of these actual flu deaths were stolen from influenza, they do not fill out the 5,579 purported covid deaths certified in Massachusetts in 2021. While I believe it is true that flu deaths were stolen from influenza in 2020–2022, and were labeled covid deaths, they only represent a small fraction of the purported covid deaths. Dwelling upon this issue as a primary source of fraud is folly and is a diversion from true and blatant fraud already established in prior chapters of this book.

Throughout this book, it has been shown that Massachusetts covid death counts were fabricated from accidental deaths such as fentanyl overdose, blunt force trauma, covid vaccination, remdesivir poisoning, flu, and other deaths. Influenza could only have contributed a minor fraction of the total fabricated deaths. Influenza theft is very low on the list of frauds but will not be forgotten in the overall schema of fraudulent overcounting.

PNI numbers games by public health officials are indeed an issue. In fact, PNI is what alerted me in April/May 2020 that the CDC data cannot be trusted. This led me to seek RLSD and obtain the Massachusetts death certificates. I knew then that they were playing games with the numbers. In early 2020, states stopped testing for flu and nearly always thereafter tested for covid even if you were seeking treatment for a hangnail. There has never been such a mass testing event in the history of mankind.

HIV testing was a dry run for this mass testing program. Government knew testing of asymptomatic people was not meant for diagnostic purposes. They knew false positives and existing background coronaviruses would yield many positive results. And they knew that positive tests would drive fear and panic.

New words such as "testdemic" and "casedemic" accurately describe what was happening in 2020 and 2021. There was a real disease in select locations at specific times; but, for the most part, covid as a "pandemic" was greatly exaggerated by using many deceptions, military behavior modification techniques, and cherry picked data. Testing was at the heart of the psychological operation of fear perpetrated on The People.

Secondly, death certificates are not restricted to one cause of death. Death certifiers can include multiple causes on a death certificate. Automated parsing systems at the CDC interpret each death certificate and assign one or more corresponding ICD-10 codes. The claim that pneumonia deaths in 2020 were stolen and coded as covid is refuted because of the massive increase in pneumonia deaths, both J18.9 unspecified and J12 viral types of pneumonia. Pneumonia is one of the leading symptoms, or causes, co-resident with covid, on many death certificates. It makes no sense to say that pneumonia deaths were stolen in favor of covid.

That does not mean that no pneumonia deaths were labeled covid and not pneumonia, but the numbers do not show that it could possibly be significant. Some of the "cardiopulmonary arrest" deaths were likely labeled covid. For certain, some of the accidental deaths were labeled covid, but not necessarily replaced by covid. It seems that if pneumonia were a symptom or cause, it was listed on the death certificate with covid.

When covid was listed alone with no other cause, we do not know if it was actually a covid vaccine death by heart attack or pulmonary embolism or some other cause.

The PNI theft premise is simply of low importance because PNI is incapable of contributing significantly to the number of covid deaths in Massachusetts data.

Bacterial pneumonia is important and interesting because antibiotics were withheld from patients and because the immune system is now known to be compromised by covid vaccines.

Look at J15 Bacterial pneumonia in the bottom left of Figure 19.12 of the montage of bar graphs. A few hundred *excess* people needlessly died involving bacterial pneumonia because of bad recommendations from the central authorities—FDA, NIH, and CDC. The J15 trend in 2020 through 2022 is completely different from the trends shared by All-Cause, "J" Codes, covid, pneumonia unspecified, and viral pneumonia.

Imagine being told by a doctor that your pneumonia is viral and that antibiotics will not help you. The thematic excuse is that they would tell you that they do not want you to become antibiotic resistant. Then you die from bacterial pneumonia. If you are dead, are you antibiotic resistant? These are not flippant, sarcastic remarks. These remarks are the brutal truth of medical practice in the 2020s in a state that claims to be the most advanced in medicine.

CONCLUSIONS

From Chapter 19, the ***seasonality profile*** proved an externality not related to covid is responsible for thousands of *excess* deaths in 2021 and 2022 in Massachusetts.

From Chapter 18, the ***age spectrum profile*** changed from 2020 to 2021 proving that an externality caused significant loss of much younger people beginning in 2021, not 2020 in Massachusetts.

OPINION

In *PRIMA PARS* and *SECUNDA PARS*, fraud was proven beyond reasonable doubt.

Real people were certified as having died involving covid as a cause or contributing condition leading to death, when covid had no causal relationship to death.

Real people, including children, died as a direct result of covid immunizations. In earlier chapters, the onset of symptoms is proven to have occurred only minutes or hours following injection; and death resulted days later. However, covid immunization, as a cause or contributing condition to death, is shown to have been purposely omitted from the death certificates, presumably to protect the gene drugs called "vaccines."

Real people, whose death certificates actually mention covid vaccination as a cause or contributing condition leading to death, were not coded by the CDC with any ICD-10 codes having to do with immunization or vaccination. This is a fraud of omission by the CDC and subsequently a fraud of omission by the MA DPH, when they were notified of the omission and did not cure the defects.

In *TERTIA PARS*, aggregated data evidence is depicted by ***symptom spectrum profile***, ***age spectrum profile***, and ***seasonality profile***. The evidence is proven beyond reasonable doubt that covid vaccines killed thousands of people in Massachusetts alone, including children through centenarians.

The covid vaccines are mass killers. Blood and circulatory deaths rise and ebb with the rise and ebb of covid immunization uptake. These are mostly short-term, acute reactions to covid vaccines.

Cancers and some of the demyelinating neurological-involved deaths caused by covid immunizations are longer term effects that take weeks to months for a vaccinated person to succumb to death, perhaps even years.

Acute renal failure (ARF)-involved deaths are an unstable system of thousands of *excess* deaths; and is still happening as of the writing of this book. The cause is speculated to be remdesivir, baricitinib, vancomycin, covid vaccines, or a combination of some or all of them.

Massachusetts is in an Acute renal failure **Health Emergency** far bigger than covid ever was.

The MA DPH and the current administration are:

Blind to the carnage, maim, and loss of life, or

Avoiding mention of the devastation to families that they know is happening all around the Commonwealth.

Government caused all these deaths and family destruction through covid immunizations and protocols recommended by central authority agencies. There is no other plausible theory.

QUARTA PARS

Solutions

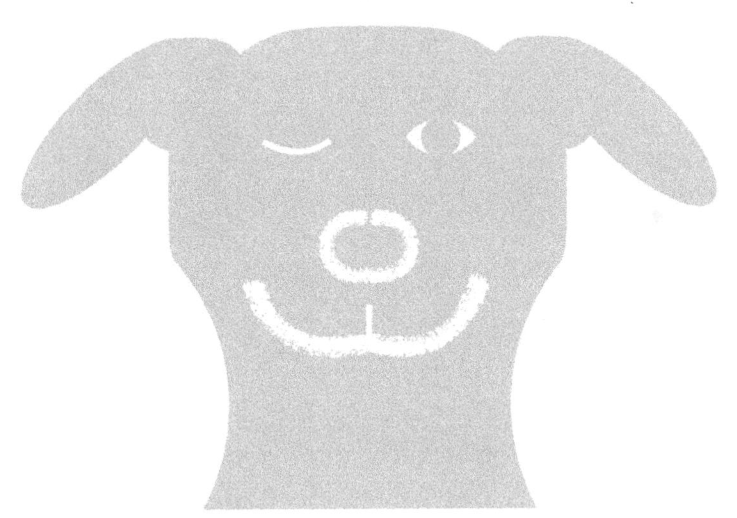

"TELL THE TRUTH TO THE PEOPLE"

~ Robert F. Kennedy, Jr.

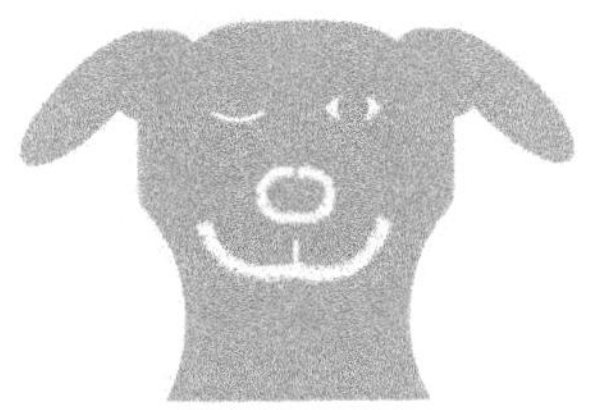

Chapter 20

Data Transparency

> As James Madison wrote, "[a] popular Government, without popular information, or the means of acquiring it, is but a Prologue to a Farce or a Tragedy; or, perhaps, both. Knowledge will forever govern ignorance: And a people who mean to be their own Governors, must arm themselves with the power which knowledge gives." *Letter from James Madison to W.T. Barry (August 4, 1822), in 9 WRITINGS OF JAMES MADISON 103 (S. Hunt ed., 1910)*

The above paragraph is taken from the January 6, 2022, order by U.S. District Court judge from the Northern District of Texas, Mark T. Pittman. The case name is *Public Health and Medical Professionals for Transparency, Plaintiff, v. Food and Drug Administration, Defendant,* Docket No. 4:21-cv-1058-P.[1]

The case was brought under the Freedom of Information Act (FOIA) seeking information enumerated in the U.S. Code of Federal Regulations 21 C.F.R. § 601.51(e) and relating to the Pfizer covid vaccine trials.

Give credit to Attorney Aaron Siri, whose name appears first on a plaintiff's brief filed in December 2021. Siri's team is trying to pry Pfizer vaccine trial data from the Food and Drug Administration (FDA).

Judge Pittman ordered the FDA to

1) Produce "more than 12,000 pages" on or before January 31, 2022,
2) Produce 55,000 pages every 30 days, the first (1st) group on or before March 1, 2022, until production is complete,
3) Redact what is privileged to be redacted, and
4) Parties shall submit a joint status report on production of documents by April 1, 2022, and every 90 days thereafter.

That is how it began. Since then, there have been multiple filings and multiple releases of information. The FDA fought against releasing information whenever possible. They wanted to drag it out for decades. A new plaintiff was added, but it seems to be a new case and not a joinder action.

The FDA proposed a document production schedule that would apparently take 23.5 years. On May 9, 2023, Judge Pittman ordered that the FDA complete the production of data by June 31, 2025.[2]

Not involved in the legal discussion is a financial analysis involving the intersection of economics and law. *Id est*, time to release the documents intersects the pecuniary cost of parsing and delivering the documents. They can do it faster, but it costs money. And the money it costs, many would gladly pay. Thus, the excuse that it takes a long time is bogus.

The above case information outlines the issue of "lacking transparency" regarding covid data. Covid data is hoarded and obscured by government agencies.

Physicians, scientists, and the general public are split on the issue of covid vaccines. There is no consensus because covid vaccine manufacturers and the FDA refused to release vaccine trial data until they were ordered to by a judge.

Frenetic social media debates persist despite governments and oligarchs, à la Bill Gates, spending billions of dollars on biased studies, media propaganda (*exempli gratia*, "*safe and effective*"), and government press briefings. **Economic inefficiency subsumes the current paradigm, which is maximum obfuscation of truth and data.**

Pfizer and Moderna studies performed in 2020 under different public health conditions are nearly useless to tell us what is happening in 2023 in any given location. Those studies are, however, good evidence to later prosecute and convict individuals and corporations for crimes of knowingly shipping products that cause maim and death to babies, children, and adults. The legal avenue of obtaining the information is not only righteous, but also very valuable for posterity. It must be done.

While researchers, politicians, and doctors are chasing the Pfizer and Moderna covid vaccine trial data, there is current data available at the fingertips of public health agency employees. This data in every state is one hundred times more robust than that of trial studies. This data can answer important questions of safety and efficacy in less than one man-week.

Id est, people are chasing tidbits in manufacturers' data, while troves of data exist in every U.S. state health department and federal agency such as the FDA and the CDC. The People are the experimental lab rats, and the governments hoard the data.

To prosecute and litigate in the future, evidence from manufacturers' trials is important to pursue. However, to prevent maiming and death now, massive amounts of government data should immediately be analyzed.

For example, if Pfizer held a trial of 100,000 participants for six months, the study may not produce a serious adverse event (SAE) if the rate of SAEs is 1 in 200,000; and the study may not produce an SAE, if the SAEs take a year to manifest.

Governments now have data representing more than one billion participants over a two year period. The Massachusetts data represents a population of seven million. Even if only half are vaccinated, that's 3.5 million participants. Most of their immunization records, the records of all death certificates, and Medicare records for those in Massachusetts are held by government agencies.

In an analysis of safety and effectiveness to determine whether covid vaccines should continue to be on the market, Option 1 is to wait for the FDA to release millions of pages over the next two years from small trials three years ago, and Option 2 is to petition the government to analyze the data it currently holds, which would take less than one man-week.

Every state collects vital records data, including births, marriages, and deaths. They also collect data comprising disease testing, miscarriages, overdoses, and many other maladies. States also collect immunization data records and Medicare information from doctor visits.

Massachusetts General Laws, Chapter 111, Sections 3 and 24M (M.G.L. c. 111 § 3 & § 24M) provide the regulatory authority for the creation of the MASSACHUSETTS IMMUNIZATION INFORMATION SYSTEM (MIIS) codified under Code of Massachusetts Regulations, Title 105, Section 222 (105 CMR 222.00).[3]

The MIIS contains the immunization records of Massachusetts citizens. The covid vaccination records of Cassidy, Eden, Brianna, Amaya, and all the others mentioned in earlier chapters can be verified in minutes by any of many clerical employees in the Massachusetts Department of Public Health (MA DPH).

The Registry of Vital Records and Statistics (RVRS) of the Commonwealth of Massachusetts is listed as being under the MA DPH.

If the reader takes one idea from this book, it is this – if any state in the nation spends one man-week of effort to correlate death certificates or Medicare physician reports to immunization records, then both sides of the debate will receive enough transparent truth to settle all debate. One man-week of effort is all it takes to end years of bickering.

In nearly all covid court actions during the covid era, the cases turn on a balance of public interest versus individual liberty. The public interest demands the safety of millions of lives hanging in the balance. On the other side of that balance scale is individual liberty, which includes privacy interest.

In the proposed database correlation, the privacy interest is of the dead, not the living. To be clear, potential vaccine-caused death and maim of millions presently yields to the privacy of the individual dead person's vaccine status. On balance, that is folly to the public interest and to family and friends left behind by the dead.

Keep in mind that governments and courts allowed strangers, working in the doorways of public access businesses, to ask visitors for their private medical information of vaccination status. That same government prevents the public from knowing the vaccination status of the dead even when the decedent died only minutes after covid vaccination.

If you live in the United States, you must be familiar with tragic automobile accident reporting in the news. The news media will tell you the toxicology report, blood alcohol level, age, gender, the name of the decedent driver, the year, make, and model of automobile, other passenger names, and what the decedent ate for breakfast before the accident. These are often made available to the press by the government after a horrific accident … but not the decedent's vaccination status.

Somehow, the legal calculus has defaulted to protecting vaccination status of a dead person over the life interest of millions.

CHAPTER THESIS

The data belongs to The People; and it is being hoarded, hidden, and under-utilized by governments.

Governments have the death data. Death certificates detail causes of death, age, gender, and other decedent information. Death certificates are required to be completed under state law in most, if not all, of the 50 U.S. states.

Most, if not all, states have an immunization registry defined by state law. Massachusetts enacted the MIIS. By the same naming convention, New Hampshire enacted the NHIIS. California enacted the California Immunization Registry (CAIR). Indiana enacted the Children and Hoosier Immunization Registry Program (CHIRP).

Governments hoard, hide, and under-utilize the data. Within this book are robust analyses that seem not to be offered by any health department of any U.S. state or U.S. federal agency. Government agencies offer bundled categories and de-identified data that no researcher in the world has been able to correlate in a search for truth regarding safety and efficacy of covid vaccines. Legitimate conclusions are obfuscated.

If one man can produce this much data, graphs, trends, and profiles in this book, imagine what 250,000 employees of state and federal government health-related agencies can provide. Analyses can be done cheaply, easily, and quickly with the data hoarded by government agencies. Why won't they do the work or let The People do it ourselves?

CONCLUSION

In the United States, our governments are of, by, and for The People. These governments are hoarding, hiding, and not using public health data to any useful extent.

The vaccine debate rages on in the absence of data transparency. Both sides of this issue should demand data transparency. Anyone who does not want truth to be told has some agenda adverse to the virtue of public health and safety.

Privacy rights can easily be enforced with a one-page agreement (contract) between any private contractor/researcher and a government agency.

There are many ways to implement solutions to this issue. One option is a law requiring state health departments to perform the correlation quarterly and report the results to The People. Another option is to allow researchers to access the data through a non-disclosure agreement or institutional review board (IRB) contracts. These two and many other options are easy, quick, and inexpensive.

Before Chapter 21 begins, next is an example bill that has been submitted to a state legislature in one state by a state representative in September 2023. Please consider enacting this in your state or nation.

IMMUNIZATION PUBLIC SAFETY BILL "CdC-1"

AN ACT IMPROVING PUBLIC SAFETY IN IMMUNIZATIONS

The bill improves immunization uptake and safety by requiring regular reporting to the public by the New Hampshire Department of Health and Human Services ("NHDHHS"). Public health records reside on multiple, disparate systems such as the New Hampshire Immunization Information System ("NHIIS"), the New Hampshire Vital Records Information system ("NHVRINweb") from the New Hampshire Department of State's Division of Vital Records Administration, and the New Hampshire Medicaid system. These records will be used to provide data vitally important to the public interest, safety, and health.

This act requires three low-cost, easy-to-implement actions to be performed by the NHDHHS: (1) require that Death Certificates include the dates and types of immunization administered within two years before the date of death, (2) require that NHDHHS provide quarterly and annual public reports, by immunization type, of the total number of people who died within 1 day, 3 days, 1 week, 3 weeks, 10 weeks, 25 weeks, and 1 year of any immunization, and (3) require that NHDHHS conduct biennial cause of death and injury studies and produce public reports within two weeks of the date that is one year before each general presidential and each general mid-term gubernatorial election.

SECTION 1: Death certificate inclusion of immunization records

Section 1. (a) "Immunization records" for this section shall include, at a minimum, for each immunization event of the decedent, the following "Vaccination Event Data Elements" to be taken from the then-current New Hampshire immunization information system such as NHIIS defined in RSA 141-C:20-f.

1) Vaccination administration date
2) Vaccine dose volume

3) Vaccine dose volume units
4) Vaccine expiration date
5) Vaccine lot number
6) Vaccine product name
7) Vaccine route of administration
8) Vaccine site of administration

(b) The Death Certificate certifier shall enter on a decedent's state death record, all Vaccination Event Data Elements available in the NHIIS, at the time the Death Certificate is certified, through and including two years prior to the date of death.

(c) For children under eighteen years of age, the entire immunization record text shall be placed into a text field such as Part II of the decedent's Death Certificate.

(d) This section shall be enforced for all deaths that occurred on or after January 1, 2020.

SECTION 2: Required Regular Public DHHS Immunization Death Reports

Section 2. (a) Within ten days after the close of each of New Hampshire's fiscal quarters, the NHDHHS shall produce a report, available to the public, that includes the prior four quarters of the following data:

(i) Total deaths that occurred within twenty-four hours of immunization, including subtotals by type of vaccine, gender, age group, race, ethnicity, and co-morbidity type, if available,

(ii) Total deaths that occurred within three days of immunization, including subtotals by type of vaccine, gender, age group, race, ethnicity, and co-morbidity type, if available,

(iii) Total deaths that occurred within one week of immunization, including subtotals by type of vaccine, gender, age group, race, ethnicity, and co-morbidity type, if available,

(iv) Total deaths that occurred within three weeks of immunization, including subtotals by type of vaccine, gender, age group, race, ethnicity, and co-morbidity type, if available,

(v) Total deaths that occurred within ten weeks of immunization, including subtotals by type of vaccine, gender, age group, race, ethnicity, and co-morbidity type, if available,

(vi) Total deaths that occurred within twenty-five weeks of immunization, including subtotals by type of vaccine, gender, age group, race, ethnicity, and co-morbidity type, if available,

(vii) Total deaths that occurred within one year of immunization, including subtotals by type of vaccine, gender, age group, race, ethnicity, and co-morbidity type, if available,

(b) Within thirty days after the close of each of New Hampshire's fiscal years, the NHDHHS shall produce a report, available to the public, that includes the prior five years of the same data enumerated under Section 2. (a) of this Act.

SECTION 3: Required Biennial DHHS Cause of Death and Injury Studies

Section 3. (a) NHDHHS shall conduct biennial cause of death and injury studies, and produce public reports, including .csv (comma separated value) files within two weeks of the date that is one year before each United States general presidential election and each general United States mid-term or gubernatorial election. The report shall include:

(i) Deaths involving cause of or contributing condition to death, *id est*, any ICD-10 code or replacement system code that appears on a death record after the CDC or an agent of NH has applied all codes to the death records,

(ii) Injuries involving anything for which an ICD-10 code or replacement system code that appears in a physician's notes for the patient,

(iii) Demographic data such as race, age, gender, occupation, and others as appropriate and not a violation of privacy,

(iv) Semi-monthly time period aggregation, which will provide a level of anonymity preservation and will reduce file size by more than an order of magnitude.

SECTION 4: Require Facilitation of Independent Audit of Reports Resulting from this Act

Section 4. (a) The NHDHHS shall select by random lottery, four public health audit proposals biennially, from a person, or persons, or organizations, not affiliated with or dependent upon any government entity, pharmaceutical industry ecosystem entity, or public official. (b) The selected auditor or auditors shall be required to sign a non-disclosure agreement to protect the privacy of individuals that the data represents, conduct themselves in accord with state and federal privacy laws, and share their findings with the NHDHHS at least two days before any public disclosure of the findings, unless life or injury might occur within those two days. (c) The NHDHHS shall provide a reasonable office or conference room space for up to 4 weeks for the auditor or auditors to conduct their work. (d) The NHDHHS shall provide the files or databases either on a portable and accessible storage device or through the NHDHHS network access. (e) Prior to the on-site engagement of the auditor or auditors, the NHDHHS shall make efforts to communicate and agree upon the format of the data files to be shared with the auditors in the on-site audit. (f) The NHDHHS will, in no way, attempt to obfuscate, frustrate, impair, unnecessarily complicate, or hinder the auditors in their mission. (g) The auditor's proposal must meet minimum standards of competence in data management, aggregation, depiction, and presentation as a result of the work to be done.

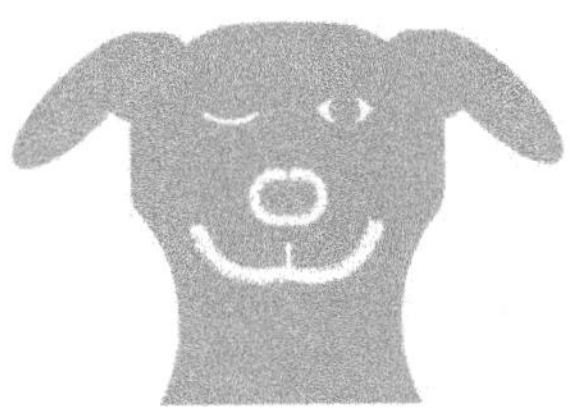

Chapter 21
Required Reporting

Breach or violation of a legal duty, through inaction or action, may be prosecuted criminally or litigated civilly.

People do not all have the same legal duties. Those who swear a public oath or have specific skills or knowledge have legal duties above the average person.

Remember the drowning child example. An average person does not have a legal duty to toss the child a lifeline. A former lifeguard, policeman, family member, or fireman does have a legal duty to toss the child a lifeline. Only those with a legal duty can be prosecuted criminally for inaction.

There is a little-known U.S. federal law. If you witness a federal felony and do not report it, your inaction may be a felony. The statute is *18 U.S. Code § 4 Misprision of felony.*

> "Whoever, having knowledge of the actual commission of a felony cognizable by a court of the United States, conceals and does not as soon as possible make known the same to some judge or other person in civil or military authority under the United States, shall be fined under this title or imprisoned not more than three years, or both."

The average citizen has a legal duty to report federal felonies, else be criminally culpable for inaction.

The legal duty to report vaccine adverse events to VAERS is explained in the beginning of Chapter 7. Aspects of the legal duty of care providers to report vaccine adverse events to VAERS is confusing. That duty may not be expressly stated in law. A good argument can be made that it is implied as an extension of prose on the VAERS website. An ultimate verdict may hinge on the mental state of the care provider. Did the care provider know of the legal duty or even VAERS *per se* at the time of the act or inaction? Generally, ignorance of law is not an excuse. It is for a judge to decide matters of law and this issue of required VAERS reporting has not yet been adjudicated criminally. *Id est*, how the legal duty to report to VAERS is defined in law is not clear, at least to this author.[1]

Even if there is a legal duty to report, there may be a defense of *excuse* or *necessity* resulting from a conflict in concurrent duties. If the amount of time for a care provider to complete a VAERS report is overly burdensome and competes with the time for care providers to otherwise save people from dying, then the excuse of conflict of duties may be proffered and accepted for innocence.

In Massachusetts, most public officials swear an oath of office to "faithfully and impartially discharge and perform all duties incumbent on me …"[2]

Another issue of legal duties is what happens after VAERS reports are made. Take the next step in a duties analysis. After the duty of a care provider to report to VAERS, there is the duty of a government agent to investigate adverse events (AEs). VAERS is a system of vigilance to protect the lives and health of The People. In the case of a serious adverse event (SAE), government agents have a legal duty to investigate, then verify or reject the SAE report being made. The report may be a signal of maiming or death causally associated with a vaccine. This is important to life and health of The People.

I first looked at VAERS data in February 2021. The VAERS system, in February 2021, had enough of a safety signal, obvious to any reasonable person, to shut down all covid vaccines in the United States. The signal was clear. The deaths were many.

Again, there is a video still on YouTube entitled "*The Hand Formula; Economics of Torts; Importance of Torts; Vax tort immunity.*"[3] In that video, at the 5 minutes 5 seconds (5m5s) mark, there is a table in the lower right. The following is a reproduction of the table in that video.

VAERS.HHS.GOV
Example
Year 2021 (thru 4/16), Vax Deaths = 3,085
Year 2020, Vax Deaths = 167
Year 2019, Vax Deaths = 184
Year 2018, Vax Deaths = 165

This table is taken from an April 2021 download of VAERS data. The historical VAERS data files at the Department of Health and Human Services (HHS) corroborate these numbers.[4]

Again, this April 2021 data alone was enough of a signal to shut down covid vaccines. At that time, Diane Dubois age 62 had died of a stroke a month earlier. Brianna McCarthy age 30 had just died of a stroke a day earlier, five miles from the law school for which that video was produced as a Torts class assignment.

Government agents, including those who work for the HHS, CDC, FDA, and MA DPH have a legal duty to investigate these reported vaccine-associated deaths. Inaction is a criminal offense of reckless disregard for human life where a concurrent duty exists to protect people from harm. They know what the VAERS system is for. They know its importance to society. Yet, they appear to ignore every aspect of VAERS. It is actually worse than that.

HHS sought to retard the use of VAERS by conspiring with social media companies to malign its own vigilance system. Their objectives are obvious—continue shipping as much covid vaccine product as possible and injecting as many people as possible as many times as they will take it. Why?

America First Legal is the organization that obtained e-mails by and between HHS and social media companies expressly stating objectives.

If government officials were held to account for their actions and inaction in context of their legal duties, then the issue of covid vaccines would have ended in February 2021. *Malum consilium quod mutari non potest*. "Bad is the plan that cannot change." Government continues to execute the same plan from years ago despite all the death and maim that resulted and results from that plan.

Deliberate indifference is a standard of recklessness that amounts to murder and is appropriately applied in this case of government actions and inaction pertaining to covid vaccines.

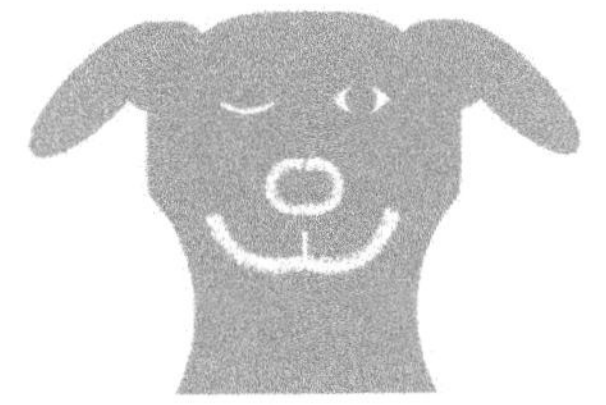

Chapter 22
Criminal versus Civil

The economist Adam Smith of 1700s Scotland put forth the idea of moral sentiment in the context of agency and trade, among other human interactions. His *rationality choice theory* boils down to the opinion that people generally, or always, act in their own self-interest. This seems cynical. Nonetheless, it is the basis of economic theory. Charity—real and true charity, not tax exemption charity—breaks many economic models because it breaks the *rationality choice theory*.[1]

Smith's trans-academic theories breached law, economics, psychology, sociology, and morality. He recognized the intersection of law and economics as important to a civil society.

In the last three years, I learned more about the current workings of U.S. federal and state justice systems than I had in the prior 56 years of my life. I recoil at how far afield our justice system now is from natural law as described by Santo Tommaso D'Aquino through Baron de Montesquieu and John Locke to Thomas Jefferson, John Adams, and other founders of our United States of America.

Anger, sadness, and disgust compete for my feelings toward the current court workings. We must right the wrongs of tyrannical covid policy deemed acceptable by our new society of the electronically zombified political cultists. 'Party before country' is not a successful strategy for the perpetuation of our nation.

Unless you have need to engage the "justice system," you may never know the injustices being perpetrated on your countrymen, whom you have a moral obligation to support in the liberal ideology of individual rights endowed by our Creator, only a few of which are enumerated in the U.S. Constitution.

If you do not stand up for your countrymen facing injustice, then who will stand up for you in the event of your need of the justice system? And your need will come, one day, perhaps through your progeny.

People in the United States, and all five eyes nations, are divided into cults of political parties where one side feels wrath toward another to a point that they will not stand up for the rights of the others simply because they are "the others."

Economics and law are tightly intertwined. To economically get through this chapter, let's only look at the U.S. District Courts. To be clear, all state and county court systems of fifty states plus U.S. Territories are not mentioned here. Thus, the numbers of cases brought are much greater than the numbers cited in the next paragraph that represents only U.S. District Courts.

In the fiscal year ending March 31, 2021, U.S. District Court (federal court) filings totaled more than 500,000 cases of which more than 460,000 were civil cases. Civil cases were up 39% year over year, which is ~130,000 civil cases more than the year before.[2] Remember that this is only the federal court system, not county or state courts, and is only April 2020 through March 2021. It does not include the year of covid vaccine mandates, April 2021 through March 2022, or the year after that.

CRIMINAL

To the best of my knowledge, there have been no criminal cases brought for fraud in connection with CARES Act payouts. The government is not prosecuting the government, which is not shocking to any thinking person. That does not mean that crimes are not being committed.

If crimes were prosecuted, the issue would be solved. The truth would be known through 'Discovery' of evidence.

Look at this one federal crime below and apply the elements to the evidence expressly stated in this book.

18 U.S. Code § 1035 - False statements relating to health care matters

(a) Whoever, in any matter involving a health care benefit program, knowingly and willfully

1) falsifies, conceals, or covers up by any trick, scheme, or device a material fact; or

2) makes any materially false, fictitious, or fraudulent statements or representations, or makes or uses any materially false writing or document knowing the same to contain any materially false, fictitious, or fraudulent statement or entry, in connection with the delivery of or payment for health care benefits, items, or services, shall be fined under this title or imprisoned not more than 5 years, or both.[3]

The CARES Act authorizes a payment schema of federal money to hospitals and care providers in exchange for covid diagnoses, deaths on a ventilator, use of remdesivir, and other qualified actions.

Again, in many companies is often heard the idiom, "*The pay plan defines the behavior*." And in the words of many economists including Walter E. Williams, Milton Friedman, and Thomas Sowell, "*if you subsidize something, you get more of it*."

If you subsidize covid diagnoses, you get more covid diagnoses. If you subsidize the use of ventilators, more ventilators are administered. If you subsidize the use of remdesivir, more remdesivir is prescribed.

The authors of the CARES Act knew the behavior that would flow from the prose when they drafted it in 2018 and introduced it on January 24, 2019, in its original form.[4] Yes, those are the right years. The plan defines the behavior, and, in this case, the plan solicits the behavior. Much of the fraud and corruption was solicited by the CARES Act and coerced by medical licensing and certification boards to be discussed in Chapter 24.

Solicitation is an inchoate crime, yet it is built into CARES Act legislation. The intent is clear. That is why no one has been prosecuted for 18 U.S. Code § 1035. The fraud is massive to an *enterprise* level across entire health care systems of all fifty states and the U.S. federal government.

> Note: Inchoate means not perfectly formed or yet completed. Inchoate crimes are conspiracy, attempt, and solicitation. An attempt is not a completion, but it is a crime in itself. For example, attempted murder. In the case of solicitation, the actor soliciting the other to commit a crime is not committing the act himself, but he is nonetheless guilty of solicitation of the crime.

One likely manifestation of these crimes formed as a result of the solicitation from the CARES Act is depicted in Figure 22.1. This is the

Minnesota N17 Acute renal failure (ARF) All ages annual bar graph similar to the other Minnesota graphs from Chapter 10.

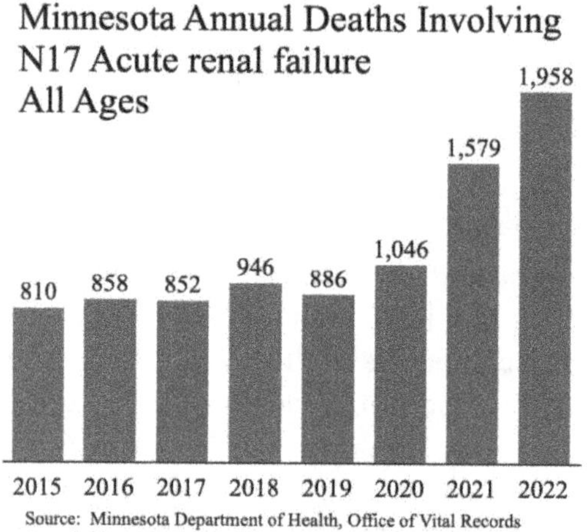

Year	Excess	Excess % over Expected
2020	104	11.0%
2021	613	63.4%
2022	968	97.7%

Figure 22.1

Minnesota is different from Massachusetts in many ways. Every region has its unique nuances of *excess* deaths and causes. USA-wide analyses are poor because they contain many Simpson's paradoxes, making it difficult to extract true signals. This is why I sought record-level source data (RLSD) by individual states.

Minnesota's ARF signal is astonishingly similar to and as stark as Massachusetts' ARF signal. Figure 22.1 depicts more than 1,600 *excess* people killed in Minnesota involving ARF beginning upon the en masse approval of remdesivir. Remdesivir use was incentivized through the NCTAP (New COVID-19 Treatments Add-On Payment) payment plan on November 2, 2020.[5]

To put this date in context, please review these timelines in Figure 22.2. The black line is 2020. Notice that the black line begins departing from the 2015–2019 bundle of gray line plots about two weeks after November 2, 2020.

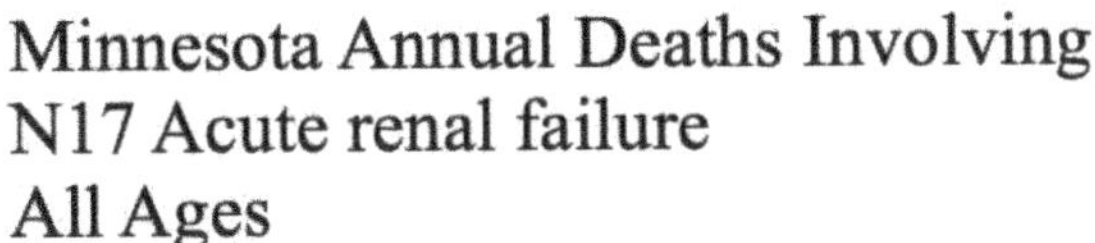

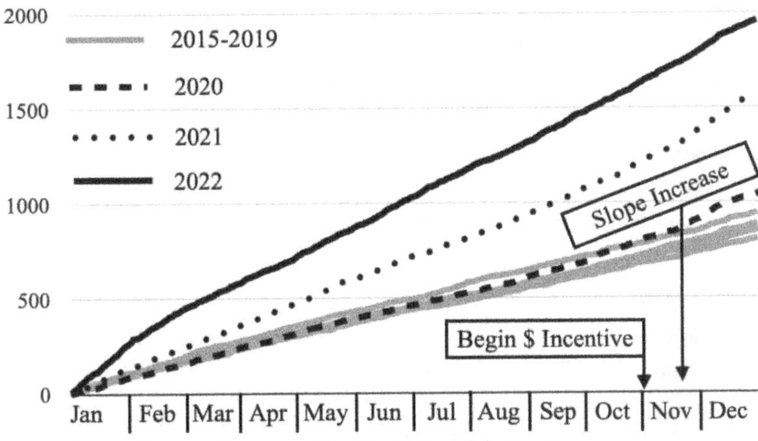

Source: Minnesota Department of Health, Office of Vital Records
Compiled by: John Paul Beaudoin, Sr. || Data Received April 2023

Figure 22.2

In addition to the § 1035 False Statements felony, there are many other federal and state felony statutes that pertain to fraud on death certificates. And in addition to fraud statutes, there are many homicide statutes that pertain to the Acute renal failure-involved deaths. Murder by premeditation and deliberation, the murder weapon possibly being remdesivir, for CARES Act money, should be investigated immediately.

There is no statute of limitations for murder. Perhaps a future administration's DoJ will hold doctors and hospital administrators criminally accountable for their actions to increase revenue through homicide.

CIVIL

Understanding that criminal prosecution will not likely ensue because the government will not investigate the government, the chapter now turns to the issues with civil litigation. Some may wish to skip this legal analysis. Lawyers, paralegals, and those interested in the Constitution versus the machinery of our courts will want to read on.

Standing Doctrine is the focus of the covid civil litigation discussion herein. Most cases against governmental entities, including covid cases, are dismissed based on lack of *standing*. This is not an exhaustive analysis as the topic could easily be a 1,000-page text book on its own.

Notwithstanding the need for brevity, it is very important for Americans to understand how rights were relegated by a doctrine created by the judicial branch from an hyperbolic interpretation of abstract Constitutional phrases.

Article III Section. 2. of the U.S. Constitution

The judicial Power shall extend to all Cases, in Law and Equity, arising under this Constitution, the Laws of the United States … to Controversies between a State … and … Citizens …

This is known as the "*cases and controversies*" clause. From this simple phraseology has been derived the power of federal courts, including U.S. District Courts, to hear a case.

What began as a delineation between the power of state courts versus federal courts to hear cases, became a subjective filter that allows U.S. District Court judges to reject a case if they do not want to get involved.

Standing Doctrine, over more than a century, became an ever-growing list of requirements to have a case heard. The case that summarizes most of the *standing* requirements is *Lujan v. Defenders of Wildlife*, 504 U.S. 555. A plaintiff must show that 1) he has an "injury-in-fact," 2) the injury is "fairly traceable" to the conduct of the defendant, and 3) that the court has the ability and power to "redress" the grievance should the plaintiff ultimately prove his case and win a favorable decision.[6]

Each of the three prongs are further expanded in legalese. An *injury-in-fact* must be a) "concrete and particularized," b) "actual or imminent," and c) "not 'conjectural' or 'hypothetical'."

Although I find this first prong of the *Lujan* decision necessary, in theory, to thwart frivolous claims that waste the court's time, the words leave too much subjectivity to a judge.

Obvious cases like a broken leg in a car accident are injuries-in-fact. However, there are cases at the margins of reason where subjectivity is required, especially regarding emotional or psychological injuries. How can you show a concrete or particularized injury before the case even begins? 'Discovery' has not yet occurred. This is the pleading stage at the very beginning of the case.

The second prong of Lujan relates to causation. There must be a causal connection between the injury and the conduct of the defendant. If the injury results from the "independent action of some third party not before the court," then it is understandable that the plaintiff does not have *standing* in the court. While these seem obvious in higher-level abstract prose, real world cases become difficult where third party doctrine is invoked.

For example, consider the following: 1) you were prevented from attending law school because 2) the school you attended threw you out for not getting a vaccine, 3) all other law schools also enacted vaccine mandates, 4) the schools expressly stated that the mandates are based upon published state health data, 5) the schools expressly stated that the vaccine mandates are also based on the state's assertions that the vaccine is safe and effective, 6) the state's data is found to be fraudulent, 7) the safety and effectiveness of vaccines were not known as the public began taking the vaccines, and 8) government agencies conspired with media to hide vaccine-caused death and maiming.

Given the above hypothetical situation, the injury is that you are deprived of the equal right to attend law school like vaccinated citizens. The traceability flows from the fact that the schools enacted mandates based on what the state published, and that the state published fraudulent data and assertions. Do you then have *standing* to sue the state to correct the fraud? Or are the school's actions those of third parties independent from the state's actions?

The third prong of *Lujan* is equally fraught with subjectivity. Does the court have the power to correct the wrong in whole or in part? Is there redressability?

The key language in this third prong is that the requested relief by the plaintiff should "likely" redress the injury. The mandate that the plaintiff is asking the judge to order should have a net positive effect on the injury cited by the plaintiff. This also sounds straightforward and reasonable. What's the point in hearing a case if the order from the judge has no bearing on the injury? That would be a waste of everyone's time.

The other legalese phrase is that it cannot be "merely speculative" that the judge's order will redress the grievance.

The subjectivity here is that, if the judge does not want to hear the case, he can simply say that it is "merely speculative" that an order for the state to correct its fraud will result in third parties (law schools) canceling their vaccine mandates, thus allowing an unvaccinated person to attend law school.

A more in-depth explanation can be found in the *Memorandum in Opposition to the Defendant's Motion to Dismiss the Plaintiff's First Amended Complaint* in the case *Beaudoin v Baker et al* (2022). If interested, please seek and read the brief.[7]

In many cases, when a judge does not want to hear a case, her subjective opinion of "likely" or "merely speculative" or "fairly traceable" can turn the decision of *standing* or *no standing* in favor of the judge's whim.

Another case, *Ashcroft v Iqbal*, 556 U.S. 662 (2009), added another layer of subjectivity allowing judges to punt cases out of court on lack of *standing*. The language in this case was that a plaintiff must plead sufficient facts to gain standing. This can be construed as conflicting with Rule 8 of the Federal Rules of Civil Procedure that a filing must be "a short and plain statement of the claim showing that the pleader is entitled to relief."

This confuses many attorneys. While sufficient facts must be in the pleading, "sufficient" is yet another word prostrated before the whim of a judge. The pleading should be a "short and plain statement," but it should include "sufficient facts" before the case ever gets to 'Discovery.' Also, the plaintiff must meet a page limit to the pleading.

It should be obvious now why so many cases are dismissed on *standing* and why people from all sections of the political spectrum are confused as to what "losing" a case on *standing* means.

Subjectivity leaves all power in the hands of a judge as to whether your First Amendment right to petition the government for redress of grievances will be upheld or whimsically flicked away.

Here now read what these two cases actually entailed from my biased and annoyed viewpoint.

In *Lujan*, the plaintiffs claimed an injury that if they traveled to Egypt sometime in the future, they might not be able to see a Nile crocodile, if the crocodiles' habitat was disturbed by Aswan Dam renovations partially funded by the United States, and the crocodile became extinct as a result of the renovations. The plaintiffs brought suit under the *Endangered Species Act of 1973* and some changes in its provisions. The Department of Interior was contributing U.S. monies toward the Egyptian Aswan Dam renovations.

You can now understand how some cases, like *Lujan*, should be tossed out based on attenuated circumstances. Would a decision favorable to the plaintiff in that lawsuit result in an order that "redressed," or had any bearing at all, on Egypt's decision to renovate the dam? Was the change in U.S. Department of Interior policy "fairly traceable" to a result in which the plaintiffs might possibly not see a crocodile at some untold future time, if they ever even went to Egypt in the future?

The *Iqbal* case also had some issues that are not mainstream. Iqbal was a Pakistani national living in New York City (NYC) at the time of the 9/11 attacks on the World Trade Center. The details are many and are not included here.

Iqbal was in a detention center in NYC after the 9/11 attacks. He claims that he was beaten badly. After being deported to Pakistan, Iqbal sued many federal employees from the guards all the way up to the Attorney General of the United States, John Ashcroft.

The government's *Motion to Dismiss* on *standing* was denied in District Court. The decision was upheld in the Second Circuit Court of Appeals. The case then went to the Supreme Court of the United States (SCOTUS).

My opinion is that this hot potato could not be allowed to go forward no matter what. The United States was at war in the Middle East. Although eight years had passed, sentiment was still strong with regard to the 9/11 attacks. SCOTUS was put in an awkward position of having to deny Iqbal his day in court. No way were they going to let a Pakistani national continue to sue the Attorney General of the United States.

Thus, SCOTUS added yet another layer of subjective prose from the *Iqbal* case to *Standing Doctrine* on top of the three prongs of *Lujan*.

Since I never got around to writing a substack article on this matter, here is a short synopsis, or thesis. *Iqbal's Revenge* (the title I'd have used) manifested in the extreme loss of rights of all American citizens because of the hurdles that the *Iqbal* case added to *Standing Doctrine.*

ECONOMIC SYSTEMS

A full economic analysis of judicial economy related to *Standing Doctrine* would be a long research paper or a large text book. Without getting too deeply into the prudential requirements of standing, which lie in wait after passing the Constitutional requirements explained above, the issue of judicial economy is important to understand.

Bear in mind that I am an engineer with an MBA and think in terms of overall system efficiency.

First, consider how lawyers (clerks and judges) might seek better economic efficiency by denying 20,000 cases out of 100,000. The system was overwhelmed over the last three years (2020–2022). For judicial economy, most of the marginal *standing* cases were tossed out on the subjective whim of a federal judge.

It is my opinion that no other doctrine is more responsible for denying citizens their First Amendment right to redress of grievances than *Standing Doctrine*.

In consideration of the whole system, I believe that if federal judges adjudicated cases fairly, Constitutionally, and liberally with regard to *standing*, then issues would settle in a Pareto efficient outcome. New cases would not be filed because substantive arguments would have been heard and mandatory authority (judge-made law) would lead to an efficient outcome, which includes avoidance of future litigation in context of settled law.

To put it simply, if a type of controversy is decided in one of the first cases brought before an Appellate Court (which includes SCOTUS), then most other controversies of that type would not be filed in court because that type of controversy will have been settled in law. Outraged people would then turn to the legislative branch to repeal such a bad law that allowed a perceived unjust outcome if outcomes were indeed unjust in such a case type.

Instead, for every legal theory and issue that was not adjudicated because it was tossed out on standing, multiples of the same or similar cases were filed, thus flooding the courts because the controversies were not resolved by a decision on the substance of the case.

Fifty thousand (50,000) cases could have been avoided by allowing fifty cases to go to trial and reach final adjudication, or decision.

***Standing Doctrine* has created an inefficient system with the negative externality of denying justice, which is contrary to the system's mission.**

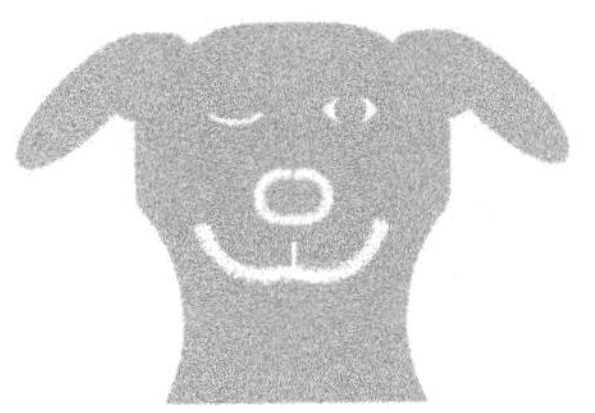

Chapter 23
Redefine Public Health

A Harvard Medical School epidemiologist said that the Massachusetts covid response plan is "one of the best examples of how to handle" the covid pandemic.[1] He was one of many to praise the Massachusetts response despite Massachusetts having one of the worst purported covid deaths as a percentage of population in the entire world.

The first statement on the MA DPH government website follows:

> "DPH keeps people healthy and communities strong. We promote the health and well-being of all residents by ensuring access to high-quality public health and healthcare services, focusing on prevention and wellness, and health equity for all." [2]

There's really not much there except the use of the word "equity" that seems to have pervaded every aspect of government and education. Ask someone what it means. Both ends of the political spectrum and the middle get it wrong most of the time.

The second most prominent paragraph on the MA DPH website follows:

> "Who we serve -
> DPH keeps people healthy and communities strong. We make it safe to eat and drink in Massachusetts, we prevent illness and disease, we give children a healthy start, we help respond to emergencies, and we promote wellness and health equity for all people. DPH also oversees a wide range of healthcare-related professions and services. Information is available for residents, providers, researchers, and stakeholders." [2]

For the grammar police, yes, the first word is grammatically incorrect. But it's the government and few know when to use the objective case interrogative pronoun, "Whom."

"Information is available for residents, ... researchers ..." The MA DPH Vital Records department did provide the death certificates necessary to perform the analyses depicted in this book. Credit the MA DPH for that delivery and transparency.

However, other important public records, such as vaccination records of the dead, are withheld, likely because these records would showcase the pervasive and continuing fraud from the MA DPH.

A Public Records Request for Cassidy Baracka's record of covid immunization was denied by MA DPH. Among other relief, *Beaudoin v Baker et al* (2022) seeks relief in the form of an order from the U.S. District Court, District of Massachusetts mandating the state actors listed as defendants to provide Cassidy's covid vaccine information to the plaintiff.

The following text is taken verbatim from the MA DPH website:

> "Highest salary at Department of Public Health in year 2022 was $349,405. Number of employees at Department of Public Health in year 2022 was 4,194. Average annual salary was $67,789 and median salary was $67,103. Department of Public Health average salary is 45 percent higher than USA average and median salary is 54 percent higher than USA median." [2]

The salaries alone comprise $284.3 Million per year. The expenses must be very high as well.

Given that the average salary computes to ~$67K, then who works for this department? Surely no doctor or biologist is working for such meager remuneration. If doctors are compensated in the higher salary range, then what functional positions are lower than average to keep the average so low? Even a seasoned lab assistant should be making at least $100,000 per year.

Public health agencies were created for the management of waste from humans and farm animals, which would otherwise result in diseases such as cholera.

Regulation of waste run-off from surface-level animal feces and urine is an important function of government to keep the public safe and to prevent property disputes from turning into family wars.

Fecal contamination can lead to cholera pandemics and contaminated wells, lakes, and other water supplies, which are now regularly tested for bacteria and other harmful substances such as lead, mercury, and toxins.

The functions of a health department should be obvious. Here is a list of bureaus and offices of the MA DPH on the main web page of the MA DPH:[2]

- Bureau of Community Health and Prevention
- Bureau of Health Care Safety and Quality
- Bureau of Infectious Disease and Laboratory Sciences
- Office of Health Equity
- Office of Preparedness and Emergency Management
- Public Health Council
- Bureau of Environmental Health
- Bureau of Health Professions Licensure
- Bureau of Substance Addiction Services
- Office of Local and Regional Health
- Office of Problem Gambling Services
- Purchase of Service Office
- Bureau of Family Health and Nutrition
- Bureau of Public Health Hospitals
- Office of Data Management and Outcomes Assessment
- Office of Population Health
- Privacy and Data Compliance Office
- Registry of Vital Records and Statistics

It is clear that the Office of Health Equity will endeavor to apportion health by race and gender, thus denying services to some based on skin color in order to try to artificially balance the results of a system regardless of the other variable inputs.

Every town has a local board of health to permit and enforce local issues. Much of the original intent of boards of health is handled at the local level.

An economically efficient system would have the state focus on engineering and science studies of externalities that affect all or large swaths of the state. Pandemics would come under this purview. The state did engage an MIT professor to test masks for effectiveness against SARS-CoV-2, but then they ignored his results and ordered masking anyway.[3]

Many of the other MA DPH bureaus and offices that taxpayers fund are not in the mission of public health. For example, The Commonwealth of Massachusetts gave gambling permits to casinos in order to shift capital from the pockets of the average citizen to the pockets of the gambling providers, the corporations. The state takes a large percentage of that in tax revenue. Having created negative externalities (gambling addiction) in society by promoting gambling, the state then takes that revenue and pays the salaries of state employees, who then create programs for gambling addicts. As in most cases, government creates the problem, then wants money from the public to grow government to solve the problem they created. This is public health?

INFECTIOUS DISEASE

After showcasing the girth of the state health department, the focus now turns to infectious disease.

The issue is simple. Something killed and maimed Massachusetts residents in thousands of *excess* deaths over the last three years 2020, 2021, and 2022.

The Bureau of Infectious Disease and Laboratory Sciences under the MA DPH is, thus, the most important bureau of the MA DPH in context of the last three years 2020–2022. What did they do?

For the first year of covid, Massachusetts was ranked third in the world for covid deaths per population for any nation or state population greater than three million. New Jersey and New York were #1 and #2, respectively.

In the three years of covid 2020–2022, Massachusetts death certificates involving covid total 20,116 deaths, while All-Cause *excess* deaths total 14,794, a discrepancy of 5,323 deaths. That's quite a large number of purported covid deaths that do not match with the expected rate of deaths in Massachusetts. Even if every single excess death was attributed to covid, they're still short by 5,323 deaths.

It was shown throughout this book that misrepresentations on death certificates are more than merely common. They are the paradigm. They seem to be the internal policy of the MA DPH.

False representations of material facts meant to induce the recipient into relying on the false representations is the policy of the MA DPH. The MA DPH personnel telephoned medical examiners and told them to add U07.1 "COVID-19" to death certificates even if covid had no causal relationship to death. They did this for cases in which a covid-positive test of the decedent occurred months earlier. This practice did happen. This is felony fraud.

Covid vaccine-caused deaths were certified without mention of covid vaccination even when the certifier knew or should have known of the causal relationship between vaccination and onset of symptoms leading to death.

Based on the evidence in this book, the internal policy, the mantra, and the paradigm of the MA DPH seems to be to hide and obfuscate covid vaccine-caused deaths in order to protect vaccines from public scrutiny. The MA DPH internal mantra does not concern the interest of protecting the public from deadly, dangerous, and poisonous vaccines.

The ***symptom spectrum profile*** in Massachusetts changed drastically from the year of covid, 2020, to the years of covid vaccine, 2021 and 2022. Does the MA DPH know this?

The ***age spectrum profile*** changed drastically from the year of covid, 2020, to the years of covid vaccine, 2021 and 2022. Does the MA DPH know this?

The ***seasonality profile*** changed drastically from the year of covid, 2020, to the years of covid vaccine 2021 and 2022. Does the MA DPH know this?

Acute renal failure is 200% of normal. Lymph node cancer is 250% of normal in 2022 and more than 400% of normal in the first half of 2023. Remdesivir is still being prescribed. Does the MA DPH know any of this?

More than 4,000 *excess* deaths, not from covid, but rather from blood and circulatory related causes, occurred in Massachusetts in the past two years, 2021 and 2022. Does the MA DPH know this?

In the most important moment of their lives, the MA DPH personnel chose to follow orders at the expense of the lives of pregnant women, babies, children, grandparents, young and old parents, sons and daughters.

If one man can compile all the data and information in this book, then what are the ~4,000 staff members at the MA DPH doing every workday for three years? They got everything wrong, and lives have been lost in order to promote and protect covid "vaccines" and remdesivir, while various causes of death are wildly out of control far more than any purported covid disease. They hide it from public view.

SOLUTIONS

Regarding both the CDC and MA DPH, one proposed solution is to remove all the bureaucrats who make unintelligent, uninformed, political decisions, and replace them with people who have utility toward the mission and objectives of actual public health. Farmers know better how to keep diseases at bay. Their livelihood and income depend on preventing disease from taking their capital investment.

The CDC should hire a team of experts in management of complex projects across multiple disciplines in order to understand the interactions of negative externalities at the margins.

For an economic example, sack 1,000 bureaucrats at $70,000/year each and replace them with fifty (50) experts at $250,000/year each. This yields a cost avoidance of $57.5 million/year and a health department that would almost immediately be the most robust and intelligent government public health team in the world.

To explain the multiple disciplines and externality avoidance, look at Figure 24.1, which is a black and white version of a slide sent to the Trump Administration in May 2020 (Coquin de Chien logo was added for this graphic and was not sent in the original).

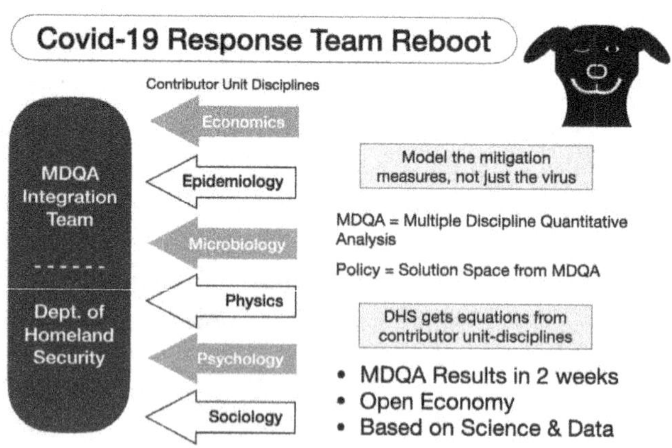

Figure 24.1

A negative externality is an economics term for unintended or unavoidable consequences that are also undesirable.

The multiple disciplines in Figure 24.1 comprise economics, epidemiology, microbiology, physics, psychology, sociology, and others, depending on the issue.

If the issue is masking, then the issue of effectiveness is more about physics and psychology than biology. Biology does come into play in the negative externalities of mask wearing. One negative externality that should be modeled is the culture of fungi and bacteria in the mask while worn for hours. Rebreathing millions of cultured fungi and bacteria aerosols from the mask deeper into the lungs is a clear and present danger never mentioned by the CDC. This is definitely occurring in mask wearing. Cassidy Baracka had to wear a mask six hours per day, five days per week in school. Please remember that Cassidy died with fungal and bacterial pleuritis as noted in Chapter 1. Was it from the mask?

The prevention of aerosol inhalation or exhalation is a function of the material property attributes of the mask and the target substance to be filtered out of the air and prevented from going into or out of the person. This is a physics problem, fluid dynamics specifically.

Why psychology? A psychologist will ascertain, through surveys and interviews, how the average person performs mask wearing. Do they touch their mask and mouth often? Do they wear a mask when no one is looking? Do they fit test the mask each and every time they don or doff the mask? The effectiveness can be modeled from psychological surveys to a sociological level.

The models are mathematical equations using variables and constants. The variables may differ by unit discipline, but shared variables at the model interfaces of unit disciplines must match. As with any simulation, naming conventions of the variables are important in order to co-simulate with other disciplines. In other words, if mask effectiveness changes based on physics, such as temperature of ambient air or velocity of HVAC air flow, then that physics model must have the same variables at the interface as does the model for psychology.

In order to model the vaccine, there are physics models that will include accidental intravenous injections and the intended intramuscular injections. The fluid dynamics models can manage dispersion, concentration, blood volume velocity, and where the Lipid Nanoparticles (LNPs) will eventually transfect the endothelium (inner lining of blood vessels). Genetics models and biological models are needed as well.

While most of the vaccine vigilance group dwells upon spike protein and myocarditis issues, equal and greater issues get comparatively little attention or airtime. Modeling and simulation would solve these biases and stress the overall harm from most of the important factors.

The vaccine vigilance group's strategy has proceeded as a hybrid of 1) ad hoc and 2) a popularity contest of grievances. There are likely more than ten times the number of covid vaccine deaths from stroke as from myocarditis in Massachusetts. Total covid vaccine deaths are likely one hundred times the rate of deaths from covid vaccine induced myocarditis.

However, myocarditis is all that anyone hears about because the FDA, CDC, and their social media and traditional media operatives allow only myocarditis to be openly talked about. Why? It's a 'limited hangout' play. That's an old spy term for agreeing to limited culpability of something small to quell the opposition, while the bigger externality lurks in the shadows, obscured by darkness and silence. The iceberg analogy works well to represent limited hangout. They admit to what's above the waterline in order to distract you from what's below.

The delivery mechanism, LNP, is possibly more deadly than the spike protein *per se*. If the market is allowed to believe that only the spike protein causes all these bleeding and clotting deaths, then the next vaccine will use the same delivery mechanism of LNPs and more people will die from anaphylaxis, anti-phospholipid syndrome, and other reactions to the LNPs. Modeling robustly across disciplines can find the best solution and the hotspots of lethality.

The net effects of arrows on floors, plexiglass everywhere, social distancing, staying at home, mask wearing, ivermectin, hydroxychloroquine, steroids, and all the government-mandated conduct during this "pandemic" could have been modeled in public view. It seems none were.

Multi-discipline quantitative analysis (MDQA) can begin with simple linear programming models and then expand to include non-linear differential equation models using something like MatLab and SimuLink from The Mathworks headquartered in Massachusetts.

The prior diagram regarding MDQA is a similar flow to how semiconductor manufacturing research and development works. They perform experiments at the unit step level of a 400-step manufacturing process. Then there are integration teams that pull the unit steps together into larger groups and then larger groups again. Eventually, the integration team simulates the interfaces between the front end-of-line and middle-of-line, then between the middle-of-line and end-of-line. Simulations are done at each step of unit development and at integration of adjacent steps and groups of steps until the process is fully modeled and simulated.

If the CDC or HHS or MA DPH had industry (non-government) management expertise, they would assemble an expert team and immediately begin MDQA.

Would the pharma lobby allow their government subordinates (politicians) to actually provide a real model? It seems that the government bureaucrats report to the pharma lobbyists who report to the pharma executives. If it were only this simple, we could fix it quickly, but, alas, there are far more players on the chess board. "We The People" are the pawns to be sacrificed in almost all government strategies.

Masking was not implemented to prevent covid. Masking was implemented as a behavioral control that would allow people to believe they could be free from masking if they took the covid vaccine. This is not my opinion. This is a fact and is expressly stated in many places, including the Massachusetts Department of Elementary and Secondary Education (DESE) memo to all parents in Massachusetts to mask children for the 2021/2022 school year. That coercive memo was dated August 2021.

The memo states that if a school reached 80% vaccination of all pupils, then covid-vaccinated students could remove their masks. There is neither data nor a scientific explanation to support this policy. It is an expressly stated behavior modification, or nudge, meant to be a carrot and stick psychological operation to coerce and solicit covid vaccination. The memo evinced that masks have nothing to do with protection from covid. The evidence is in the prose of the DESE "order." Press releases stating the aforementioned DESE orders can be found at the Massachusetts Department of Education website.[4] The August 20, 2021 DESE Press Release describes how the education commissioner asked the DESE board for the authority to mandate masks for all school students and staff statewide.[5] This was challenged in court. The judge sided with the state in a comical decision. The judge equated mandating students to wear snow pants during recess in wintertime to prevent frostbite, to requiring students to wear masks to prevent covid.[6] What Judge Snowpants didn't consider is that DESE has no authority to give the Education Commissioner authority to prescribe medical devices be worn by the entire population of students and school staff statewide. DESE cited neither an expert opinion nor the statutory authority to give such guidance or a mandate. Remember that the CDC sidestepped their own NIOSH and OSHA personnel, who have subject matter expertise. The entire fiasco landed at the feet of an obviously biased judge who opted for status quo rather than for equity and justice. He is one of the greatest disgraces in all of this. Judge Snowpants should be removed and disbarred for the deaths of children that occurred because he chose the popular decision rather than the just and equitable decision.

SOLUTIONS

The MA DPH, CDC, FDA, NIH, and other organizations purporting to be experts at public health administration are dangerous to The People.

Sack most of the management of these organizations to reset the culture. Hire industry experts near retirement who agree to never interact with industry for compensation in any way. Until a great American reset, such as deployment of these ideas, occurs, people should ignore all government orders surrounding public health, vaccines, masks, arrows on floors, and other dangerous and ridiculous orders. The government will kill you and then go out for a sushi lunch to laugh about it.

Civil disobedience is the only way to protect yourself from the deadly and injurious mandates imposed upon us by government.

When government health departments are serious about working for The People rather than working for the oligarchs, politicians, and pharmaceutical industry lobbyists, then an implementation plan using an MDQA approach can be executed.

Within weeks, a government agency can have a new, robust, revolutionary, and, most importantly, effective process in place to serve the public health needs of The People.

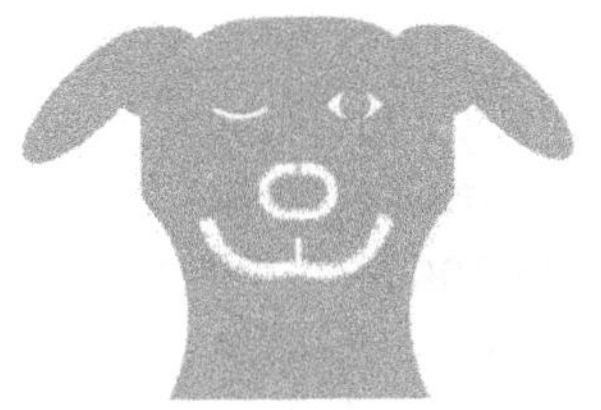

Chapter 24
Redefine Epidemiology

Epidemiology is known to be the study of infectious diseases and perhaps how to control them.[1] While some believe one has to be a medical doctor to be an epidemiologist, there does not seem to be a requirement specific to MD degrees. There are PhD microbiologists and biologists who call themselves epidemiologists. There are virologists and immunologists who also call themselves epidemiologists. Some degrees for those who call themselves epidemiologists are merely Masters in Public Health (MPH).

Epidemiology seems to be a looser discipline than one might expect. Epidemiologists often put forth models of disease spread and virulence. For example, that guy in England, whose name should not ever be mentioned, put forth models of the H1N1 influenza pandemic, covid pandemic, and others. How someone can be so wrong throughout his entire career and still be listened to is an enigma. A track record that bad in the private sector would be grounds for dismissal and public ridicule, not a platform from which to preach doom and recommend restrictions on individual liberties. The only reason people know his name is because the media's output is controlled by government intelligence agencies.

How do epidemiologists create their models? Most models found on the internet seem to be based on a Gompertz curve, which was referenced earlier in this book. The SIR curve represents *susceptible*, *infected*, and *recovered*. The curves are mostly adherent to Gompertz shapes.

Other than Gompertz and SIR, throw out all the recent models and begin from scratch using data, reasoning, logic, and signal analysis by modeling in both the time domain and frequency domain. Apply algorithms in software to detect anomalies across variables, including time, age, gender, cause of death, and place of death, to name a few.

The Gompertz curves will visually pop out of the page when there is a real infectious disease or externality. Chapter 14 shows nearly perfect

Gompertz and first derivative Gompertz curves in the covid cause of death in Figure 14.10. The ideal Gompertz curve in Figure 14.11 follows immediately to demonstrate the near perfection.

The compute power now exists to be able to feed all the data collected from the past one hundred years into a set of algorithms. Such a system can determine when anomalies occurred in the past. Such a system would also provide an early warning system that will find an unknown, hidden issue weeks or months earlier than would otherwise be found. These massive computer systems can find a low signal of food poisoning by manufacturing location or a hotspot of cancer due to limestone radiation.

With signal analysis algorithms, epidemiology will be revolutionized to provide faster time to results and more robust results from more accurate models.

In other words, from methods used to create graphs in this book, a new epidemiological system can look into the past and find anomalous ailments. Those ailments can be traced to causes such as food, air, water, or human genetic lineage.

Trajectories of waveforms in real-time can alert a society that a disease is brewing before anyone knows it is coming. Certain causes of death or ailments might be coded in excess of 300% of normal rate and doctors around a state would not know it. But a system tuned to find anomalies in public health data would find the negative externality before humans would.

Details are avoided for brevity and for the typical reader of this book. Be aware, however, that the work in this book found signals and symptoms patterns like no one else in the world. And it was done by one man in a short time using a simple spreadsheet program, about thirty sheets linked in a file, and a few days of writing code for all the cells.

COMMENTS

Some "experts" and politicians will say that these last two chapters contain ideas that cannot be accomplished. In one week, I listened to three politicians on separate video conference calls, a member of British Parliament, a Senator from Australia, and a former gubernatorial candidate and state legislator from the United States. During the following week, I video-conferenced with three staff members of the United States Congress.

What I learned from that experience is consistent with what someone told me days after my video conferences. He asked if I knew what the biggest caucus in the U.S. Congress is. I guessed at something well-known like the "Freedom Caucus." He answered, "It's the '*That's impossible*' caucus." I laughed, though he is absolutely correct. The common attitude of lawmakers is not limited to the United States. Lawmakers from three continents responded to me the same way. "That's impossible."

Many politicians never, in their careers, put together teams of engineers to attack an issue, win a large contract, and provide value to all parties of an engagement. Everything is possible with the right vision and leadership. Leadership rarely manifests in those who first respond with, "That's impossible."

Reforming public health and redefining epidemiology can be done. An efficient system is not that difficult to implement if politicians get out of the way, or if there exists at least one who is a good leader. Given access to authority, any state can be righted.

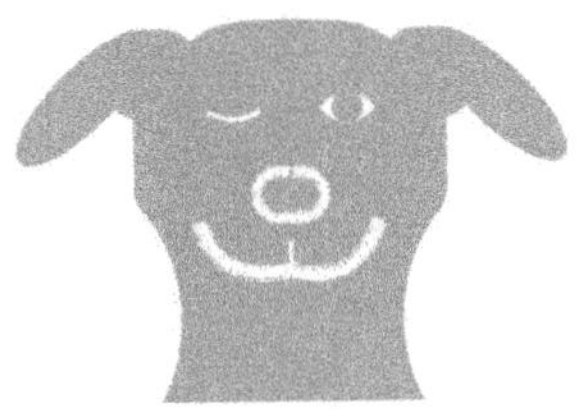

Chapter 25
International Medical Ethics Forum (IMEF)

This chapter is a high-level outline of the U.S. healthcare services market, regulatory governmental agencies, and non-governmental organization (NGO) certification boards. The closing suggests an International Medical Ethics Forum (IMEF) in order to reaffirm existing medical ethics codes, add new ethical constraints to manage telemedicine, and especially to ensure that governments and pharmaceutical companies never get between a patient and his doctor, which was the paradigm during the covid era.

ISSUES

Dr. Meryl Nass is an accomplished 40-year career medical doctor, general internist, and an epidemic and anthrax expert. In 1978, she determined that the Zimbabwe anthrax epidemic was indeed the result of biological warfare.

Between 1999 and 2009, Dr. Nass testified before numerous U.S. Senate and House committees and subcommittees as a subject matter expert. She also practiced as a physician for decades.

Dr. Nass had her license to practice medicine suspended by the Maine Board of Licensure in Medicine ("the board") pending investigation. Hearings on the issue were held—two in October 2022, one in January 2023, and one in March 2023. The suspensions were upheld in each hearing as the issue had not been resolved. As of the time of this writing, the issue is still not resolved.

This single case demonstrates the issue of corruption and tyranny manifesting from centralized power in the modern healthcare services market. Examples of centralized power include, among others, professional licensing boards, which are state governmental bodies, and the parallel system of NGO medical certification boards such as the American Board of Internal Medicine (ABIM).

Over the past decade, state licensing boards and NGOs became more politicized, corrupt, and inefficient with regard to what is just. These boards now exercise their power to suspend or revoke the license or board certification of many professionals based on political biases and edicts rather than based upon violations of ethics or good practices, which is their charter.

In Maine, the Office of Professional and Occupational Regulation (OPOR) holds the power to license funeral practitioners, pharmacists, nurses and nurse practitioners, physicians, veterinarians, and many other professionals outside health care.

Tyranny, through the administrative state, is happening all over the United States, Canada, and other nations. If any professional speaks against government covid "recommendations" regardless of truth, regardless of the life, health, or safety of a patient, or regardless of positive outcome, the state boards are attacking the professionals by suspending or revoking their license and investigating the practitioner.

Any physician or other professional who speaks against a politician is now in the crosshairs of government boards. *Exempli gratia*, if a doctor draws ire from someone connected to an influential board member, that doctor should worry that his or her license to practice medicine will be suspended.

In one case, the board found that Dr. Nass discussed the medical history and prescriptions of an elderly couple with their son who was caring for his elderly parents. He was not a formal care provider but was involved in their care. Neither of these patients nor any other patient filed a complaint against Dr. Nass. The board is claiming that Dr. Nass violated the elderly couple's health privacy for those discussions with their son about their treatment.

In another case, the board found that Dr. Nass admitted to lying to a pharmacist about a prescription in order to effect the treatment that she (Dr. Nass) deemed necessary. The pharmacist was likely under coercion from the state "recommendations" not to fill prescriptions of ivermectin (IVM) or hydroxychloroquine (HCQ) for covid patients. Dr. Nass knew this and skirted truth to effect righteous treatment of a patient. *Id est*, Dr. Nass did the right thing in order to effect treatment around a likely corporate edict or around the pharmacist's personal fear of retribution from the government licensing board. This is coercion.

It seems highly unethical for a pharmacist to deny patient care prescribed by a practicing physician in good standing, if the prescription is safe and effective, which these two drugs are.

Government will not intervene to reprimand the pharmacist in this matter because the pharmacist is following the coercion from the government. The government has already intervened to cause this issue, with purposeful intent, to achieve the results that flow from their actions. The government uses not only the state licensing boards to effect their plan, but also the pharmacists, their corporations, and social media censorship and coercion. The *enterprise* of government agencies and corporations act in a *pattern* of illegal, illicit, and unethical behavior, to the detriment of patients, doctors, and the public interest.

Dr. Nass believes that IVM and HCQ may have therapeutic effect in those infected by SARS-CoV-2 virus. She spoke about the two drugs on a radio show.

Around the time of the first board hearing involving Dr. Nass, the sister of the governor of Maine, having heard Dr. Nass on the radio show, then filed a complaint against Dr. Nass via e-mail to the board. She complained that Dr. Nass was spreading medical misinformation. The board was thus influenced by a political activist closely connected to the Governor of the State of Maine. This has been documented in the news media.[1]

The board continued to seek anything derogatory that they could find against Dr. Nass. She was obviously targeted for behavior deviant from government edict, though perfectly in line with her Oaths and good medical practice. The government of Maine effectively stepped between tens or hundreds of Dr. Nass's patients and their doctor for political reasons. Imagine her many patients needing to find a new doctor at the last minute for a new issue, or for an ongoing issue. The government displaced, inconvenienced, and potentially placed in danger tens or hundreds of Dr. Nass's regular patients. Why? The government's reason was nothing more than a political administrative agency muscle flex to demand conformance to failed government recommendations.

Remdesivir could not be prescribed under Emergency Use Authorization (EUA) if effective alternative treatments existed.

21 U.S. Code § 360bbb–3 - Authorization for medical products for use in emergencies

(c) Criteria for issuance of authorization

The Secretary may issue an authorization under this section with respect to the emergency use of a product only if … the Secretary concludes -

(3) that there is no adequate, approved, and available alternative to the product for diagnosing, preventing, or treating such disease or condition;[2]

The EUA law was opportunistically used by government to promote remdesivir by soliciting hospitals and doctors with exorbitant compensation for prescribing remdesivir at the taxpayers' expense and to the negative health consequences of patients.[3]

The government needed to prevent IVM and HCQ, two medicines with the highest safety profiles for decades via billions of doses administered, from being used in order for the remuneration to flow through remdesivir under EUA. Government planned and conspired to denigrate IVM and HCQ in order to effect the planned remdesivir windfall of billions of dollars.

Those two examples brought forth by the board in Dr. Nass's case, the elderly couple and the IVM prescription falsity, along with the governor's activist sister's strange call for censorship of free speech, seem to comprise all the evidence that the Maine licensing board has on Dr. Nass. "The process is the punishment" is a well-known and understood idiom.

Dr. Nass, who was still practicing in a distinguished and exemplary career, is being attacked by bureaucrats and doctors who seek power over other doctors. I was shocked to see how the board members conducted themselves in an official hearing. The display was quite disgraceful.

One board member smirked when derogatory statements were made by the State Attorney about Dr. Nass. That same board member also was not attentive during parts of the hearing. After glancing at a laptop or desktop computer next to her, she then turned to type while the official state hearing was in session and people were speaking. This breach of duty is actionable.

To fathom a guess as to why such a case is happening, note that Dr. Nass is closely connected to a well-known physician and biochemist, Dr. Robert Malone. Malone spoke out strongly against covid "vaccines" on perhaps the largest English speaking podcast in the world, *The Joe Rogan Experience*.[4] A price had to be paid for speaking counter to government propaganda. It is suspected that Dr. Nass is paying that price.

The targeting of Dr. Nass is believed to be a message to all physicians that if they go against the recommendations of the central authority government, whether the CDC or FDA or another agency, then their license to practice medicine will be suspended or revoked by a state licensing board. Government will smear a physician in the media, take her ability to earn a living, and then laugh about it over a sushi lunch.

The Maine licensing board went so far as to order psychiatric testing of Dr. Nass, a common cold-war era communist tactic against divergent citizens. The message is clear. "Conform!" Else be put through an inquisition, psychiatric testing, multiple hearings, hyperbolic evidence to gaslight the public, and have your career and reputation sullied.

There is an obvious generational battle occurring between hubris-filled youth who seek power and the steadfast, stalwart, stoic and honorable of all ages, who do not cringe before power. The younger should be doing, not judging, especially if they are politically biased. Young activists like those on the Maine licensing board are wrong for the public interest. They do not care that they are stepping between patients and their physicians.

Though Dr. Nass is used as the main example in this chapter, other high-profile physicians around the United States and the world were attacked by licensing boards. The government sent purposeful messages in obvious attempts to chill free speech, thwart individualized medical practice, and suppress individual thinking that is contrary to the central authority CDC, NIH, and FDA recommendations.

Dr. Scott Jensen is a former Minnesota State senator and gubernatorial candidate. He is also a physician. Dr. Jensen was attacked by the Minnesota Board of Medical Practice in what appears to be an obvious political and bureaucratic move to silence or embarrass him for speaking against government central authority recommendations.

The Canadian government acted even more disgracefully in a full-on totalitarian communist manner reminiscent of the Cold War era Soviet Union. The College of Physicians and Surgeons of Ontario (CPSO) raided doctors' offices to confiscate patients' private medical files and did so without notice or warrant. They combed through files looking for evidence of malpractice. They threatened and chilled doctors into conforming to government recommendations, else be accused by the college, subjected to jail time, and prevented from earning an income.

Drs. Daniel Nagase, Patrick Phillips, Ira Bernstein, Mark Trozzi, Mary O'Connor, Kulvinder Gill, and so many others whose stories could fill a book were and are being attacked for performing their medical and legal duties righteously. They saved patients from dying from covid. And because they did so in a manner that contradicted government recommendations, they had their licenses suspended or revoked.

Though these harsher examples are not in the USA, they are on our border. And they are evidence that more centralization and control manifests in more tyranny. If 'The People' of Canada knew the truth about their government, they would revolt and throw that little puppet dictator wannabe in Lac Saint Louis de Le Fleuve Saint Laurent.

Stalin's secret police chief, Lavrentiy Beria, is famous for saying (translated), "Show me the man and I'll show you the crime." Is not this exactly what the Maine licensing board is doing to Dr. Nass and what the colleges are doing to doctors in Canada?

The doctors, who are the recipients of such treatment, are those who prescribed ivermectin. In Canada, some of the doctors who disagreed with government central medical authority were jailed.

These truthful accounts culminate in a situation of the government standing between patients and their health care providers. The government has no conscience. Individuals do. And when authority is centralized, there is no individual making decisions using scruples and conscience. Rules are followed notwithstanding compassion and humanity. Then people die.

HOW IT ALL HAPPENED

Evidence-based medicine (EBM) pervades the practice of medicine in the western world. A few details and history of EBM adoption are noted in Chapter 9.

Since the early 1990s, all medical doctors in North America have been indoctrinated into the "EBM way." Doctors under age 50 generally defer to EBM as the only true paradigm, or the archetype.

The short version of EBM is that the most important deciding factor in how to treat a patient is found in the most recent literature. Doctors now abdicate thinking to the central authority of EBM. "What does the literature say?" This is religious mantra for them.

The EBM way is contrary to all medical practice since the beginning of medical practice. Surely, the most important evidence is the patient presenting to the physician. *Id est*, the person standing in front of the physician is the highest form of evidence. The patient tells the physician directly his symptoms, location of pain, length of time of illness, or other specifics. These are the most important evidence, not "the literature."

Days ago, a friend told of her interaction with her physician. She had pneumonia. Her doctor said that most doctors today would not do simple back tapping and listening. He said they would not ask certain questions or take into consideration nuances of the individual. Her physician told her that younger physicians nowadays would follow what the laptop told them after they typed the symptoms into the laptop. Medical students and residents are taught to follow the laptop, else be liable for malpractice, because doing what the laptop says is indemnification from malpractice accusations.

This case of my friend is important because it is the explanation of how EBM corrupted the practice of medicine thirty years ago. My friend has bacterial pneumonia. The laptop would say that cold symptoms during cold, flu, and covid season should be treated with antivirals and not antibiotics. Antibiotics were withheld from many patients during the first two years of covid. The central authority EBM literature said not to use antibiotics. More than three hundred *excess* bacterial pneumonia deaths occurred in Massachusetts alone in the past three years 2020–2022, likely because antibiotics were withheld due to EBM religious mantra.

Doctors abdicated their thinking to the laptops on the little tables they wheel around among patient rooms.

Only thirty years ago, family doctors worked in small to medium sized groups, or practices. Each practice comprised a core group of one to ten (1–10) doctors. The young docs would ask the wise older docs about anomalous and rare symptoms in patients. The wise old docs would know the issue because of experience and knowledge of local differences such as food, water, genetic origin, or externalities such as smoke stacks, mining, or other local pollutants.

Small practices are now rare as most have consolidated into a system of hundreds of doctors in a practice under a large corporation. The corporation is not a personalized care firm.

Wisdom and personalized medicine are lost under EBM. EBM will save the bulk of the patients, as was happening before EBM, but those at the margins of normalcy will be misdiagnosed, leading to suffering, maiming, or death. EBM resulted in central authority and processing, which is nearly always the least efficient system, though it may be the most profitable. Profit efficiency is contradictory to life and health efficiency outcomes. Profits rank above life and health in the centralized government system.

There is no nuance in EBM. Central processing, deferred thinking, deferred theorizing, and deferred discerning to the central authority results in lives lost at the margins of every disease, congenital defect, and other health issues.

The laptop will tell a doctor to treat according to the highest probability of root cause and based upon the symptoms that the doctor typed into the laptop. Nuanced thinking is lost, or maybe just overridden by fear of opposing the central authority EBM laptop.

Centralization of any system also creates a single point of failure, greater harm from failure, and loss of signal fidelity and effectiveness at the margins. 'Acceptable losses' makes for good profits, but not for those who have the child with the rare disease or young parent with the rare disorder. Those at the margins are left behind, dead, unhealthy, or maimed. Government actuaries calculate whether you will get the transplant or get the $1,500/dose medicine without which you will die in weeks or months. In the eyes of the government, you are just a variable in an equation to determine whether you are worth saving.

On a social media audio platform with a few thousand people listening live, Steve Kirsch presented a political activist physician with a hypothetical situation. Given: the physician injects twenty of his patients with covid vaccines and ten of them die within a week. Steve then presented his question. "Would you stop injecting people with covid vaccine or continue?" Shockingly, the physician answered on an open platform for thousands to hear, "I would have to consult the literature first." No more needed to be said. The physician is an EBM, government drone physician without scruples or an ability to think for himself as physicians used to do before EBM.

The centralization of information allowed the central power brokers to step in and take over the medical marketplace.

The government takeover that followed the entrance of SARS-CoV-2 into society could not have happened 30 years ago. Doctors would not have gone along with it. There were still enough older doctors not infected by EBM cultist mantra. Doctors would have thought for themselves and then fought the centralized government narrative.

Most of those doctors from 30 years ago are now retired, leaving us with automatons and their laptop gods on wheely tables, reciting EBM mantra from the 2D screen to the patients' ears.

WHO BENEFITS

"Who benefits?" or "W.H.O. benefits." Both interpretations of the subsection title work well.

18 U.S. Code § 1962 - Prohibited Activities

> "(b) It shall be unlawful for any person through a pattern of racketeering activity ... to acquire or maintain, directly or indirectly, ... control of any enterprise which is engaged in, or the activities of which affect, interstate or foreign commerce." [5]

A "*pattern*" has different meanings in different jurisdictions. One interpretation from a recent SCOTUS case throws a rope around the idea to mean "*at least two predicates committed within 10 years of each other*." [6] By predicates, they mean predicate acts, or underlying crimes.

"*Racketeering*" includes bribery, extortion, mail fraud, wire fraud, obstruction of criminal investigations, and many others. These example predicates apply to what is happening in the healthcare marketplace.

The other important legal prose is that the actor or actors take "*control of any enterprise*" and "*which is engaged in, or the activities of which affect, interstate or foreign commerce*" means that this federal Racketeer Influenced and Corrupt Organizations (RICO) Act § 1962 pertains to interstate or international activities where the actors are in control of the enterprise, which comprises multiple entities.

Now imagine that the following entities operate as an enterprise: HHS, FDA, CDC, NIH, CMS, FSMB, ABIM, ABFM, ABP, BORIM, BOLIM, CPSO, Pfizer, Moderna, DoD, Military Intelligence, CIA, NSA, FBI, Twitter, Facebook, CNN, MSNBC, Fox News, MNBOMP, CBC, and many others. Further imagine that they are controlled by one or a few heads of those listed.

Are two or more of these entities engaged in extortion of doctors by illegal threat, under color of law, to take away a doctor's ability to practice medicine? If more than a single act occurred, then it is a "*pattern of racketeering activity*."

Are two or more of these entities engaged in censoring speech in conspiracy with governmental or NGO entities? This violates federal felonies **18 U.S. Code § 241 Conspiracy against rights** and **18 U.S. Code § 242 Deprivation of rights under color of law**, which also satisfy predicate acts, occur among two or more entities listed, and occur as a "*pattern*" being more than one act committed of valid predicate crimes.

Doctors are coerced, hospital administrators are solicited, The People are misinformed, censored, some are even jailed. Canada is acting beyond the limits of civil society. All Five Eyes nations (Australia, Canada, New Zealand, United Kingdom, and United States) acted in lock-step and against the contract that governments have with The People. The U.S. Constitution is a social contract. Breaching it is acting against The People and usurping power for the governmental ruling class.

There is no hyperbole in this chapter. All these factual accounts occurred. Evidence was produced through various FOIA requests such as America First Legal's receipt of internal HHS e-mails and presentations detailing conspiracy against rights of U.S. citizens.

Governmental and NGO entities conspired with pharmaceutical companies and media to deprive citizens of rights, squash free speech, threaten and coerce citizens, including doctors, which resulted in a massive transfer of wealth from the middle class to the holders of certain securities—the upper class and politicians.

This happened, in part, because of the changes that occurred in the past thirty years in the healthcare services market. They happened slowly over time like the frog in the pot and most of The People now do not even remember when healthcare was better, freer, and a marketplace of progress, ideas, and services.

Many doctors privately know that the system is broken, and that the government is responsible for the deaths of hundreds of thousands of people in the United States during the covid era. Only a few spoke up and were summarily attacked. Many remain quiet in order to keep their jobs and their incomes. I personally spoke to doctors who left the Commonwealth in order to avoid harming patients at the demand of hospital administrators acting on plan from centralized government. Others know they are harming patients but do it anyway in order for their life to go on without governmental confrontation such as suspension or revocation of their license to practice.

The CEOs from the American Board of Internal Medicine (ABIM), American Board of Family Medicine (ABFM), and American Board of Pediatrics (ABP) published an open letter and e-mailed it to all physicians in their national network of certified physicians. The letter stated that any doctor spreading misinformation will have his license or board certification suspended or revoked.[7]

The coercion is palpable. There is no definition of misinformation in that ABIM, ABFM, and ABP coercion letter. We know from Dr. Nass, Dr. Jensen, Dr. Marble, Dr. Nagase, and others that "misinformation" means anything central authorities want it to mean if a doctor merely has an opinion different from the central authority.

Government doctors at the central authority usually did poorly in medical school and opted for a government salary half of what they could have made in private practice. Centralized power creates a single point of failure. If the weakest link in the chain is the government at the top (central authority), then all other links down the chain are doomed to fail if they are compelled to attach to government rather than have the freedom to attach to stronger, independent sources of information and guidance.

ISSUES REITERATED

Government takeover and centralized healthcare would not have happened but for the indoctrination of most medical doctors into the twisted ethos of EBM and central authority.

Doctors abdicated their duty to diagnose and treat patients to the laptop god on the wheely table.

Medical schools seduced decades of graduating medical doctors into subjugating and relegating the true morality embodied in express medical ethics such as the Hippocratic Oath[8], Nuremberg Code[9], and the Declaration of Helsinki[10].

The ethos of the healthcare services market and its forebear, medical research, must be wrought plumb again.

The issue is a moral one. The healthcare market system must undergo a change at its core ethos to correct those decades of seemingly banal, but actually destructive, elevation of EBM and centralization.

SOLUTION

INTERNATIONAL MEDICAL ETHICS FORUM

The IMEF is a concept proposal. Planning would start if enough grassroots interest manifests.

Begin with a solid moral foundation.

The solution proposed is a mere spark to kindling; and if all goes well, the spark will become a righteous conflagration that will incinerate EBM and reaffirm truly moral medical ethics that existed before EBM.

Solution
Form a new ethical medical culture:

- Reaffirm the Hippocratic Oath
- Reaffirm the Nuremberg Code
- Reaffirm the Declaration of Helsinki
- Adopt new electronic era and telemedicine ethical standards
- Add protections against governmental interference in medical practice and research
- Propose codified versions of the new summary of medical ethics for nations to adopt

In the autumn of 2024, the International Medical Ethics Forum (IMEF) can be held at the Mount Washington Hotel, site of the historic Bretton Woods Agreement that created the International Monetary Fund and the World Bank.[11]

Representatives from around the world would come together, verify a code of ethics that had been architected over the prior twelve months, and sign an agreement to promote codifying the declaration into law wherever possible.

No medical certification boards, state licensing boards, public health entities, corporations, or other entities would be invited to participate. Doctors and other practitioners who focus on patients would challenge their biases and objectivity to remain focused on ethics in the context of the doctor-patient relationship.

DR. NASS CASE UPDATE

On August 16, 2023, Dr. Nass filed a complaint against the Maine Board of Licensure in Medicine (BOLIM) and board members individually in the United States District Court, District of Maine.[12]

The complaint relies on the U.S. Constitution and other laws, including civil action for deprivation of rights, violation of first amendment free speech rights, overuse and constructive error of state law relative to disciplinary sanctions by BOLIM, void for vagueness, retaliation for free exercise of free speech that BOLIM members did not like, and state Constitution violations of free speech and freedom of the press.

Dr. Nass is taking to offense. She deserves to win and the BOLIM members deserve criminal investigation for racketeering, RICO, and many other crimes.

EPILOGUE

The adventures of Coquin de Chien will be further memorialized in the next book, *The Real CdC Does Minnesota - The Pandemic is Moral, Not Viral.*

Whereas the thesis in *The Real CdC - Public Health Crimes 2020-2022* states,

> "The ***symptom spectrum profile***, ***age spectrum profile***, and ***seasonality profile*** of excess deaths all changed starkly on a year boundary coincident with the introduction of covid vaccines."

The thesis of *The Real CdC Does Minnesota* will likely further the notion of profile changes at the margins and investigate the veracity of vital records. What killed people? When were they killed? At what ages?

Acute renal failure (ARF) is also a mass killer in Minnesota, which is partly shown in the Chapter 10. *Excess* ARF deaths total more than one thousand six hundred in Minnesota in 2021 and 2022. Like in Massachusetts, ARF is also a **health emergency** in Minnesota; and the Minnesota Department of Health (MDH) does not seem to know or care.

Coquin de Chien already generated more than four hundred graphs using Minnesota's death certificate data. More than one thousand two hundred total graphs will be generated from the Minnesota data in order to robustly analyze what happened in Minnesota in 2020–2023. The more pertinent graphs and facts from the thousands will be selected and included in *The Real CdC Does Minnesota.*

Another author and researcher, Ashmedai (from Asmodeus, or אַשְׁמְדָאי), has begun providing analyses of the Minnesota data through his substack found at https://ashmedai.substack.com/. He found instances of Fraud of Omission and Fraud of Commission in the Minnesota data similar to those found by Coquin de Chien in the Massachusetts data.

On the other hand, Coquin de Chien and Ashmedai also found that Minnesota death certificate signals are very different from Massachusetts death certificate signals. Misrepresentations, or falsities, are not nearly as prevalent in Minnesota in the early 2020 records. Thus far, Massachusetts seems to be the worst offender of all U.S. states with regard to false statements on vital records at the very beginning of the covid era.

In *The Real CdC - COVID Facts for Regular People*, Coquin de Chien evinced enterprise crimes of murder, fraud, and conspiracy involving multiple governments, NGOs, corporations, and individuals.

In the next book involving Minnesota data, Coquin de Chien will amble beyond law and economics, beyond data analysis, and beyond individual cases. In the *The Real CdC Does Minnesota*, Coquin de Chien will ask the reader to explore his or her own morality and that of our society. In the context of covid vaccines imposed upon society by government, what obligation does each citizen have to defy authority and reject vaccines, masks, and the other edicts propagandized to bend society to the will of a tyrannical government?

Coquin de Chien will examine the moral calculus of what is now known to be a Death Lottery. A Death Lottery is explored through deductive syllogism in the short substack article *The Moral Calculus of a Death Lottery.*[1]

In a Death Lottery, everyone knows that someone will die. They draw lots hoping not to win. Given the option to not enter, they would not enter. Threat of being killed is the usual reason that someone chooses to enter a Death Lottery.

Does your belief system require that you forego self-harm in order to maintain the integrity of your soul?

If the government will not stop, and it appears they will not, then do not participate in the Death Lottery. You may save the lives of many sons and daughters, brothers and sisters, mothers and fathers, by living the following imperative.

DO NOT COMPLY

REFERENCES

Praefatio

1) *Beaudoin v Baker et al. (2022)*. U.S. District Court, District of Massachusetts. Docket No. 1:22-cv-11356-NMG. Pending as of August 6, 2023.

Introduction

1) Note that the CDC URLs for these data have since been changed by the CDC. Centers for Disease Control and Prevention. (2020). *Weekly Counts of Deaths by State and Select Causes 2014–2018.* And *Weekly Counts of Deaths by State and Select Causes 2019–2020.* Found at https://data.cdc.gov/browse in April and May 2020.

2) Template example letter. Names of senders were removed for privacy reasons.

<NAME>
<Street Address>
<City, ST zicode>
<Telephone Number>
<email address>

January 31, 2022

Department of Public Health
Attn: Records Access Officer - Helen Rush-Lloyd and Jennifer K. Soivilien
1 Ashburton Place
Boston, MA 02108

NOTE:
The following request was also submitted using the website:
https://www.mass.gov/forms/request-public-records-from-the-department-of-public-health

Dear Ms. Rush-Lloyd and Ms. Soivilien:
This request is made pursuant to Massachusetts General Law Chapter 66: *Public Records*, Section 10: *Inspection and copies of public records; requests; written responses; extension of time; fees.*

Please compile the following records and send to one of the physical or email address herein provided: **each individual record of every death recorded in Massachusetts in the years 2015 through 2021, inclusive.**

To be clear, I understand that proprietary and personal information such as name, address, social security number, and other proprietary information will be withheld.

All other fields, including but not limited to **age, gender, race, ethnicity, date of death, cause of death (including but not limited to R00-R99), other contributing causes of death, conditions noted but not causing death, dates of covid vaccinations, and death narratives** should be included.

At approximately 60,000 deaths per year in Massachusetts and 7 years requested, the estimated total is 420,000 records. Using the Vitals Information Partnership (VIP) system or other system used by MA DPH, it is estimated to be 10 to 15 minutes of work by DPH personnel to hide the personal information fields, then save the remaining fields to a file and email it to me.

A written response is required within within 10 business days, else you are statutorily required to provide an explanation in writing. Massachusetts General Law Chapter 66, Section 15 describes the punishments for any attempt to hide, alter, deface, mutilate, or destroy records.

Regards,
<Name>

3) (2020). Patriots plane arrives in Boston from China with 1.2 million masks for local health care workers. *WCVB5 Boston's News Leader*. Found at https://www.wcvb.com/article/robert-kraft-using-patriots-plane-to-get-protective-equipment-from-china/32014916# on August 4, 2023. Updated April 2, 2020.

4) Coquin de Chien. (March 27, 2022). The Baker Knew. *Substack*. Found here https://open.substack.com/pub/coquindechien/p/the-baker-knew?r=1d6m3v&utm_campaign=post&utm_medium=web on August 4, 2023.

5) Baker, C. (May 1, 2020). ORDER REQUIRING FACE COVERINGS IN PUBLIC PLACES WHERE SOICAL DISTANCING IS NTO POSSIBLE. *Office of the Governor. Commonwealth of Massachusetts*. Found here https://www.mass.gov/doc/may-1-2020-masks-and-face-coverings/download on August 4, 2023.

6) Levitt, M. (July 31, 2021). Twitter post found here https://twitter.com/MLevitt_NP2013/status/1421321431418277892

7) (February 11, 2021). Operation Warp Speed: Accelerated COVID-19 Vaccine Development Status and Efforts to Address Manufacturing Challenges. *U.S. Government Accountability Office*. Found here https://www.gao.gov/products/gao-21-319

8) Beaudoin, J. (April 2021). The Hand Formula; Economics of Torts; Importance of Torts; Vax tort immunity. Written and produced for Torts class. Found here https://www.youtube.com/watch?v=JObGnOCD6mI

9) Office of Public Affairs. (May 31, 2017). Electronic Health Records Vendor to Pay $155 Million to Settle False Claims Act Allegations. *U.S. Department of Justice*. Found here https://www.justice.gov/opa/pr/electronic-health-records-vendor-pay-155-million-settle-false-claims-act-allegations

10) CDC. (August 2004). Instructions for Completing the Cause-of-Death Section of the Death Certificate. *U.S. DEPARTMENT OF HEALTH AND HUMAN SERVICES. Centers for Disease Control and Prevention. National Center for Health Statistics*. Found here https://www.cdc.gov/nchs/data/dvs/blue_form.pdf

11) (2019). International Statistical Classification of Diseases and Related Health Problems 10th Revision - ICD-10 Version:2019. Found here https://icd.who.int/browse10/2019/en on August 7, 2023.

Chapter 1

1) (January 18, 2022). Cassidy Patrice Baracka Obituary. *Badger Funeral Home of Littleton*. Found here https://www.legacy.com/us/obituaries/name/cassidy-baracka-obituary?pid=201289667 on August 6, 2023.

2) Bass, C. (February 8, 2022). Family's heartbreak as girl, 7, 'dies from Covid complications.' *yahoo!news*. Found here https://au.news.yahoo.com/family-heartbreak-girl-7-dies-covid-complications-us-060823080.html on August 6, 2023.

3) (February 3, 2022). Pink ribbons dot community remembering 7-year-old who died of COVID-19. *WCVB5 Boston's News Leader*. Found here https://www.wcvb.com/article/cassidy-baracka-covid-death-7-year-old-groton-massachusetts/38975512 on August 6, 2023.

4) (February 10, 2022). Cassidy Patrice Baracka, 7. *The Groton Herald*. Found here https://grotonherald.com/cassidy-patrice-baracka-7 on August 6, 2023.

5) Schwartz, S. (March 24, 2020). COVID-19 Alert No. 2 New ICD code introduced for COVID-19 deaths. *NVSS National Vital Statistics System, National Center for Health Statistics*. Found here https://www.cdc.gov/nchs/data/nvss/coronavirus/Alert-2-New-ICD-code-introduced-for-COVID-19-deaths.pdf on August 6, 2023.

6) (April 2020). (Expanded February 2023). Report No. 3 Guidance for Certifying Deaths Due to Coronavirus Disease 2019 (COVID-19) Expanded in February 2023 to Include Guidance for Certifying Deaths Due to Post-acute Sequelae of COVID-19. *NVSS National Vital Statistics System, National Center for Health Statistics*. Found here https://www.cdc.gov/nchs/data/nvss/vsrg/vsrg03-508.pdf on August 6, 2023.

7) VAERS Vaccine Adverse Event Reporting System. *VAERS is co-sponsored by the Centers for Disease Control and Prevention (CDC), and the Food and Drug Administration (FDA), agencies of the U.S. Department of Health and Human Services (HHS)*. Found here https://vaers.hhs.gov/data.html on August 6, 2023.

8) (January 15, 2022). VAERS Event Details. Details for VAERS ID: 2038120-1. *CDC Wonder*. Found here https://wonder.cdc.gov/controller/datarequest/D8;jsessionid=777585F67A9D4BEED49519FB78F3 on August 12, 2023.

9) Coquin de Chien. (March 24, 2022). Tragedy in Groton, Massachusetts. *Substack*. Found here https://open.substack.com/pub/coquindechien/p/tragedy-in-groton-massachusetts?r=1d6m3v&utm_campaign=post&utm_medium=web on August 6, 2023.

10) *Beaudoin v Baker et al.* (2022). U.S. District Court, District of Massachusetts. Docket No. 1:22-cv-11356-NMG. Pending as of August 6, 2023.

Chapter 2

1) Coquin de Chien. (January 7, 2023). Massachusetts Anecdrokes. Substack. Found here https://coquindechien.substack.com/p/massachusetts-anecdrokes on August 6, 2023.

2) (June 2, 2021). VAERS Event Details. Details for VAERS ID: 1368271-1. *CDC Wonder*. Found here https://wonder.cdc.gov/controller/datarequest/D8;jsessionid=777585F67A9D4BEED49519FB78F3 on August 12, 2023.

3) Kirk, B. (March 9, 2021). Methuen teachers to get vaccine next week. *The Eagle-Tribune*. Found here https://www.eagletribune.com/news/merrimack_valley/methuen-teachers-to-get-vaccine-next-week/article_907e7e30-336b-5eb5-b181-d779f5f20476.html on August 6, 2023.

4) Coquin de Chien. (January 7, 2023). Massachusetts Anecdrokes. *Substack*. Found here https://coquindechien.substack.com/p/massachusetts-anecdrokes?utm_source=profile&utm_medium=reader2 on August 6, 2023.

5) (June 10, 2021). VAERS Event Details. Details for VAERS ID: 1388042-1. *CDC Wonder*. Found here https://wonder.cdc.gov/controller/datarequest/D8;jsessionid=777585F67A9D4BEED49519FB78F3 on August 12, 2023.

6) McMillan, N. (December 5, 2022). Fatal Post COVID mRNA-Vaccine Associated Cerebral Ischemia. *The Neurohospitalist*. Found here https://journals.sagepub.com/doi/10.1177/19418744221136898 on August 6, 2023.

Chapter 3

1) (2021). Holly Hodgdon Obituary. Found here https://www.legacy.com/us/obituaries/atholdailynews/name/holly-hodgdon-obituary?id=23177040 on August 6, 2023.

2) (2021). Daniel "Dan" L. Earley. *Cheshire Family Funeral Home*. Found here https://cheshirefamilyfuneralhome.com/daniel-dan-l-earley/ on August 6, 2023.

3) (February 14, 2023). VAERS Event Details. Details for VAERS ID: 2582749-1. *CDC Wonder*. Found here https://wonder.cdc.gov/controller/datarequest/D8;jsessionid=777585F67A9D4BEED49519FB78F3 on August 12, 2023.

Chapter 4

4) (2021). Karyn Samantha Slack. *Day Funeral Home*. Found here https://www.dayfunerals.com/obituary/karyn-slack on August 7, 2023.

5) (June 13, 2022). VAERS Event Details. Details for VAERS ID: 2317423-1. *CDC Wonder*. Found here https://wonder.cdc.gov/controller/datarequest/D8;jsessionid=D37C6621B763B28B9FC08010DD55 on August 11, 2023.

6) (April 25, 2021). Martin Aloysius Joyce IV - Obituary. *Caledonian Record Since 1837*. Found here https://www.caledonianrecord.com/community/deaths/martin-aloysius-joyce-iv---obituary/article_f4eef74c-7389-5a1c-a4ba-5f285492cefb.html on August 7, 2023.

7) (April 23, 2021). VAERS Event Details. Details for VAERS ID: 1247687-1. *CDC Wonder*. Found here https://wonder.cdc.gov/controller/datarequest/D8;jsessionid=777585F67A9D4BEED49519FB78F3 on August 11, 2023.

Chapter 5

1) (May 2020). fraud. *Cornell Law School Legal Information Institute*. Found here https://www.law.cornell.edu/wex/fraud on August 7, 2023.

2) *Beaudoin v Baker et al.* (2022). U.S. District Court, District of Massachusetts. Docket No. 1:22-cv-11356-NMG. Pending as of August 6, 2023.

Chapter 6

There are no references for this chapter

Chapter 7

1) (2023). Investigation of safety signals. *World Health Organization*. Found here https://www.who.int/initiatives/the-global-vaccine-safety-initiative/investigation-of-safety-signals on August 11, 2023.

2) (September 8, 2022). Vaccine Adverse Event Reporting System (VAERS). *Centers for Disease Control and Prevention*. Found here https://www.cdc.gov/vaccinesafety/ensuringsafety/monitoring/vaers/index.html on August 6, 2023.

3) (June 1, 2023). Reporting Adverse Events Following Vaccination. *Centers for Disease Control and Prevention*. Found here https://www.cdc.gov/vaccinesafety/hcproviders/reportingadverseevents.html on August 11, 2023.

4) (March 13, 2023). How to Report Adverse Events to VAERS. *Centers for Disease Control and Prevention*. Found here https://www.cdc.gov/

vaccinesafety/ensuringsafety/monitoring/vaers/reportingaes.html on August 11, 2023.

5) (August 13, 2021). Vaccine Adverse Event Reporting System (VAERS) Questions and Answers. *U.S. Food & Drug Administration.* Found here https://www.fda.gov/vaccines-blood-biologics/vaccine-adverse-events/vaccine-adverse-event-reporting-system-vaers-questions-and-answers on August 8, 2023

6) McMillan, N. (December 5, 2022). Fatal Post COVID mRNA-Vaccine Associated Cerebral Ischemia. *The Neurohospitalist.* Found here https://journals.sagepub.com/doi/10.1177/19418744221136898 on August 6, 2023.

7) *Beaudoin v Baker et al.* (2022). U.S. District Court, District of Massachusetts. Docket No. 1:22-cv-11356-NMG. Pending as of August 6, 2023.

8) (2023). Fighting Back. *American First Legal.* Found here https://aflegal.org/ on August 11, 2023.

9) Beaudoin, J. (April 2021). The Hand Formula; Economics of Torts; Importance of Torts; Vax tort immunity. Written and produced for Torts class - then placed on *YouTube.* Found here https://www.youtube.com/watch?v=JObGnOCD6mI

10) (March 8, 2021). VAERS Event Details. Details for VAERS ID: 1080840-1. *CDC Wonder.* Found here https://wonder.cdc.gov/controller/datarequest/D8;jsessionid=68C4B74E6BE017EC5B1835349D4B on August 11, 2023.

11) (March 8, 2021). VAERS Event Details. Details for VAERS ID: 1243791-1. *CDC Wonder.* Found here https://wonder.cdc.gov/controller/datarequest/D8;jsessionid=68C4B74E6BE017EC5B1835349D4B on August 11, 2023.

12) Unacceptable Jessica. Found here https://jessicar.substack.com/ on August 11, 2023.

13) Anandamide. (August 13, 2022). Peer Review = Pharma Gatekeeping. *Nepetalactone Newsletter. Substack.* Found here https://anandamide.substack.com/p/peer-review-pharma-gatekeeping on August 11, 2023.

Chapter 8

1) Fischer, M. (May 28, 2021). COVID-19 Vaccine Breakthrough Infections Reported to CDC — United States, January 1–April 30, 2021. *Morbidity and Mortality Weekly Report (MMWR). Centers for Disease Control and Prevention.* Found here https://www.cdc.gov/mmwr/volumes/70/wr/mm7021e3.htm on August 11, 2023.

2) (January 18, 2021). VAERS Event Details. Details for VAERS ID: 0953922-1. *CDC Wonder*. Found here https://wonder.cdc.gov/controller/datarequest/D8;jsessionid=777585F67A9D4BEED49519FB78F3 on August 11, 2023.

Chapter 9

1) (June 15, 2016). The history of evidence-based medicine. National Library of Medicine. *National Center for Biotechnology Information*. Found here https://www.ncbi.nlm.nih.gov/books/NBK390299/ on August 13, 2023.

2) Evidence-Based Medicine Working Group (1992). Evidence-based medicine. A new approach to teaching the practice of medicine. *JAMA, 268(17), 2420–2425*. Found here https://doi.org/10.1001/jama.1992.03490170092032 on August 13, 2023.

3) Zimerman, A. (January 2013). Evidence-Based Medicine: A Short History of a Modern Medical Movement. *AMA Journal of Ethics*. Found here https://journalofethics.ama-assn.org/article/evidence-based-medicine-short-history-modern-medical-movement/2013-01 on August 13, 2023.

4) Druzin, R. (August 3, 2016). Crossing the Border for Care. *U.S. News*. Found here https://www.usnews.com/news/best-countries/articles/2016-08-03/canadians-increasingly-come-to-us-for-health-care on August 13, 2023.

Chapter 10

1) (April 25, 2022). Revocation of Emergency Use of a Drug During the COVID-19 Pandemic; Availability. *Federal Register*. Found here https://www.federalregister.gov/documents/2022/07/26/2022-15956/revocation-of-emergency-use-of-a-drug-during-the-covid-19-pandemic-availability on August 15, 2023.

2) (June 20, 2023). New COVID-19 Treatments Add-On Payment (NCTAP). *Centers for Medicare & Medicaid Services*. Found here https://www.cms.gov/medicare/covid-19/new-covid-19-treatments-add-payment-nctap on August 15, 2023.

3) Beaudoin, J. (June 22, 2023). MEMORANDUM: NOTICE OF HEALTH EMERGENCY REQUIRING IMMEDIATE INVESTIGATION OF DEATHS BY ACUTE RENAL FAILURE IN MINNESOTA. *ViaVeraVita*. Found here https://viaveravita.com/minnesota-memorandum on August 14, 2023.

Chapter 11

1) Beaudoin, J. (May 19, 2023). MEMORANDUM: NOTICE OF MISREPRESENTATION REQUIRING PUBLIC ADMISSION AND CORRECTION OF VITAL RECORDS. *ViaVeraVita*. Found here https://viaveravita.com/vermont-memorandum-exhibits on August 12, 2023.

2) Beaudoin, J. (May 19, 2023). Vermont EXHIBITS. *ViaVeraVita*. Found here https://viaveravita.com/vermont-memorandum-exhibits on August 12, 2023.

3) Beaudoin, J. (May 19, 2023). VT Memo USPS Tracking Receipts and Delivery Confirmation. *ViaVeraVita*. Found here https://viaveravita.com/vermont-memorandum-exhibits on August 12, 2023.

4) (January 13, 2021). VAERS Event Details. Details for VAERS ID: 0942072-1. *CDC Wonder*. Found here https://wonder.cdc.gov/controller/datarequest/D8;jsessionid=D37C6621B763B28B9FC08010DD55 on August 12, 2023.

5) (March 4, 2021). *VAERS Event Details. Details for VAERS ID: 1072218-1*. CDC Wonder. Found here https://wonder.cdc.gov/controller/datarequest/D8;jsessionid=D37C6621B763B28B9FC08010DD55 on August 12, 2023.

6) (April 5, 2021). *VAERS Event Details. Details for VAERS ID: 1169181-1*. CDC Wonder. Found here https://wonder.cdc.gov/controller/datarequest/D8;jsessionid=D37C6621B763B28B9FC08010DD55 on August 12, 2023.

7) (April 23, 2021). *VAERS Event Details. Details for VAERS ID: 1247687-1*. CDC Wonder. Found here https://wonder.cdc.gov/controller/datarequest/D8;jsessionid=D37C6621B763B28B9FC08010DD55 on August 12, 2023.

8) (April 28, 2021). *VAERS Event Details. Details for VAERS ID: 1267587-1*. CDC Wonder. Found here https://wonder.cdc.gov/controller/datarequest/D8;jsessionid=D37C6621B763B28B9FC08010DD55 on August 12, 2023.

9) (May 24, 2021). *VAERS Event Details. Details for VAERS ID: 1343614-1*. CDC Wonder. Found here https://wonder.cdc.gov/controller/datarequest/D8;jsessionid=D37C6621B763B28B9FC08010DD55 on August 12, 2023.

10) (June 13, 2022). *VAERS Event Details. Details for VAERS ID: 2317423-1*. CDC Wonder. Found here https://wonder.cdc.gov/controller/datarequest/D8;jsessionid=D37C6621B763B28B9FC08010DD55 on August 12, 2023.

11) O'Neill, N. (April 2, 2021). *CDC walks back claim that vaccinated people can't carry COVID-19*. New York Post. Found here https://nypost.com/2021/04/02/cdc-walks-back-claim-that-vaccinated-people-cant-carry-covid/ on August 12, 2023.

12) (July 27, 2021). *VAERS Event Details. Details for VAERS ID: 1505017-1*. CDC Wonder. Found here https://wonder.cdc.gov/controller/datarequest/D8;jsessionid=E909E5E4787DEF5C0AA465FD92AF on August 12, 2023.

13) (January 3, 2022). *VAERS Event Details. Details for VAERS ID: 1999297-1*. CDC Wonder. Found here https://wonder.cdc.gov/controller/datarequest/D8;jsessionid=E909E5E4787DEF5C0AA465FD92AF on August 12, 2023.

14) (March 29, 2021). *VAERS Event Details. Details for VAERS ID: 1150385-1*. CDC Wonder. Found here https://wonder.cdc.gov/controller/datarequest/D8;jsessionid=E909E5E4787DEF5C0AA465FD92AF on August 12, 2023.

15) (December 22, 2022). *VAERS Event Details. Details for VAERS ID: 2540777-1*. CDC Wonder. Found here https://wonder.cdc.gov/controller/datarequest/D8;jsessionid=E909E5E4787DEF5C0AA465FD92AF on August 12, 2023.

16) (February 15, 2022). *VAERS Event Details. Details for VAERS ID: 2122755-1*. CDC Wonder. Found here https://wonder.cdc.gov/controller/datarequest/D8;jsessionid=E909E5E4787DEF5C0AA465FD92AF on August 12, 2023.

Chapter 12

1) (July 11, 2023). COVID-19 Funeral Assistance. *FEMA*. Found here https://www.fema.gov/disaster/historic/coronavirus/economic/funeral-assistance on August 12, 2023.

Chapter 13

1) (2023). Centers for Disease Control and Prevention Salaries of 2022. *FederalPay.org*. Found here https://www.federalpay.org/employees/centers-for-disease-control-and-preventn on November 17, 2023.

2) (2023). Department of Public Health (Dph) Salaries. *GovSalaries*. Found here https://govsalaries.com/salaries/MA/department-of-public-health-dph on November 27, 2023.

3) Smalley, J. (February 24, 2022). The Definitive Guide to COVID and COVID vaccine deaths. Dead Man Talking. *Substack*. Found here https://open.substack.com/pub/metatron/p/the-definitive-guide-to-covid-and?r=1d6m3v&utm_campaign=post&utm_medium=web

4) Sobey, R. (March 10, 2022). Massachusetts' coronavirus death count is dropping by nearly 4,000 deaths based on new definition. *Boston Herald*. Found here https://www.bostonherald.com/2022/03/10/massachusetts-coronavirus-death-count-is-dropping-by-nearly-4000-deaths-based-on-new-definition/

5) Baker, C. (May 1, 2020). ORDER REQUIRING FACE COVERINGS IN PUBLIC PLACES WHERE SOICAL DISTANCING IS NTO POSSIBLE. *Office of the Governor. Commonwealth of Massachusetts.* Found here https://www.mass.gov/doc/may-1-2020-masks-and-face-coverings/download on August 4, 2023.

Chapter 14

1) McConnell M. (March 19, 2020). S.3548 - 116th Congress (2019-2020). *Library of Congress*. Found here https://www.congress.gov/bill/116th-congress/senate-bill/3548 on August 31, 2023.

2) Zonta F, Scaiewicz A, Levitt M. *The Gompertz Growth of COVID-19 Outbreaks is Caused by Super-Spreaders*. ArXiv [Preprint]. 2021 Nov 3:arXiv:2111.02962v2. PMID: 34981031; PMCID: PMC8722603. Found here https://www.ncbi.nlm.nih.gov/pmc/articles/PMC8722603/ on August 23, 2023.

3) (December 31, 2021). Daily COVID-19 Vaccine Report. *Massachusetts Department of Public Health COVID-19 Vaccine Data.* Found here https://www.mass.gov/doc/daily-covid-19-vaccine-report-december-31-2021/download on August 23, 2023.

4) (December 28, 2022). Weekly COVID-19 Vaccination Report. *Massachusetts Department of Public Health COVID-19 Dashboard.* Found here https://www.mass.gov/doc/weekly-covid-19-vaccination-report-december-28-2022/download on August 23, 2023.

5) Beaudoin, J. (2022). Multiple articles from nom de plume author, Coquin de Chien, found here coquindechien.substack.com on August 26, 2023.

6) Richards L. (May 23, 2021). Why do we get shots in the arm? It's all about the muscle. *The Conversation. North Carolina Health News*. Found here https://www.northcarolinahealthnews.org/2021/05/23/why-do-we-get-shots-in-the-arm-its-all-about-the-muscle/ on August 26, 2023.

7) Hanna N, Heffes-Doon A, Lin X, et al. (2022). Detection of Messenger RNA COVID-19 Vaccines in Human Breast Milk. *JAMA Pediatr.* 2022;176(12):1268–1270. doi:10.1001/jamapediatrics.2022.3581

8) Fox A, Martin J, Beilharz T. (June 24, 2021). Can the Pfizer of Moderna mRNA vaccines affect my genetic code? *The Conversation.* Found here https://theconversation.com/can-the-pfizer-or-moderna-mrna-vaccines-affect-my-genetic-code-162590 on August 26, 2023.

9) Sagili Anthony, D. P., Sivakumar, K., Venugopal, P., Sriram, D. K., & George, M. (2021). Can mRNA Vaccines Turn the Tables During the COVID-19 Pandemic? Current Status and Challenges. *Clinical drug investigation*, 41(6), 499–509. https://doi.org/10.1007/s40261-021-01022-9 Also found here https://www.ncbi.nlm.nih.gov/pmc/articles/PMC7985228/ on August 26, 2023.

10) (December 11, 2020). Learn About the New mRNA COVID-19 Vaccines. The first two COVID-19 vaccines expected to receive authorization for use in the United States are what is known as messenger RNA vaccines—also called "mRNA" vaccines. *CDC | NCIRD*. Found here https://www.cdc.gov/vaccines/covid-19/downloads/healthcare-professionals-mRNA.pdf on August 26, 2023.

11) Tomita, T., Kato, M., Mishima, T. et al. (June 16, 201). Extracellular mRNA transported to the nucleus exerts translation-independent function. *Nature Communications*. 12, 3655 (2021). Found here https://doi.org/10.1038/s41467-021-23969-1 on August 26, 2023.

12) Anandamide. (July 12, 2023). BNT162b2 vials tested in South Carolina deliver qPCR CTs in the 18-19 range. *Nepetalactone Newsletter. Substack*. Found here https://anandamide.substack.com/p/bnt162b2-vials-tested-in-south-carolina on August 26, 2023.

13) McMillan, N. (December 5, 2022). Fatal Post COVID mRNA-Vaccine Associated Cerebral Ischemia. *The Neurohospitalist*. Found here https://journals.sagepub.com/doi/10.1177/19418744221136898 on August 6, 2023.

Chapter 15

1) Sing, C. (January 26, 2022). COVID-19 vaccines and risks of hematological abnormalities: Nested case–control and self-controlled case series study. *American Journal of Hematology*. Wiley Online Library. Found here https://onlinelibrary.wiley.com/doi/10.1002/ajh.26478 on November 27, 2023.

2) Tu W. (April 9, 2021). COVID-19 Vaccination–related Lymphadenopathy: What To Be Aware Of. *Radiological Society of North America*. Found here https://pubs.rsna.org/doi/10.1148/rycan.2021210038 on September 23, 2023.

Chapter 16

1) (2023). dysautonomia. *Google Trends*. Found here https://trends.google.com/trends/explore?date=2013-07-28%20 2023-08-28&geo=US&q=dysautonomia&hl=en on August 28, 2023.

2) International Statistical Classification of Diseases and Related Health Problems 10th Revision (ICD-10). *WHO Version for ;2019-covid-expanded.*

Found here https://icd.who.int/browse10/2019/en#/G90.9 on August 26, 2023.

3) Burgess L. (December 15, 2018). What to know about encephalopathy. *MedicalNewsToday*. Found here https://www.medicalnewstoday.com/articles/324008 on August 28, 2023.

Chapter 17

1) (June 20, 2023). New COVID-19 Treatments Add-On Payment (NCTAP). *Centers for Medicare & Medicaid Services*. Found here https://www.cms.gov/medicare/payment/covid-19/new-covid-19-treatments-add-payment-nctap on August 15, 2023.

2) Pardo, J., Shukla, A. M., Chamarthi, G., & Gupte, A. (2020). The journey of remdesivir: from Ebola to COVID-19. *Drugs in context*, 9, 2020-4-14. https://doi.org/10.7573/dic.2020-4-14. Found here https://www.ncbi.nlm.nih.gov/pmc/articles/PMC7250494/ on October 8, 2023.

3) Yan, V. C., & Muller, F. L. (2021). Why Remdesivir Failed: Preclinical Assumptions Overestimate the Clinical Efficacy of Remdesivir for COVID-19 and Ebola. *Antimicrobial agents and chemotherapy*, 65(10), e0111721. https://doi.org/10.1128/AAC.01117-21. Found here https://www.ncbi.nlm.nih.gov/pmc/articles/PMC8448091/ on October 8, 2023.

4) Eldridge A. (July 3, 2023). Jonestown. *Britannica*. Found here https://www.britannica.com/event/Jonestown on August 29, 2023.

5) (Page last reviewed: October 03, 2023). CDC Wonder. *Centers for Disease Control and Prevention*. Found here https://wonder.cdc.gov/ on October 8, 2023.

6) (August 16, 2022). Christine Grady, M.S.N., Ph.D. Senior Investigator. Department of Bioethics. *NIH Clinical Center*. NIH Intramural Research Program. Found here https://irp.nih.gov/pi/christine-grady on August 29, 2023.

7) Myrick H. (August 26, 2021). Success of some disproves systemic racism. *Gaston Gazette*. Found here https://www.gastongazette.com/story/opinion/2021/08/26/success-some-disproves-systemic-racism/5598271001/ on August 29, 2023.

Chapter 18

1) (2020). Positive Tests by Age Group. *Massachusetts Department of Public Health COVID-19 Dashboard*. Thursday, December 31, 2020. Found here

https://www.mass.gov/doc/covid-19-dashboard-december-31-2020/download on September 29, 2023.

2) (2022). US Coronavirus vaccine tracker. Compare states' vaccination progress or select a state to see detailed information. *USA FACTS*. Found here https://usafacts.org/visualizations/covid-vaccine-tracker-states on September 6, 2023.

Chapter 19

There are no references for this chapter

Chapter 20

1) *Public Health and Medical Professionals for Transparency, Plaintiff, v. Food and Drug Administration, Defendant. (2021)*. U.S. District Court, Northern District of Texas. Docket No. 4:21-cv-1058-P. Found here https://fingfx.thomsonreuters.com/gfx/legaldocs/gdvzykdllpw/Pittman%20FOIA%20Order.pdf on August 31, 2023.

2) *Public Health and Medical Professionals for Transparency, Plaintiff, v. Food and Drug Administration, Defendant. (2021)*. U.S. District Court, Northern District of Texas. Docket No. 4:21-cv-1058-P. FindLaw. Found here https://caselaw.findlaw.com/court/us-dis-crt-n-d-tex-for-wor-div/2200023.html on August 31, 2023.

3) The General Court of the Commonwealth of Massachusetts. (2023). General Laws. *The 193rd General Court of the Commonwealth of Massachusetts*. Found here https://malegislature.gov/Laws/GeneralLaws on August 31, 2023.

Chapter 21

1) See Chapter 7 references 2., 3., 4., and 5.

2) The General Court of the Commonwealth of Massachusetts. (2023). General Laws. Part I. Title XVIII. Chapter 125. Section 10. Oaths of officers; administration. *The 193rd General Court of the Commonwealth of Massachusetts*. Found here https://malegislature.gov/Laws/GeneralLaws/PartI/TitleXVIII/Chapter125/Section10 on August 31, 2023.

3) Beaudoin, J. (April 2021). The Hand Formula; Economics of Torts; Importance of Torts; Vax tort immunity. Written and produced for Torts class. Found here https://www.youtube.com/watch?v=JObGnOCD6mI on November 27, 2023.

4) VAERS Vaccine Adverse Event Reporting System. *VAERS is co-sponsored by the Centers for Disease Control and Prevention (CDC), and the Food*

and Drug Administration (FDA), agencies of the U.S. Department of Health and Human Services (HHS). Found here https://vaers.hhs.gov/data.html on August 6, 2023.

Chapter 22

1) Nickerson C. (April 13, 2023). Rational Choice Theory: What It Is In Economics, With Examples. *SimplyPsychology*. Found here https://www.simplypsychology.org/rational-choice-theory.html on September 1, 2023.

2) Administrative Office of the U.S. Courts. (2023). Federal Judicial Caseload Statistics 2021. *United States Courts*. Found here https://www.uscourts.gov/statistics-reports/federal-judicial-caseload-statistics-2021 on September 1, 2023.

3) False statements relating to health care matters. 18 U.S. Code § 1035. Found here https://www.law.cornell.edu/uscode/text/18/1035 on September 1, 2023.

4) H.R. 748 - CARES Act. (2019-2020). Congress.Gov. Found here https://www.congress.gov/bill/116th-congress/house-bill/748 on September 1, 2023.

5) (June 20, 2023). New COVID-19 Treatments Add-On Payment (NCTAP). *Centers for Medicare & Medicaid Services*. Found here https://www.cms.gov/medicare/covid-19/new-covid-19-treatments-add-payment-nctap on August 15, 2023.

6) *Lujan v. Defenders of Wildlife*, 504 U.S. 555 (1992). Found here https://scholar.google.com/scholar_case?case=10150124802357408838&q=lujan+v+defenders+of+wildlife&hl=en&as_sdt=40000006 on November 27, 2023.

7) Beaudoin J. (2023). Memorandum in Opposition to the Defendant's Motion to Dismiss the Plaintiff's First Amended Complaint. *Beaudoin v Baker et al* (2022). Found here https://viaveravita.com/covid-19-vaccine-lawsuit-filings on September 1, 2023.

Chapter 23

1) Reilly A. (May 25, 2020). What Massachusetts Got Right In Its Pandemic Response. *GBH*. Found here https://www.wgbh.org/news/local/2020-05-25/what-massachusetts-got-right-in-its-pandemic-response on September 1, 2023.

2) Commonwealth of Massachusetts. (2023). Department of Public Health. Found here https://www.mass.gov/orgs/department-of-public-health on September 1, 2023.

3) Coquin de Chien. (March 27, 2022). The Baker Knew. *Coquin de Chien's Newsletter on Substack*. Found here https://coquindechien.substack.com/p/the-baker-knew on September 1, 2023.

4) Massachusetts Department of Elementary and Secondary Education. (2023). COVID-19 Information and Resources. DESE. Found here https://www.doe.mass.edu/covid19/ on September 2, 2023.

5) Massachusetts Department of Elementary and Secondary Education. (August 20, 2021). Education Commissioner Riley to Ask Board to Grant Him Authority to Mandate Masks for All K-12 Public Schools to Provide Time to Increase Vaccinations. *DESE Press Release*. Found here https://mailchi.mp/doe.mass.edu/press-releaseeducation-commissioner-to-ask-board-for-authority-to-mandate-masks-in-public-schoolsto-provide-time-to-increase-vaccinations?e=583fc2bc03 on September 2, 2023.

6) Fernandes M. and Cowperthwaite W. (January 30, 2022). Judge upholds suspension for lawyer suing South Shore schools over mask mandates. *The Patriot Ledger*. Found here https://www.patriotledger.com/story/news/2022/01/30/nh-upholds-anti-mask-attorney-robert-fojo-suspension-over-100-k-mishandled-funds-lawsuits/9253132002/ on September 2, 2023.

Chapter 24

1) Merriam-Webster, Incorporated. (2023). epidemiology noun. *Merriam-Webster*. Found here https://www.merriam-webster.com/dictionary/epidemiology on September 2, 2023.

Chapter 25

1) Robinson S. (October 11, 2022). State agency defends punishment for Ellsworth doctor who criticized COVID-19 policies. *Maine Wire*. Found here https://www.themainewire.com/2022/10/state-agency-defends-punishment-for-ellsworth-doctor-who-criticized-covid-19-policies/ on September 2, 2023.

2) U.S. Code. Title 21. Chapter 9. Subchapter V. Part E. 21 U.S. Code § 360bbb–3 - Authorization for medical products for use in emergencies. Found here https://www.law.cornell.edu/uscode/text/21/360bbb-3 on September 2, 2023.

3) (June 20, 2023). New COVID-19 Treatments Add-On Payment (NCTAP). *Centers for Medicare & Medicaid Services*. Found here https://www.cms.gov/medicare/payment/covid-19/new-covid-19-treatments-add-payment-nctap on August 15, 2023.

4) (December 2021). Podcast Episode #1757 - Dr. Robert Malone, MD. *The Joe Rogan Experience Podcast* on Spotify. Found here https://open.spotify.com/episode/3SCsueX2bZdbEzRtKOCEyT on November 2, 2023.

5) 18 U.S. Code § 1962 - Prohibited Activities. Found here https://www.law.cornell.edu/uscode/text/18/1962 on September 2, 2023.

6) *RJR Nabisco, Inc. v. European Community*, 136 S. Ct. 2090 (2016). Found here https://scholar.google.com/scholar_case?case=6251342729543315 82&q=R-JR+Nabisco,+Inc.+v.+European+Community,+136+S.+Ct.+2090+(2016)&hl=en&as_sdt=40000006 on November 27, 2023.

7) Newton W., Baron R., Nichols D. (September 9, 2021). Joint Statement on Dissemination of Misinformation. *American Board of Internal Medicine*. Found here https://www.abim.org/media-center/press-releases/joint-statement-on-dissemination-of-misinformation/ on September 2, 2023.

8) The Editors of Encyclopedia Britannica. Hippocratic oath ethical code. *Britannica*. Found here https://www.britannica.com/topic/Hippocratic-oath on September 2, 2023.

9) Berenbaum M. (August 22, 2023). Nürnberg Laws German history. *Britannica*. Found here https://www.britannica.com/topic/Nurnberg-Laws on September 2, 2023.

10) Doenges T., Dik B. Declaration of Helsinki 1964. *Britannica*. Found here https://www.britannica.com/topic/Declaration-of-Helsinki on September 2, 2023.

11) Chen J. (March 21, 2022). Bretton Woods Agreement and the Institutions It Created Explained. *Investopedia*. Found here https://www.investopedia.com/terms/b/brettonwoodsagreement.asp on September 2, 2023.

12) *Nass v Maine Board of Licensure in Medicine et al.* (2023). U.S. District Court, District of Maine. Docket No. 1:23-cv-00321-JDL. Found here https://childrenshealthdefense.org/wp-content/uploads/Meryl_Nass_Complaint.pdf and found from here https://www.themainewire.com/2023/08/dr-meryl-nass-sues-maine-medical-board-over-suspension-alleges-first-amendment-violation/ on November 2, 2023.

Epilogue

1) Coquin de Chien. (March 11, 2022). The Moral Calculus of a Death Lottery. *Substack*. Found here https://coquindechien.substack.com/p/the-moral-calculus-of-a-death-lottery?r=1d6m3v&utm_campaign=post&utm_medium=web on September 2, 2023.

INDEX

ABOUT THE AUTHOR

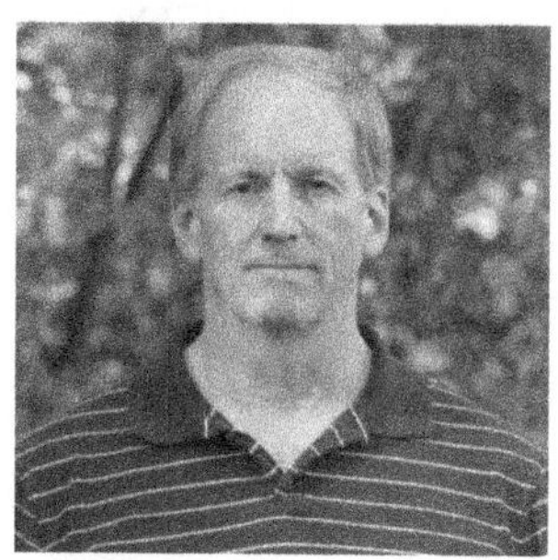

John Paul Beaudoin, Sr. is a Christian and father of three sons. He spent his first 18 years in Windsor, Connecticut, obtained a BS in Systems Engineering, worked 30 years in the semiconductor research and design industry, and obtained an MBA in Management. In July 2018, John's eldest son died in a motorcycle accident at the age of 20. The fraudulent Covid narrative gave John a purpose again, which is to save children from harm. He enrolled in law school at 56-years-old, attended for two semesters, and was unenrolled due to his Covid "vaccination status." John now uses engineering, economics, morality, law, and philosophy to find evidence and bring TRUTH to The People.